W9-BNP-916

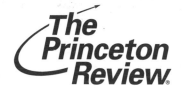

The Princeton Review.

MCAT®

General Chemistry Review

For MCAT 2015

The Staff of The Princeton Review

PENGUIN RANDOM HOUSE

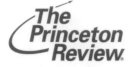

The Princeton Review
24 Prime Parkway, Suite 201
Natick, MA 01760
E-mail: editorialsupport@review.com

Copyright © 2014 by TPR Education IP Holdings, LLC

Published in the United States by Random House LLC,
New York, a Penguin Random House Company, and in
Canada by Random House of Canada Limited, Toronto,
A Penguin Random House Company.

Terms of Service: The Princeton Review Online
Companion Tools ["Online Companion Tools"] for the
Cracking book series and MCAT General Chemistry
Review are available for the most recent edition. Online
Companion Tools may be activated only once per
eligible book purchased. Activation of Online Companion
Tools more than once per book is in direct violation of
these Terms of Service and may result in discontinua-
tion of access to Online Companion Tools Services.

ISBN: 978-0-8041-2506-2
ISSN: 2150-8879

The Princeton Review is not affiliated with Princeton
University.

MCAT is a registered trademark of the Association of
American Medical Colleges, which does not sponsor or
endorse this product.

Editor: Selena Coppock
Production Artist: Deborah A. Silvestrini
Production Editor: Kiley Pulliam

Printed in the United States of America.

10 9 8 7 6 5 4 3 2 1

Editorial

Rob Franek, Senior VP, Publisher
Casey Cornelius, VP, Content Development
Mary Beth Garrick, Director of Production
Selena Coppock, Senior Editor
Calvin Cato, Editor
Kristen O'Toole, Editor
Meave Shelton, Editor
Alyssa Wolff, Editorial Assistant

Random House Publishing Team

Tom Russell, Publisher
Alison Stoltzfus, Publishing Manager
Dawn Ryan, Associate Managing Editor
Ellen Reed, Production Manager
Erika Pepe, Associate Production Manager
Kristin Lindner, Production Supervisor
Andrea Lau, Designer

CONTRIBUTORS

Steven A. Leduc
     Senior Author
Kendra Bowman
     Ph.D., Senior Author

TPR MCAT G-Chem Development Team:
Bethany Blackwell, M.S., William Ewing, Ph.D., Chris Fortenbach, B.S.

Senior Editor, Lead Developer
Bethany Blackwell, M.S.

Edited for Production by:
Judene Wright, M.S., M.A.Ed.
     National Content Director, MCAT Program, The Princeton Review

The TPR MCAT G-Chem Team and Judene would like to thank the following people for their contributions to this book :

Patrick Abulencia, Ph.D., Kashif Anwar, M.D., M.M.S., Argun Can, Brian Cato, Nita Chauhan, H.BSc, MSc, Rob Fong, M.D., Ph.D., Neil Maluste, B.S., Chris Manuel, M.P.H., Douglas K. McLemore, B.S., Marion-Vincent L. Mempin, B.S., Donna Memran, Brian Mikolasko, M.D., M.BA, Katherine Miller, Ph. D., Steven Rines, Ph.D., Andrew Snyder, Daniah Vaiyani, Christopher Volpe, Ph.D.

Periodic Table of the Elements

1 H 1.0																	2 He 4.0
3 Li 6.9	4 Be 9.0											5 B 10.8	6 C 12.0	7 N 14.0	8 O 16.0	9 F 19.0	10 Ne 20.2
11 Na 23.0	12 Mg 24.3											13 Al 27.0	14 Si 28.1	15 P 31.0	16 S 32.1	17 Cl 35.5	18 Ar 39.9
19 K 39.1	20 Ca 40.1	21 Sc 45.0	22 Ti 47.9	23 V 50.9	24 Cr 52.0	25 Mn 54.9	26 Fe 55.8	27 Co 58.9	28 Ni 58.7	29 Cu 63.5	30 Zn 65.4	31 Ga 69.7	32 Ge 72.6	33 As 74.9	34 Se 79.0	35 Br 79.9	36 Kr 83.8
37 Rb 85.5	38 Sr 87.6	39 Y 88.9	40 Zr 91.2	41 Nb 92.9	42 Mo 95.9	43 Tc (98)	44 Ru 101.1	45 Rh 102.9	46 Pd 106.4	47 Ag 107.9	48 Cd 112.4	49 In 114.8	50 Sn 118.7	51 Sb 121.8	52 Te 127.6	53 I 126.9	54 Xe 131.3
55 Cs 132.9	56 Ba 137.3	57 *La 138.9	72 Hf 178.5	73 Ta 180.9	74 W 183.9	75 Re 186.2	76 Os 190.2	77 Ir 192.2	78 Pt 195.1	79 Au 197.0	80 Hg 200.6	81 Tl 204.4	82 Pb 207.2	83 Bi 209.0	84 Po (209)	85 At (210)	86 Rn (222)
87 Fr (223)	88 Ra 226.0	89 †Ac 227.0	104 Rf (261)	105 Db (262)	106 Sg (266)	107 Bh (264)	108 Hs (277)	109 Mt (268)	110 Ds (281)	111 Rg (272)	112 Cn (285)	113 Uut (286)	114 Fl (289)	115 Uup (288)	116 Lv (293)	117 Uus (294)	118 Uuo (294)

*Lanthanide Series:

58 Ce 140.1	59 Pr 140.9	60 Nd 144.2	61 Pm (145)	62 Sm 150.4	63 Eu 152.0	64 Gd 157.3	65 Tb 158.9	66 Dy 162.5	67 Ho 164.9	68 Er 167.3	69 Tm 168.9	70 Yb 173.0	71 Lu 175.0

†Actinide Series:

90 Th 232.0	91 Pa (231)	92 U 238.0	93 Np (237)	94 Pu (244)	95 Am (243)	96 Cm (247)	97 Bk (247)	98 Cf (251)	99 Es (252)	100 Fm (257)	101 Md (258)	102 No (259)	103 Lr (260)

MCAT GENERAL CHEMISTRY CONTENTS

CONTENTS

MCAT MATH FOR GENERAL CHEMISTRY

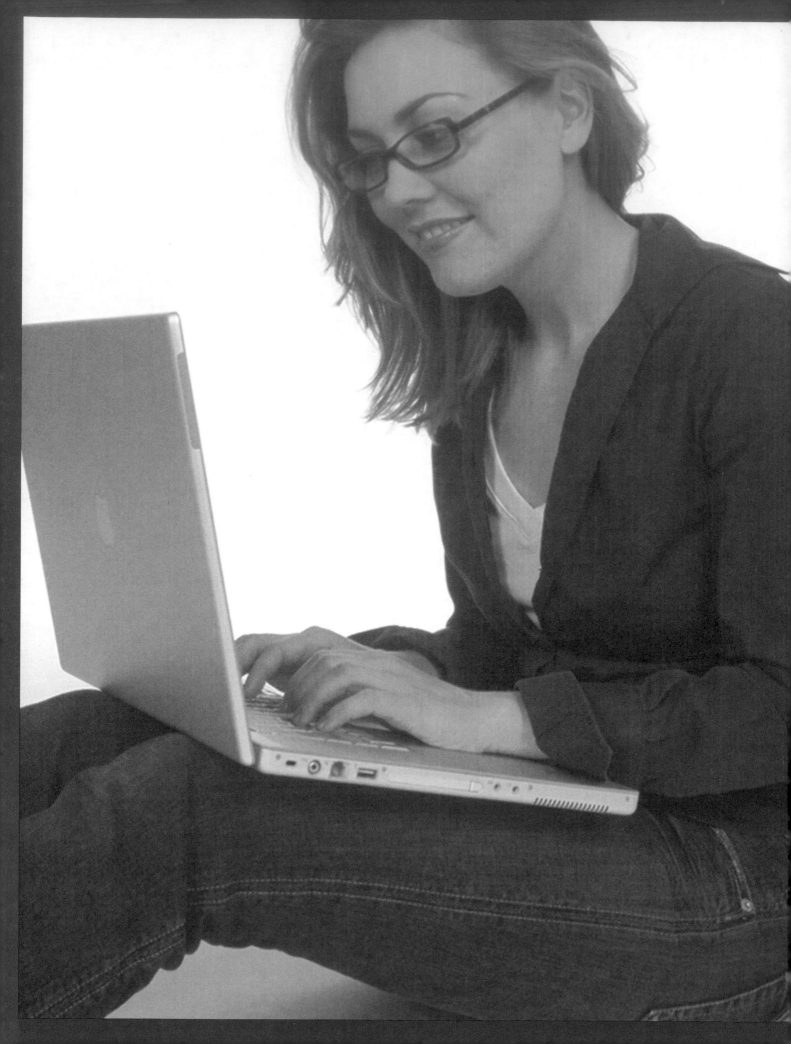

...So Much More Online!

Register your book now!

- Go to www.PrincetonReview.com/cracking

- You'll see a welcome page where you should register your book using the ISBN. Type in the ISBN of your book (the hardcopy book ISBN is: 9780804125062) and create a username and password so that next time you can log into www.PrincetonReview.com easily.

- Now you're good to go!

Once you've registered, you can...

- Take 3 full-length practice MCAT exams

- Find useful information about taking the MCAT and applying to medical school

Offline Resources

If you are looking for more review or medical school advice, please feel free to pick up these books in stores right now!

- *Medical School Essays That Made a Difference*

- *The Best 167 Medical Schools*

- *The Princeton Review Complete MCAT 2015*

princetonreview.com/cracking

Chapter 1
MCAT 2015 Basics

SO YOU WANT TO BE A DOCTOR

So...you want to be a doctor. If you're like most premeds, you've wanted to be a doctor since you were pretty young. When people asked you what you wanted to be when you grew up, you always answered "a doctor." You had toy medical kits, bandaged up your dog or cat, and played "hospital." You probably read your parents' home medical guides for fun.

When you got to high school you took the honors and AP classes. You studied hard, got straight A's (or at least really good grades!), and participated in extracurricular activities so you could get into a good college. And you succeeded!

At college you knew exactly what to do. You took your classes seriously, studied hard, and got a great GPA. You talked to your professors and hung out at office hours to get good letters of recommendation. You were a member of the premed society on campus, volunteered at hospitals, and shadowed doctors. All that's left to do now is get a good MCAT score.

Just the MCAT.

Just the most confidence-shattering, most demoralizing, longest, most brutal entrance exam for any graduate program. At about 7.5 hours (including breaks), the MCAT tops the list...even the closest runners up, the LSAT and GMAT, are only about 4 hours long. The MCAT tests significant science content knowledge along with the ability to think quickly, reason logically, and read comprehensively, all under the pressure of a timed exam.

The path to a good MCAT score is not as easy to see as the path to a good GPA or the path to a good letter of recommendation. The MCAT is less about what you know, and more about how to apply what you know...and how to apply it quickly to new situations. Because the path might not be so clear, you might be worried. That's why you picked up this book.

We promise to demystify the MCAT for you, with clear descriptions of the different sections, how the test is scored, and what the test experience is like. We will help you understand general test-taking techniques as well as provide you with specific techniques for each section. We will review the science content you need to know as well as give you strategies for the Critical Analysis and Reasoning Skills (CARS) section. We'll show you the path to a good MCAT score and help you walk the path.

After all...you want to be a doctor. And we want you to succeed.

WHAT IS THE MCAT...REALLY?

Most test-takers approach the MCAT as though it were a typical college science test, one in which facts and knowledge simply need to be regurgitated in order to do well. They study for the MCAT the same way they did for their college tests, by memorizing facts and details, formulas and equations. And when they get to the MCAT they are surprised...and disappointed.

It's a myth that the MCAT is purely a content-knowledge test. If medical school admission committees want to see what you know, all they have to do is look at your transcripts. What they really want to see, though, is how you *think*. Especially, how you think under pressure. And *that's* what your MCAT score will tell them.

The MCAT is really a test of your ability to apply basic knowledge to different, possibly new, situations. It's a test of your ability to reason out and evaluate arguments. Do you still need to know your science content? Absolutely. But not at the level that most test-takers think they need to know it. Furthermore, your science knowledge won't help you on the Critical Analysis and Reasoning Skills (CARS) section. So how do you study for a test like this?

You study for the science sections by reviewing the basics and then applying them to MCAT practice questions. You study for the CARS section by learning how to adapt your existing reading and analytical skills to the nature of the test (more information about the CARS section can be found in the *MCAT Critical Analysis and Reasoning Skills Review*).

The book you are holding will review all the relevant MCAT General Chemistry content you will need for the test, and a little bit more. It includes hundreds of questions designed to make you think about the material in a deeper way, along with full explanations to clarify the logical thought process needed to get to the answer. It also comes with access to three full-length online practice exams to further hone your skills; see below.

GO ONLINE!

In addition to the review material you'll find in this book, there is a wealth of practice content available online at **PrincetonReview.com/cracking**. There you'll find:

- 3 full-length practice MCATs
- Useful information about taking the MCAT and applying to medical school

To register your book, go to **PrincetonReview.com/cracking**. You'll see a welcome page where you can register your book by its ISBN number (found on the back cover above the barcode). Set up an account using this number and your email address, then you can access all of your online content.

MCAT NUTS AND BOLTS

Overview

The MCAT is a computer-based test (CBT) that is *not* adaptive. Adaptive tests base your next question on whether or not you've answered the current question correctly. The MCAT is *linear*, or *fixed-form*, meaning that the questions are in a predetermined order and do not change based on your answers. However, there are many versions of the test, so that on a given test day, different people will see different versions. The following table highlights the features of the MCAT exam.

Registration	Online via www.aamc.org. Begins as early as six months prior to test date; available up until week of test (subject to seat availability).
Testing Centers	Administered at small, secure, climate-controlled computer testing rooms.
Security	Photo ID with signature, electronic fingerprint, electronic signature verification, assigned seat.
Proctoring	None. Test administrator checks examinee in and assigns seat at computer. All testing instructions are given on the computer.
Frequency of Test	28 times per year distributed over January, March, April, May, June, July, August, and September.
Format	Exclusively computer-based. NOT an adaptive test.
Length of Test Day	7.5 hours
Breaks	Optional 10-minute breaks between sections, with a longer break for lunch.
Section Names	1. Biological and Biochemical Foundations of Living Systems (Bio/Biochem) 2. Critical Analysis and Reasoning Skills (CARS) 3. Chemical and Physical Foundations of Biological Systems (Chem/Phys) 4. Psychological, Social, and Biological Foundations of Behavior (Psych/Soc)
Number of Questions and Timing	67 Bio/Biochem questions, 95 minutes 60 CARS questions, 90 minutes 67 Chem/Phys questions, 95 minutes 67 Psych/Soc questions, 95 minutes
Scoring	Test is scaled. Several forms per administration.
Allowed/Not allowed	No timers/watches. Noise reduction headphones available. Scratch paper and pencils given at start of test and taken at end of test. Locker or secure area provided for personal items.
Results: Timing and Delivery	Approximately 30 days. Electronic scores only, available online through AAMC login. Examinees can print official score reports.
Maximum Number of Retakes	Can be taken a maximum of three times per year, but an examinee can be registered for only one date at a time.

Registration

Registration for the exam is completed online at https://www.aamc.org/students/applying/mcat/reserving. The AAMC opens registration for a given test date at least two months in advance of the date, often earlier. It's a good idea to register well in advance of your desired test date to make sure that you get a seat.

Sections

There are four sections on the MCAT exam: Biological and Biochemical Foundations of Living Systems (Bio/Biochem), Critical Analysis and Reasoning Skills (CARS), Chemical and Physical Foundations of Biological Systems (Chem/Phys), and Psychological, Social, and Biological Foundations of Behavior (Psych/Soc). All sections consist of multiple-choice questions.

Section	Concepts Tested	Number of Questions and Timing
Biological and Biochemical Foundations of Living Systems	Basic concepts in biology and biochemistry, scientific inquiry, reasoning, research methods, and statistics.	67 questions, 95 minutes
Critical Analysis and Reasoning Skills	Critical analysis of information drawn from a wide range of social science and humanities disciplines.	60 questions, 90 minutes
Chemical and Physical Foundations of Biological Systems	Basic concepts in chemical and physical sciences, scientific inquiry, reasoning, research methods, and statistics.	67 questions, 95 minutes
Psychological, Social, and Biological Foundations of Behavior	Basic concepts in psychology, sociology, and biology, scientific inquiry, reasoning, research methods, and statistics.	67 questions, 95 minutes

Most questions on the MCAT (approximately 3/4 of the science sections, all 60 in the CARS section) are **passage-based**, and each section of the test will have about 9–10 passages. A passage consists of a few paragraphs of information on which several following questions are based. In the science sections, passages often include equations or reactions, tables, graphs, figures, and experiments to analyze. CARS passages come from literature in the social sciences, humanities, ethics, philosophy, cultural studies, and population health, and do not test content knowledge in any way.

Some questions in the science sections are *freestanding questions* (FSQs). These questions are independent of any passage information. These questions appear in several groups of about four to five questions, and are interspersed throughout the passages. About 1/4 of the questions in the sciences sections are free-standing, and the remainder are passage-based.

Each section on the MCAT is separated by either a 10-minute break or a longer lunch break:

Section	Time
Test Center Check-In	Variable, can take up to 40 minutes if center is busy.
Tutorial	10 minutes
Biological and Biochemical Foundations of Living Systems	95 minutes
Break	10 minutes
Critical Analysis and Reasoning Skills	90 minutes
Lunch Break	May be 30–45 minutes
Chemical and Physical Foundations of Biological Systems	95 minutes
Break	10 minutes
Psychological, Social, and Biological Foundations of Behavior	95 minutes
Void Option	5 minutes
Survey	10 minutes

The survey includes questions about your satisfaction with the overall MCAT experience, including registration, check-in, etc., as well as questions about how you prepared for the test.

Scoring

The MCAT is a scaled exam, meaning that your raw score will be converted into a scaled score that takes into account the difficulty of the questions. There is no guessing penalty. Because different versions of the test have varying levels of difficulty, the scale will be different from one exam to the next. Thus, there is no "magic number" of questions to get right in order to get a particular score. Plus, some of the questions on the test are considered "experimental" and do not count toward your score; they are just there to be evaluated for possible future inclusion in a test.

At the end of the test (after you complete the Psychological, Social, and Biological Foundations of Behavior section), you will be asked to choose one of the following two options, "I wish to have my MCAT exam scored" or "I wish to VOID my MCAT exam." You have five minutes to make a decision, and if you do not select one of the options in that time, the test will automatically be scored. If you choose the VOID option, your test will not be scored (you will not now, or ever, get a numerical score for this test), medical schools will not know you took the test, and no refunds will be granted. You cannot "unvoid" your scores at a later time.

So, what's a good score? If your GPA is on the low side, you'll need higher MCAT scores to compensate, and if you have a strong GPA, you can get away with lower MCAT scores. But the reality is that your chances of acceptance depend on a lot more than just your MCAT scores. It's a combination of your GPA, your MCAT scores, your undergraduate coursework, letters of recommendation, experience related to the medical field (such as volunteer work or research), extracurricular activities, your personal statement, etc. Medical schools are looking for a complete package, not just good scores and a good GPA.

GENERAL TEST-TAKING STRATEGIES

CBT Tools

There are a number of tools available on the test, including highlighting, strike-outs, the Mark button, the Review button, the Exhibit button, and of course, scratch paper. The following is a brief description of each tool.

1) **Highlighting:** This is done in passage text (including table entries and some equations, but excluding figures and molecular structures) by clicking and dragging the cursor over the desired text. To remove the highlighted portion, just click over the highlighted text. Note that highlights DO NOT persist once you leave the passage.

2) **Strike-outs:** This is done on the various answer choices by clicking over the answer choice that you wish to eliminate. As a result, the entire set of text associated with that answer choice is crossed out. The strike-out can be removed by clicking again. Note that you cannot strike-out figures or molecular structures, and strike-outs DO persist after leaving the passage.

3) **Mark button:** This is available for each question and allows you to flag the question as one you would like to review later if time permits. When clicked, the "Mark" button turns red and says "Marked."

4) **Review button:** This button is found near the bottom of the screen, and when clicked, brings up a new screen showing all questions and their status (either "answered," "unanswered," or "marked"). You can then choose one of three options: "review all," "review unanswered," or "review marked." You can only review questions in the section of the MCAT you are currently taking, but this button can be clicked at any time during the allotted time for that section; you do NOT have to wait until the end of the section to click it.

5) **Exhibit button:** Clicking this button will open a periodic table. Note that the periodic table is originally large, covering most of the screen. However, this window can be resized to see the questions and a portion of the periodic table at the same time. The table text will not decrease, but scroll bars will appear on the window so you can center the section of the table of interest in the window.

6) **Scratch paper:** You will be given four pages (8 faces) of scratch paper at the start of the test. While you may ask for more at any point during the test, your first set of paper will be collected before you receive fresh paper. Scratch paper is only useful if it is kept organized; do not give in to the tendency to write on the first available open space! Good organization will be very helpful when/if you wish to review a question. Indicate the passage number in a box near the top of your scratch work, and indicate which question you are working on in a circle to the left of the notes for that question. Draw a line under your scratch work when you change passages to keep the work separate. Do not erase or scribble over any previous work. If you do not think it is correct, draw one line through the work and start again. You may have already done some useful work without realizing it.

Pacing

Since the MCAT is a timed test, you must keep an eye on the timer and adjust your pacing as necessary. It would be terrible to run out of time at the end to discover that the last few questions could have been easily answered in just a few seconds each.

If you complete every question, in the science sections you will have about one minute and twenty-five seconds (1:25) per question, and in the CARS section you will have about one minute and thirty seconds per question (1:30).

Section	# of Questions in passage	Approximate time (including reading the passage)
Bio/Biochem, Chem/Phys, and Psych/Soc	5	7 minutes
	6	8.5 minutes
	7	10 minutes
CARS	5	7.5 minutes
	6	9 minutes
	7	10.5 minutes

When starting a passage in the science sections, make note of how much time you will allot for it, and the starting time on the timer. Jot down on your scratch paper what the timer should say at the end of the passage. Then just keep an eye on it as you work through the questions. If you are near the end of the time for that passage, guess on any remaining questions, make some notes on your scratch paper (remember that highlighting disappears), Mark the questions, and move on. Come back to those questions if you have time.

For the CARS section, one important thing to keep in mind is that most people will maximize their score by *not* trying to complete every question, or every passage, in the section. A good strategy for a majority of test takers is to complete all but one of the passages, and randomly guess on that last one. This allows you to have good accuracy on the passages you complete, and to maximize your total percent correct in the section as a whole. To complete all but one of the passages, you should spend about ten minutes on each passage. This is an approximation, of course—you should spend a bit more time on difficult passages or passages with more questions, and a bit less on easier passages or passages with fewer questions.

To help maximize your number of correct answer choices in any section, do the questions and passages within that section in the order *you* want to do them in. Skip over the more difficult passages your first time through the section (mark the first question of the passage and randomly guess on all the questions before moving on), and work the passages you feel most comfortable with first.

Process of Elimination

Process of elimination (POE) is probably the most useful technique you have to tackle MCAT questions. Since there is no guessing penalty, POE allows you to increase your probability of choosing the correct answer by eliminating those you are sure are wrong. If you are guessing between a couple of choices, use the CBT tools to your advantage:

1) Strike out any choices that you are sure are incorrect or that do not address the issue raised in the question.

2) Jot down some notes on your scratch paper to help clarify your thoughts if you return to the question.

3) Use the "Mark" button to flag the question for review at a later time. (Note, however, that in the CARS section, you generally should not be returning to rethink questions once you have moved on to a new passage.)

4) Do not leave it blank! If you are not sure and you have already spent more than 60 seconds on that question, just pick one of the remaining choices. If you have time to review it at the end, you can always debate the remaining choices based on your previous notes.

5) Special Note: if three of the four answer choices have been eliminated, the remaining choice must be the correct answer. Don't waste time pondering *why* it is correct, just click it and move on. The MCAT doesn't care if you truly understand why it's the right answer, only that you have the right answer selected.

6) More subject-specific information on techniques will be presented in the next chapter.

Guessing

Remember, there is NO guessing penalty on the MCAT. NEVER leave a question blank!

QUESTION TYPES

In the science sections of the MCAT, the questions fall into one of three main categories.

1) Memory questions: These questions can be answered directly from prior knowledge and represent about 25 percent of the total number of questions.

2) Explicit questions: These questions are those for which the answer is explicitly stated in the passage. To answer them correctly, for example, may just require finding a definition, or reading a graph, or making a simple connection. Explicit questions represent about 35 percent of the total number of questions.

3) Implicit questions: These questions require you to apply knowledge to a new situation; the answer is typically implied by the information in the passage. These questions often start "if.... then...." (for example, "if we modify the experiment in the passage like this, then what result would we expect?"). Implicit style questions make up about 40 percent of the total number of questions.

In the CARS section, the questions fall into four main categories:

1) Specific questions: These questions either ask you for facts from the passage (Retrieval questions) or require you to deduce what is most likely to be true based on the passage (Inference questions).

2) General questions: These questions ask you to summarize themes (main idea and primary purpose questions) or evaluate an author's opinion (tone/attitude questions).

3) Reasoning questions: These questions ask you to describe the purpose of, or support provided for, a statement made in the passage (Structure questions) or to judge how well the author supports his or her argument (Evaluate questions).

4) Application questions: These questions ask you to apply new information from either the question stem itself (New Information questions) or from the answer choices (Strengthen, Weaken, and Analogy questions) to the passage.

More detail on question types and strategies can be found in Chapter 2.

TESTING TIPS

Before Test Day

- Take a trip to the test center a day or two before your actual test date so that you can easily find the building and room on test day. This will also allow you to gauge traffic, and see if you need money for parking or anything like that. Knowing this type of information ahead of time will greatly reduce your stress on the day of your test.
- Don't do any heavy studying the day before the test. Try to get a good amount of sleep during the nights leading up to the test.
- Eat well. Try to avoid excessive caffeine and sugar. Ideally, in the weeks leading up to the actual test you should experiment a little bit with foods and practice tests to see which foods give you the most endurance. Aim for steady blood sugar levels during the test: sports drinks, peanut-butter crackers, and trail mix make good snacks for your breaks and lunch.

General Test Day Info and Tips

- On the day of the test, you'll want to arrive at the test center at least a half hour prior to the starting time of your test.
- Examinees will be checked in to the center in the order in which they arrive.
- You will be assigned a locker or secure area in which to put your personal items. Textbooks and study notes are not allowed, so there is no need to bring them with you to the test center.
- Your ID will be checked, a digital image of your fingerprint will be taken, and you will be asked to sign in.
- You will be given scratch paper and a couple of pencils, and the test center administrator will take you to the computer on which you will complete the test. (If a white-board and erasable marker is provided, you can specifically request scratch paper at the start of the test.) You may not choose a computer; you must use the computer assigned to you.
- Nothing is allowed at the computer station except your photo ID, your locker key (if provided), and a factory sealed packet of ear plugs; not even your watch.
- If you choose to leave the testing room at the breaks, you will have your fingerprint checked again, and you will have to sign in and out.
- You are allowed to access the items in your locker except for notes and cell phones. (Check your test center's policy on cell phones ahead of time: some centers do not even allow them to be kept in your locker.)
- Don't forget to bring the snack foods and lunch you experimented with in your practice tests.
- At the end of the test, the test administrator will collect your scratch paper and shred it.
- Definitely take the breaks! Get up and walk around. It's a good way to clear your head between sections and get the blood (and oxygen!) flowing to your brain.
- Ask for new scratch paper at the breaks if you use it all up.

Chapter 2
General Chemistry
Strategy for the MCAT

2.1 SCIENCE SECTIONS OVERVIEW

There are three science sections on the MCAT:

- Biological and Biochemical Foundations of Living Systems
- Chemical and Physical Foundations of Biological Systems
- Psychological, Social, and Biological Foundations of Behavior

The Biological and Biochemical Foundations of Living Systems section (Bio/Biochem) is the first section on the test. Approximately 65% of the questions in this section come from biology, approximately 25% come from biochemistry, and approximately 10% come from Organic and General Chemistry. Math calculations are generally not required on this section of the test, however a basic understanding of statistics as used in biological research is helpful.

The Chemical and Physical Foundations of Biological Systems section (Chem/Phys) is the third section on the test. It includes questions from General Chemistry (about 35%), Physics (about 25%), Organic Chemistry (about 15%), and Biochemistry (about 25%). Further, the questions often test chemical and physical concepts within a biological setting, for example, pressure and fluid flow in blood vessels. A solid grasp of math fundamentals is required (arithmetic, algebra, graphs, trigonometry, vectors, proportions, and logarithms), however there are no calculus-based questions.

The Psychological, Social, and Biological Foundations of Behavior section (Psych/Soc) is the fourth and final section on the test. About 60% of the questions will be drawn from Psychology, about 30% from Sociology, and about 10% from Biology. As with the Bio/Biochem section, calculations are generally not required, however a basic understanding of statistics as used in research is helpful.

Most of the questions in the science sections (about 75%) are passage-based, and each section will likely have about nine or ten passages. Passages consist of a few paragraphs of information and include equations, reactions, graphs, figures, tables, experiments, and data. Five to seven questions will be associated with each passage.

The remaining 25% of the questions in each science section are freestanding questions (FSQs). These questions appear in groups interspersed between the passages. Each group contains four to five questions.

95 minutes are allotted to each of the science sections. This breaks down to approximately one minute and 25 seconds per question.

2.2 GENERAL SCIENCE PASSAGE TYPES

The passages in the science sections fall into one of three main categories: Information and/or Situation Presentation, Experiment/Research Presentation, or Persuasive Reasoning.

Information and/or Situation Presentation

These passages either present straightforward scientific information or they describe a particular event or occurrence. Generally, questions associated with these passages test basic science facts or ask you to predict outcomes given new variables or new information. Here is an example of an Information/Situation Presentation passage:

Figure 1 shows a portion of the inner mechanism of a typical home smoke detector. It consists of a pair of capacitor plates which are charged by a 9-volt battery (not shown). The capacitor plates (electrodes) are connected to a sensor device, D; the resistor R denotes the internal resistance of the sensor. Normally, air acts as an insulator and no current would flow in the circuit shown. However, inside the smoke detector is a small sample of an artificially produced radioactive element, americium-241, which decays primarily by emitting alpha particles, with a half-life of approximately 430 years. The daughter nucleus of the decay has a half-life in excess of two million years and therefore poses virtually no biohazard.

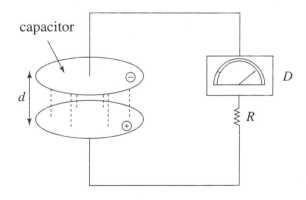

Figure 1   Smoke detector mechanism

The decay products (alpha particles and gamma rays) from the ^{241}Am sample ionize air molecules between the plates and thus provide a conducting pathway which allows current to flow in the circuit shown in Figure 1. A steady-state current is quickly established and remains as long as the battery continues to maintain a 9-volt potential difference between its terminals. However, if smoke particles enter the space between the capacitor plates and thereby interrupt the flow, the current is reduced, and the sensor responds to this change by triggering the alarm. (Furthermore, as the battery starts to "die out," the resulting drop in current is also detected to alert the homeowner to replace the battery.)

$$C = \varepsilon_0 \frac{A}{d}$$

Equation 1

where ε_0 is the universal permittivity constant, equal to 8.85×10^{-12} $C^2/(N\ m^2)$. Since the area A of each capacitor plate in the smoke detector is 20 cm^2 and the plates are separated by a distance d of 5 mm, the capacitance is 3.5×10^{-12} F = 3.5 pF.

Experiment/Research Presentation

These passages present the details of experiments and research procedures. They often include data tables and graphs. Generally, questions associated with these passages ask you to interpret data, draw conclusions, and make inferences. Here is an example of an Experiment/Research Presentation passage:

The development of sexual characteristics depends upon various factors, the most important of which are hormonal control, environmental stimuli, and the genetic makeup of the individual. The hormones that contribute to the development include the steroid hormones estrogen, progesterone, and testosterone, as well as the pituitary hormones FSH (follicle-stimulating hormone) and LH (luteinizing hormone).

To study the mechanism by which estrogen exerts its effects, a researcher performed the following experiments using cell culture assays.

Experiment 1:

Human embryonic placental mesenchyme (HEPM) cells were grown for 48 hours in Dulbecco's Modified Eagle Medium (DMEM), with media change every 12 hours. Upon confluent growth, cells were exposed to a 10 mg per mL solution of green fluorescent-labeled estrogen for 1 hour. Cells were rinsed with DMEM and observed under confocal fluorescent microscopy.

Experiment 2:

HEPM cells were grown to confluence as in Experiment 1. Cells were exposed to Pesticide A for 1 hour, followed by the 10 mg/mL solution of labeled estrogen, rinsed as in Experiment 1, and observed under confocal fluorescent microscopy.

Experiment 3:

Experiment 1 was repeated with Chinese Hamster Ovary (CHO) cells instead of HEPM cells.

Experiment 4:

CHO cells injected with cytoplasmic extracts of HEPM cells were grown to confluence, exposed to the 10 mg/mL solution of labeled estrogen for 1 hour, and observed under confocal fluorescent microscopy.

The results of these experiments are given in Table 1.

Table 1 Detection of Estrogen (+ indicates presence of Estrogen)

Experiment	Media	Cytoplasm	Nucleus
1	+	+	+
2	+	+	+
3	+	+	+
4	+	+	+

After observing the cells in each experiment, the researcher bathed the cells in a solution containing 10 mg per mL of a red fluorescent probe that binds specifically to the estrogen receptor only when its active site is occupied. After 1 hour, the cells were rinsed with DMEM and observed under confocal fluorescent microscopy. The results are presented in Table 2.

The researcher also repeated Experiment 2 using Pesticide B, an estrogen analog, instead of Pesticide A. Results from other researchers had shown that Pesticide B binds to the active site of the cytosolic estrogen receptor (with an affinity 10,000 times greater than that of estrogen) and causes increased transcription of mRNA.

Table 2 Observed Fluorescence and Estrogen Effects (G = green, R = red)

Experiment	Media	Cytoplasm	Nucleus	Estrogen effects observed?
1	G only	G and R	G and R	Yes
2	G only	G only	G only	No
3	G only	G only	G only	No
4	G only	G and R	G and R	Yes

Based on these results, the researcher determined that estrogen had no effect when not bound to a cytosolic, estrogen-specific receptor.

Persuasive Reasoning

These passages typically present a scientific phenomenon along with a hypothesis that explains the phenomenon, and may include counter-arguments as well. Questions associated with these passages ask you to evaluate the hypothesis or arguments. Persuasive Reasoning passages in the science sections of the MCAT tend to be less common than Information Presentation or Experiment-based passages. Here is an example of a Persuasive Reasoning passage:

Two theoretical chemists attempted to explain the observed trends of acidity by applying two interpretations of molecular orbital theory. Consider the pK_a values of some common acids listed along the conjugate base:

acid	pK_a	conjugate base
H_2SO_4	< 0	HSO_4^-
H_2CrO_4	5.0	$HCrO_4^-$
H_2PO_4	2.1	$H_2PO_4^-$
HF	3.9	F^-
HOCl	7.8	ClO^-
HCN	9.5	CN^-
HIO_3	1.2	IO_3^-

Recall that acids with a $pK_a < 0$ are called strong acids, and those with a $pK_a > 0$ are called weak acids. The arguments of the chemists are given below.

Chemist #1:

"The acidity of a compound is proportional to the polarization of the H—X bond, where X is some nonmetal element. Complex acids, such as H_2SO_4, $HClO_4$, and HNO_3 are strong acids because the H—O bonding electrons are strongly drawn towards the oxygen. It is generally true that a covalent bond weakens as its polarization increases. Therefore, one can conclude that the strength of an acid is proportional to the number of electronegative atoms in that acid."

Chemist #2:

"The acidity of a compound is proportional to the number of stable resonance structures of that acid's conjugate base. H_2SO_4, $HClO_4$, and HNO_3 are all strong acids because their respective conjugate bases exhibit a high degree of resonance stabilization."

MAPPING OUT A PASSAGE

"Mapping a passage" refers to the combination of on-screen highlighting and scratch paper notes that you take while working through a passage. Typically, good things to highlight include the overall topic of a paragraph, familiar terms, unusual terms, numerical values, hypothesis, and results. Scratch paper notes can be used to summarize the paragraphs and to jot down important facts and connections that are made when reading the passage. Remember that highlighting disappears once you leave the passage, so a good set of scratch paper notes can be extremely useful if you have to return to the passage. More details on passage mapping will be presented in Section 2.5.

2.3   GENERAL SCIENCE QUESTION TYPES

Question in the science sections are generally one of three main types: Memory, Explicit, or Implicit.

Memory Questions

These questions can be answered directly from prior knowledge, with no need to reference the passage or question text. Memory questions represent approximately 25 percent of the science questions on the MCAT. Usually, Memory questions are found as FSQs, but they can also be tucked into a passage. Here's an example of a Memory question:

Which of the following acetylating conditions will convert diethylamine into an amide at the fastest rate?

A) Acetic acid / HCl
B) Acetic anhydride
C) Acetyl chloride
D) Ethyl acetate

Explicit Questions

Explicit questions can be answered primarily with information from the passage, along with prior knowledge. They may require data retrieval, graph analysis, or making a simple connection. Explicit questions make up approximately 35–40 percent of the science questions on the MCAT; here's an example (taken from the Information/Situation Presentation passage above):

The sensor device D shown in Figure 1 performs its function by acting as:

A)   an ohmmeter.
B)   a voltmeter.
C)   a potentiometer.
D)   an ammeter.

Implicit Questions

These questions require you to take information from the passage, combine it with your prior knowledge, apply it to a new situation, and come to some logical conclusion. They typically require more complex connections than do Explicit questions, and may also require data retrieval, graph analysis, etc. Implicit questions usually require a solid understanding of the passage information. They make up approximately 35–40 percent of the science questions on the MCAT; here's an example (taken from the Experiment/ Research Presentation passage above):

If Experiment 2 were repeated, but this time exposing the cells first to Pesticide A and then to Pesticide B before exposing them to the green fluorescent-labeled estrogen and the red fluorescent probe, which of the following statements will most likely be true?

A)   Pesticide A and Pesticide B bind to the same site on the estrogen receptor.
B)   Estrogen effects would be observed.
C)   Only green fluorescence would be observed.
D)   Both green and red fluorescence would be observed.

2.4 GENERAL CHEMISTRY ON THE MCAT

Although general chemistry is sometimes remembered as a daunting topic from college, the MCAT does not test the fine details of general chemistry. Rather, the focus of this section is on having a strong knowledge of chemistry fundamentals, and manipulating that knowledge to adapt to different scenarios presented in passages and questions. The passages often contain information that recapitulates basic chemistry knowledge, and may present additional information that builds on fundamental concepts.

The majority of the G-Chem questions will not be based on rote memory, but will require you to retrieve information from the passage and use some deductive reasoning skills. Thus, in order to succeed in this section, you not only need solid knowledge of fundamental principles of chemistry, but also strong critical reasoning and reading comprehension skills. These three components may be stressed differently depending on the passage type.

MCAT 2015 is likely to have around 9-10 passages and about 17 freestanding questions (FSQs) in each of the science sections. General Chemistry will make up about a third of the questions in the Chemical and Physical Foundations of Biological Systems section. The remaining questions will be on Physics (25%), Organic Chemistry (15%), and Biochemistry (25%). In addition, about 5% of the questions on the Biological and Biochemical Foundations of Living Systems section will be General Chemistry.

2.5 PASSAGE TYPES AS THEY APPLY TO GENERAL CHEMISTRY

Information/Situation Presentation: G-Chem

These passages assume knowledge of basic scientific concepts, and also present new information that builds on these basic concepts. The new information may be presented in a way that is very similar to how it would appear in a textbook or other scientific reference. The questions may be about basic scientific facts that you already know, but often the passage will present topics or subtopics with which you are unfamiliar. Information/Situation Presentation passages can be intimidating, as they often explore topics in a greater level of detail than the scope of your MCAT preparation. However, keep in mind that the whole point of these types of passages is to force you to use critical reasoning and apply your basic scientific knowledge to new topics. It is not to see how much advanced scientific coursework you have memorized. Therefore, it is important when you see a passage on, say, molecular orbital theory, that you don't think to yourself, "Oh no!! I forgot to study molecular orbital theory!!!" Rather, look at the information in the passage, and consider how your knowledge about more basic chemical concepts, such as electron configurations, can be applied in order to answer the questions. The new information in the passage can supplement your basic knowledge.

This type of passage may also present information in the context of a specific situation, such as the results of a research study or an experiment. In this case, the questions may ask you to distinguish between data that supports or refutes the result being presented. In some passages, an apparently contradictory or erroneous result is presented and questions may ask what mistakes could have been made over the course of the experiment to cause such a result. Thus, these passages require to you think critically about the importance of each chemical and physical element of an experiment. Note however, that they do not present the steps of an experiment in great detail; that style is reserved for Experiment/Research Presentation passages.

Experiment/Research Presentation: G-Chem

These passages present an experimental set up in great detail; they describe the rationale behind an experiment, how it is set up and executed, and its results. In these passages you are often asked to analyze data given in the form of charts and graphs. In addition, questions may ask you how the results of the experiment would differ if a certain variable were changed; this requires you to think critically about the role of each element of the experiment. In this passage type, be careful not to gloss over important experimental details as you retrieve information from the passage. Be aware that details such as units can make the difference between answering a question correctly or incorrectly, and be vigilant about these experimental details as you work through the questions and look back to the passage.

Persuasive Argument: G-Chem

In a Persuasive Argument passage, two perspectives on a problem are presented. It may be different researchers putting forth two different methodologies for conducting an experiment, or two different explanations for an experimental result or phenomenon.

The questions may ask how the authors came to develop different perspectives, or ask you to evaluate the credibility of each of their arguments. Persuasive Argument passages are the least common passage type in G-Chem.

READING A GENERAL CHEMISTRY PASSAGE

Reading a G-Chem passage is not like reading a scientific paper or a textbook. That is, you are not reading thoroughly and trying to understand the relevance of each sentence, as the passage will likely contain details beyond the scope of the questions. In fact, many of the questions can be answered without using any information from the passage.

Instead, your goal is to take no more than 30 to 60 seconds and skim the passage in order to determine the general topic area being tested and create a brief passage map before moving on to the questions. To do this as efficiently as possible, focus on the first sentence of each paragraph and any bolded or italicized words. In addition, chemical equations and figures may provide insight as to the general topic of the passage. For example, if you see a titration curve, it is likely that the passage will test acid-base chemistry.

G-Chem passages often include complex graphs and data tables. Avoid the temptation to analyze this data on your first pass through the passage. Rather, wait until you find a question that requires the use of the data in the graph or table, then analyze the data in the context of that question. This approach is more efficient and productive than trying to preemptively interpret data.

The bottom line: You can always go back and reread more details from the passage. Furthermore, not all of the details from the passage are necessary to answer the questions. Therefore, it is a waste of your time to read and attempt to thoroughly understand the passage the first time you read it.

MAPPING A G-CHEM PASSAGE

As you skim through a G-Chem passage to get a feel for the type of questions that might follow, take note of the general location of information within the passage. The highlighter is a useful way to visually note a few key words that relate to the general topic of the passage or some unusual or new term that is introduced. Use the highlighter sparingly, and keep in mind that any highlighting you do will not persist as you move from passage to passage. If you want to make more permanent notes, use the scratch paper. An example of a highlighted passage is shown below. This is an Information Presentation passage:

The batteries that start an automobile or power flashlights are devices that convert chemical energy into electrical energy. These devices use spontaneous oxidation-reduction reactions (called half-reactions) that take place at the electrodes to create an electric current. The strength of the battery, or electromotive force, is determined by the difference in electric potential between the half cells, expressed in volts. This voltage depends on which reactions occur at the anode and the cathode, the concentrations of the solutions in the cells, and the temperature. The cell voltage, E, at a temperature of 25°C and nonstandard conditions, can be calculated from the Nernst equation, where $E°$ is the standard potential, n denotes the number of electrons transferred in the balanced half reaction, and Q is the reaction quotient.

$$E = E° - \frac{0.0592}{n} \log_{10} Q$$

Equation 1

The lead storage battery used in automobiles is composed of six identical cells joined in series. The anode is solid lead, the cathode is lead dioxide, and the electrodes are immersed in a solution of sulfuric acid. As each cell discharges during normal operation, the sulfate ion is consumed as it is deposited in the form of lead sulfate on both electrodes, as shown in Reaction 1:

Reaction 1:

$$Pb(s) + PbO_2(s) + 4\,H^+(aq) + 2\,SO_4{}^{2-}(aq)$$
$$\downarrow$$
$$2\,PbSO_4(s) + 2\,H_2O(l)$$

Each cell produces 2 V, for a total of 12 V for the typical car battery. Unlike many batteries, however, the lead storage battery can be recharged by applying an external voltage. Because the redox reaction in the battery consumes sulfate ions, the degree of discharge of the battery can be checked by measuring the density of the battery fluid with a hydrometer. The fluid density in a fully charged battery is 1.2 g/cm^3.

Table 1 Standard Reduction Potentials at T = 25°C

Half-reaction	E° (V)
$F_2(g) + 2e^- \rightarrow 2F^-(aq)$	+2.87
$Cl_2(g) + 2e^- \rightarrow 2Cl^-(aq)$	+1.36
$Cu^+(aq) + e^- \rightarrow Cu(s)$	+0.52
$Cu^{2+}(aq) + 2e^- \rightarrow Cu(s)$	+0.34
$Zn^{2+}(aq) + 2e^- \rightarrow Zn(s)$	−0.76
$Al^{3+}(aq) + 3e^- \rightarrow Al(s)$	−1.66
$Li^+(aq) + e^- \rightarrow Li(s)$	−3.05

Note that only a few words are highlighted. In the first paragraph, "batteries" and "spontaneous oxidation-reduction" relate to the general topic of the passage, and serve as a reminder that batteries contain a spontaneous redox reaction. The second paragraph identifies the two electrodes in the battery and, in the last paragraph, the voltage of a car battery is highlighted. Since this is a specific and unusual piece of information, it is likely to come up in a question.

Rather than highlighting large portions of the passage as you skim it, use your scratch paper to create a simple passage map to help organize where different types of information are in the passage. Scratch paper is only useful if it is kept organized! Make sure that your notes for each passage are clearly delineated and marked with the passage number on your scratch paper. This will allow you to easily read your notes when you come back to review a marked question. Resist the temptation to write in the first available blank space, as this makes it much more difficult to refer back to your work.

As you skim the passage, note the subject of each paragraph and any key words or values. A well-constructed passage map makes it easier and more efficient to go back and retrieve specific information as you work through the questions. Here is an example of a passage map for the passage shown above:

> P1 – Batteries, general information, background
> P2 – Automobile batteries, more specific information about them
> P3 – Recharging car battery, Reduction Potentials in Table 1

As you can see, your passage map does not need to be particularly detailed, nor should it be, as reading and mapping the passage should only take a minute of your time. However, this does provide a valuable framework for efficiently locating information within the passage.

Let's look at another passage and how to map it. This is an Experiment/Research Presentation passage from The Princeton Review's free online demo MCAT:

Two cube-shaped compartments, X and Y, each with a volume of one cubic meter, were used in several experiments to study the properties of gases. Compartment X was fitted with a piston of negligible mass which fit snugly against the walls of the container. The compartments were connected by a pinhole which could be opened or closed at will (see Figure 1). The pressure and temperature could be measured in either compartment. At the start of each experiment, Compartment X contained equal molar quantities of four gases (helium, oxygen, nitrogen, and carbon dioxide), the temperature in Compartment X was 25°C and the pressure was 1 atm. Initially, Compartment Y was evacuated. The behavior of all the gases can be assumed to be ideal. (Note: 1 atm ≈ 105 Pa.)

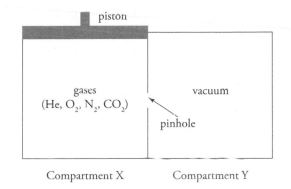

Figure 1   Experimental apparatus

Experiment 1:

With the pinhole closed, the temperature of the gases in Compartment X was gradually increased to 50°C, and the pressure of the gas inside the compartment was measured.

Experiment 2:

With the pinhole closed, the piston was gradually lowered into Compartment X until it had dropped a distance of 0.5 m. The pressure of the gas in the container was then measured.

Experiment 3:

The pinhole was opened, and the pressure change in each compartment was measured until equilibrium was reached.

2.5

Here, the highlighter tool can be used to emphasize that this passage is about the behavior of gases. Any time a passage is about gases, it's useful to know if the gas behaves in a real or ideal manner; therefore the phrase "assumed to be ideal" is also highlighted. In experimental passages, if important details jump out at you on your initial skim of the passage, it's useful to highlight them. For example, Figure 1 makes it fairly obvious that compartment X contains four gases, while compartment Y is a vacuum with no gas, however the "equal molar quantities" of the four gases in compartment X is a useful detail to highlight. Here's how you might map this passage on your scratch paper:

P1 – Experimental setup
E1 – Temp change
E2 – Pressure change
E3 – Pressure change, equilibrium

As was true of our last passage map, the main purpose is to create an outline so that it will be easier to re-trieve necessary information as you work through the questions. Since this is an Experiment Presentation passage, the map points out the location of the main experimental details. Note that on the first pass, it is not important to note the specific details of each individual experiment on your scratch paper, though quickly highlighting new experimental conditions, like temperature, etc. can be helpful. If possible, how-ever, it may be helpful to note the general variable being changed.

Let's look at one more example of passage mapping. This passage is a Persuasive Argument Passage:

Two theoretical chemists attempted to explain the observed trends of acidity by applying two interpretations of molecular orbital theory. Consider the pK_a values of some common acids listed along with the conjugate base of each acid:

acid	pK_a	conjugate base
H_2SO_4	< 0	HSO_4^-
H_2CrO_4	5.0	$HCrO_4^-$
H_3PO_4	2.1	$H_2PO_4^-$
HF	3.9	F^-
HOCl	7.8	ClO^-
HCN	9.5	CN^-
HIO_3	1.2	IO_3^-

Recall that acids with a $pK_a < 0$ are called strong acids, and those with a $pK_a > 0$ are called weak acids. The arguments of the chemists are given below.

Chemist #1:

"The acidity of a compound is proportional to the polarization of the H—X bond, where X is some nonmetal element. Complex acids, such as H_2SO_4, $HClO_4$, and HNO_3 are strong acids because the H—O bonding electrons are strongly drawn towards the oxygen. It is generally true that a covalent bond weakens as its polarization increases. Therefore, one can conclude that the strength of an acid is proportional to the number of electronegative atoms in that acid."

Chemist #2:

> "The acidity of a compound is proportional to the number
> of stable resonance structures of that acid's conjugate base.
> H_2SO_4, $HClO_4$, and HNO_3 are all strong acids because their
> respective conjugate bases exhibit a high degree of resonance
> stabilization."

For a Persuasive Argument passage, the goal of passage mapping and highlighting is to identify the issue being addressed, and the main points of each of the opposing lines of reasoning. This can be accomplished using the highlighter tool to emphasize that the passage is about "trends of acidity", and that Chemist #1 attributes the behavior of acids to "polarization of the H—X bond," while Chemist #2 focuses on "stable resonance structures."

In this case, a passage map would be very similar to the results achieved by highlighting. However, keep in mind that while highlighting does not persist as you move from passage to passage, a passage map can permanently be referred to on well-organized scratch paper. Also, the very act of writing things down helps clarify it in your head:

P1/Main issue: Trends of acidity, interpretation of molecular orbital theory
Chemist #1: acidity $\propto$ polarization of H—X bond
Chemist #2: acidity $\propto$ # of stable resonance structures for conjugate base.

As you can see from the examples above, effective passage-mapping requires a combination of highlighting and jotting down notes in an organized fashion on your scratch paper. The best way to improve your passage mapping, and to determine which combination of these skills works best for you, is to practice, practice, practice.

2.8 TACKLING THE QUESTIONS

In general, G-Chem questions require a combination of basic knowledge, passage retrieval, and critical reasoning. The more difficult G-Chem questions tend to weigh the last two skills more heavily. Therefore, if you have a sound basis in the fundamental principles of General Chemistry, it is safe to assume that a tough question will be best addressed by looking back to the passage for information that is either explicitly stated or implied.

In the section on passage mapping, we reviewed an Information/Situation Presentation passage on batteries and redox reactions. We will draw on questions from this passage in order to illustrate the different question types.

G-Chem Memory Questions

These questions test background knowledge and require you to recall a specific definition or relationship. Memory questions are often freestanding questions, either on their own or within a set of questions that accompany a passage. In the latter instance, the information they require is not given in the passage. For example, a question from the car battery passage shown above asked:

If the reaction in a concentration cell is spontaneous in the reverse direction, then:

A) $Q < K$, ΔG for the forward reaction is negative, and the cell voltage is positive.

B) $Q < K$, ΔG for the forward reaction is positive, and the cell voltage is negative.

C) $Q > K$, ΔG for the forward reaction is negative, and the cell voltage is positive.

D) $Q > K$, ΔG for the forward reaction is positive, and the cell voltage is negative.

In order to answer this question correctly, you need to know the connection between ΔG and spontaneity. A spontaneous reaction has a negative ΔG, and a nonspontaneous reaction has a positive ΔG. Since the reaction is spontaneous in the reverse direction, it must be nonspontaneous in the forward direction. Therefore, the ΔG of the forward reaction is positive, eliminating choices A and C. Alternatively, you could know that cell voltage applies to the forward direction, and that a nonspontaneous cell has a negative voltage, also eliminating choices A and C.

To distinguish between choices B and D, you must have a fundamental understanding of equilibrium and Le Châtelier's Principle. The reaction quotient, Q, always approaches the equilibrium constant, K, and if $Q > K$ the reaction will be pushed in the reverse direction, toward the reactants side of the equilibrium, in order to decrease the value of Q. Thus, since the question says the reaction is spontaneous in the reverse direction, Q must be greater than K. This makes choice D the best answer.

Also, note that this question asks about concentration cells, which are not mentioned in the passage, and therefore this problem is essentially a free-standing question.

G-Chem Explicit Questions

Explicit questions require direct retrieval of information from the passage. Sometimes, the answers to Explicit questions are definitions or relationships that are clearly stated in the passage. However, these types of questions may also require some background knowledge or a simple step of logical reasoning. Here is another example from the car battery redox passage shown above:

Of the following, which is the best reducing agent?

A) Li^+

B) Li

C) Cl^-

D) F^-

To answer this question, you must have fundamental knowledge of redox definitions and relationships, but you also need to retrieve information from the passage. The best reducing agent is the species that has the highest oxidizing potential, and Table 1 gives the reduction potentials for these reagents. However, you also need the knowledge that the oxidation potential is the same as the reduction potential, but with the opposite sign. Since the oxidation of Li has the highest positive potential (3.05 V), Li is the strongest reducing agent.

The best way to approach Explicit questions is to refer to your passage map to find the location of the information you need. Then, go back to the passage and read that section in greater detail. There are two instances when retrieval of information for Explicit questions can be especially tricky. First, in research study passages, be cautious when retrieving information from tables and graphs. Rather than simply pulling data directly from the figures, be sure to read the text just before and after the figures as well, as it may contain important information that changes the way the data should be interpreted. Second, when a passage goes into greater detail about a subject that you already have fundamental knowledge of, avoid the temptation to answer questions directly from memory. Often, these types of passages will provide some obscure detail or anomalous situation that will be tested in the questions, and require you to retrieve information from the passage in order to select the correct answer.

G-Chem Implicit Questions

Implicit questions require you to work through two or more steps of critical reasoning based on your background knowledge and information given in the passage. In other words, the answer is not directly stated in the passage, but is implied by the information provided. The distinction between an Implicit and an Explicit question can be subtle, as both require you to retrieve information from the passage, and Explicit questions may also require you to make a simple critical reasoning decision. The difference is that in Implicit questions, the reasoning step required is not as direct or obvious, and more than one step is usually required. For example:

> When a lead storage battery recharges, what happens to
> the density of the battery fluid?
>
> A) It decreases to 1.0 g/cm^3.
> B) It increases to 1.0 g/cm^3.
> C) It decreases to 1.2 g/cm^3.
> D) It increases to 1.2 g/cm^3.

First, information on the density of the battery fluid must be retrieved from the passage. Our passage map tells us that specific information on car batteries can be found in paragraphs two and three. Re-skimming these sections reveals that in the third paragraph of the passage, it states that the density of fluid in a fully charged battery is 1.2 g/cm^3. Therefore, as the battery is recharging, its density is approaching this value, eliminating choices A and B.

The difference between choices C and D is whether the density of the solution is increasing or decreasing to 1.2 g/cm^3 during recharge. To determine this, we can look for additional information in the passage that may relate to changing density of the battery fluid. The second paragraph of the passage states that as the battery discharges, sulfate ions are consumed and deposited in the form of lead sulfate. The removal of ions from solution implies that the amount of mass in the solution is going down, and therefore its density is also decreasing. Therefore, density is decreasing during discharge, and increasing during recharge. This makes choice D the best answer.

The key step here is focusing on the differences among answer choices. What can be difficult about approaching implicit questions is that it often hard to determine which information is supposed to "imply" something about the answer. Zeroing in on differences among the answer choices can help you determine which information from the passage is most relevant, and may help you rephrase what the question is really asking. Also, note that the first step of our analysis, eliminating the choices with 1.0 g/cm³ density, was basically just answering an explicit question via direct passage retrieval. Many implicit questions begin this way, and it is much easier to eliminate answer choices first based on explicit information than it is to try to make a decision based on implicit information.

2.7 SUMMARY OF THE APPROACH TO GENERAL CHEMISTRY

How to Map the Passage and Use Scratch Paper

1) The passage should not be read like textbook material, with the intent of learning something from every sentence (science majors especially will be tempted to read this way). Skim through the paragraphs to get a feel for the type of questions that will follow, and to get a general idea of the location of information within the passage. For example, you might jot down on your scratch paper that paragraph 1 discusses properties of buffers, and that equation 1 is the Henderson-Hasselbach equation. These observations tip you off that the questions will likely relate to acid/base properties, and that if you need more information about the specific properties of buffers, you can refer to paragraph 1.

2) Highlighting—Use this tool sparingly, or you will end up with a passage that is completely covered in yellow highlighter! Keep in mind that highlighting does not persist as you move from passage to passage within the section. If you want to make more permanent notes, use the scratch paper. Highlighting in a General Chemistry passage should be used to draw attention to a few words that demonstrate one of the following:

   - The main theme of a paragraph
   - A general chemistry principle that has been taught (i.e., familiar terms)
   - An unusual or unfamiliar term that is defined specifically for that passage (e.g., something that is italicized)

3) Pay brief attention to equations, figures, and experiments, noting only what information they deal with. Do not spend a lot of time analyzing at this point, as you can come back and look more closely at this information if a question requires it.

4) Scratch paper is only useful if it is kept organized! Make sure that your notes for each passage are clearly delineated and marked with the passage number on your scratch paper. This will allow you to easily read your notes when you come back to review a marked question. Resist the temptation to write in the first available blank space, as this makes it much more difficult to refer back to your work.

General Chemistry Question Strategies

1) Remember that Process of Elimination is paramount! The strikeout tool allows you to eliminate answer choices; this will improve your chances of guessing the correct answer if you are unable to narrow it down to one choice.

2) Answer the straightforward questions first. Leave questions that require analysis of experiments and graphs for later.

3) Make sure that the answer you choose actually answers the question, and isn't just a true statement.

4) I-II-III questions: Always work between the I-II-III statements and the answer choices. Unfortunately, it is not possible to strike out the Roman numerals, but this is a great use for scratch paper notes. Once a statement is determined to be true (or false), strike out answer choices that do not contain (or do contain) that statement.

5) LEAST/EXCEPT/NOT questions: Don't get tricked by these questions that ask you to pick the answer that doesn't fit (the incorrect or false statement). It's often good to use your scratch paper and write a T or F next to answer choices A–D. The one that stands out as different is the correct answer!

6) 2 x 2 style questions: These questions require you to know two pieces of information to get the correct answer, and are easily identified by their answer choices, which commonly take the form A because X, B because X, A because Y, B because Y. Tackle one piece of information at a time, which should allow you to quickly eliminate two answer choices.

7) Ranking questions: When asked to rank items, look for an extreme—either the greatest or the smallest item—and eliminate answer choices that do not have that item shown at the correct end of the ranking. This is often enough to eliminate one to three answer choices. Based on the remaining choices, look for the other extreme at the other end of the ranking and use POE again.

8) If you read a question and do not know how to answer it, look to the passage for help. It is likely that the passage contains information pertinent to answering the question, either within the text or in the form of experimental data.

9) If a question requires a lengthy calculation, mark it and return to it later, particularly if you are slow with arithmetic or dimensional analysis.

10) Again, don't leave any question blank.

2.7

A NOTE ABOUT FLASHCARDS

Contrary to popular belief, flashcards are NOT the best way to study for the MCAT. For most of the exams you've taken previously, flashcards were probably helpful. This was because those exams mostly required you to regurgitate information, and flashcards are pretty good at helping you memorize facts. Remember, however, that the most challenging aspect of the MCAT is not that it requires you to memorize the fine details of content knowledge, but that it requires you to apply your basic scientific knowledge to unfamiliar situations. Flashcards won't help you do that.

There is only one situation in which flashcards can be beneficial, and that's if your basic content knowledge is deficient in some area. For example, if you don't know the strong acids and bases, flashcards can help you memorize these facts. Or, maybe you are unsure of some of molecular geometries and shapes from the VSEPR theory. You might find that flashcards can help you memorize these. (And remember that part of what makes flashcards useful is that you *make them yourself.* Not only are they customized for your personal areas of weakness, but the very act of writing down facts on a flashcard helps that information stick in your brain.) But if you are not trying to memorize basic facts in your personal weak areas, you are better off doing and analyzing practice passages than carrying around a stack of flashcards.

Chapter 3
Chemistry
Fundamentals

3.1 METRIC UNITS

Before we begin our study of chemistry, we will briefly go over metric units. Scientists use the *Système International d'Unitès* (the International System of Units), abbreviated SI, to express measurements of physical quantities. Six of the seven **base units** of SI are given below:

SI Base Unit	Abbreviation	Measures
meter	m	length
kilogram	kg	mass
second	s	time
mole	mol	amount of substance
kelvin	K	temperature
ampere	A	electric current

(The seventh SI base unit, the candela [cd], measures luminous intensity, but we will not need to worry about this one.) The units of any physical quantity can be written in terms of the SI base units. For example, the SI unit of speed is meters per second (m/s), the SI unit of energy (the joule) is kilograms times meters^2 per second^2 ($kg \cdot m^2/s^2$), and so forth.

Multiples of the base units that are powers of ten are often abbreviated and precede the symbol for the unit. For example, m is the symbol for milli-, which means 10^{-3} (one thousandth). So, one thousandth of a second, 1 millisecond, would be written as 1 ms. The letter M is the symbol for mega-, which means 10^6 (one million); a distance of one million meters, 1 megameter, would be abbreviated as 1 Mm. Some of the most common power-of-ten prefixes are given in the list below:

Prefix	Symbol	Multiple
nano-	n	10^{-9}
micro-	μ	10^{-6}
milli-	m	10^{-3}
centi	c	10^{-2}
kilo-	k	10^3
mega-	M	10^6

Two other units, ones that are common in chemistry, are the liter and the angstrom. The liter (abbreviated L) is a unit of volume equal to 1/1000 of a cubic meter:

$$1000 \text{ L} = 1 \text{ m}^3$$

$$1 \text{ L} = 1000 \text{ cm}^3$$

The standard SI unit of volume, the cubic meter, is inconveniently large for most laboratory work. The liter is a smaller unit. Furthermore, the most common way of expressing solution concentrations, **molarity** (*M*), uses the liter in its definition: *M* = moles of solute per liter of solution.

In addition, you will see the milliliter (mL) as often as you will see the liter. A simple consequence of the definition of a liter is the fact that one milliliter is the same volume as one cubic centimeter:

$$1 \text{ mL} = 1 \text{ cm}^3 = 1 \text{ cc}$$

While the volume of any substance can, strictly speaking, be expressed in liters, you rarely hear of a milliliter of gold, for example. Ordinarily, the liter is used to express the volumes of liquids and gases, but not solids.

The **angstrom**, abbreviated Å, is a unit of length equal to 10^{-10} m. The angstrom is convenient because atomic radii and bond lengths are typically around 1 to 3 Å.

Example 3-1: By how many orders of magnitude is a centimeter longer than an angstrom?

Solution: An **order of magnitude** is a factor of ten. Since 1 cm = 10^{-2} m and 1 Å = 10^{-10} m, a centimeter is 8 factors of ten, or 8 orders of magnitude, greater than an angstrom.

3.2 DENSITY

The **density** of a substance is its mass per volume:

$$\text{Density: } \rho = \frac{\text{mass}}{\text{volume}} = \frac{m}{V}$$

In SI units, density is expressed in kilograms per cubic meter (kg/m^3). However, in chemistry, densities are more often expressed in grams per cubic centimeter (g/cm^3). This unit of density is convenient because most liquids and solids have a density of around 1 to 20 g/cm^3. Here is the conversion between these two sets of density units:

$$g/cm^3 \rightarrow \text{multiply by } 1000 \rightarrow kg/m^3$$

$$g/cm^3 \leftarrow \text{divide by } 1000 \leftarrow kg/m^3$$

For example, water has a density of 1 g/cm^3 (it varies slightly with temperature, but this is the value the MCAT will expect you to use). To write this density in kg/m^3, we would multiply by 1000. The density of water is 1000 kg/m^3. As another example, the density of copper is about 9000 kg/m^3, so to express this density in g/cm^3, we would divide by 1000: The density of copper is 9 g/cm^3.

Example 3-2: Diamond has a density of 3500 kg/m^3. What is the volume, in cm^3, of a 1 3/4-carat diamond (where, by definition, 1 carat = 0.2 g)?

Solution: If we divide mass by density, we get volume, so, converting 3500 kg/m^3 into 3.5 g/cm^3, we find that

$$V = \frac{m}{\rho} = \frac{1.75 \ (0.2 \text{ g})}{3.5 \text{ g}/\text{cm}} = \frac{0.35 \text{ g}}{3.5 \text{ g}/\text{cm}} = 0.1 \text{ cm}^3$$

3.3 MOLECULAR FORMULAS

When two or more atoms form a covalent bond they create a **molecule**. For example, when two atoms of hydrogen (H) bond with one atom of oxygen (O), the resulting molecule is H_2O, water. A compound's **molecular formula** gives the identities and numbers of the atoms in the molecule. For example, the formula $C_4H_4N_2$ tells us that this molecule contains 4 carbon atoms, 4 hydrogen atoms, and 2 nitrogen atoms.

Example 3-3: What is the molecular formula of *para*-nitrotoluene?

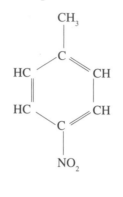

A) $C_6H_5NO_2$
B) $C_7H_7NO_2$
C) $C_7H_8NO_2$
D) $C_7H_9NO_2$

Solution: There are a total of seven C's, seven H's, one N, and two O's, so choice B is the correct answer.

3.4 EMPIRICAL FORMULAS

Let's look again at the molecule $C_4H_4N_2$. There are four atoms each of carbon and hydrogen, and half as many (two) nitrogen atoms. Therefore, the smallest whole numbers that give the same *ratio* of atoms (carbon to hydrogen to nitrogen) in this molecule are 2:2:1. If we use *these* numbers for the atoms, we get the molecule's **empirical formula**: C_2H_2N. In general, to reduce a molecular formula to the empirical formula, divide all the subscripts by their greatest common factor. Here are a few more examples:

Molecular Formula	Empirical Formula
$C_6H_{12}O_6$	CH_2O
$K_2S_2O_8$	KSO_4
$Fe_4Na_8O_{35}P_{10}$	$Fe_4Na_8O_{35}P_{10}$
$C_{30}H_{27}N_3O_{15}$	$C_{10}H_9NO_5$

Example 3-4: What is the empirical formula for ethylene glycol, $C_2H_6O_2$?

A) CH_3O
B) CH_4O
C) CH_6O
D) $C_2H_6O_2$

Solution: Dividing each of the subscripts of $C_2H_6O_2$ by 2, we get CH_3O, choice A.

3.5   FORMULA AND MOLECULAR WEIGHT

If we know the chemical formula, we can figure out the **formula weight**, which is the sum of the atomic weights of all the atoms in the molecule. The unit for atomic weight is the **atomic mass unit**, abbreviated **amu**. (Note: Although *weight* is the popular term, it should really be *mass*.) One atomic mass unit is, by definition, equal to exactly 1/12 the mass of an atom of carbon-12 (^{12}C), the most abundant naturally occurring form of carbon. The periodic table lists the mass of each element; it is actually a weighted average of the atomic masses of all its naturally occurring forms (isotopes) based on their relative abundance. For example, the atomic mass of hydrogen is listed as 1.0 (amu), and that of nitrogen as 14.0 (amu). Therefore, the formula weight for $C_4H_4N_2$ is

$$4(12) + 4(1) + 2(14) = 80$$

(The unit *amu* is often not explicitly included.) When a compound exists as discrete molecules, the term **molecular weight (MW)** is usually used instead of formula weight. For example, the molecular weight of water, H_2O, is $2(1) + 16 = 18$. The term formula weight is usually used for *ionic* compounds, such as NaCl. The formula weight of NaCl is $23 + 35.5 = 58.5$.

Example 3-5: What is the formula weight of calcium phosphate, $Ca_3(PO_4)_2$?

A)   310 amu
B)   350 amu
C)   405 amu
D)   450 amu

Solution: The masses of the elements are Ca = 40 amu, P = 31 amu, and O = 16 amu. Therefore, the formula weight of calcium phosphate is

$$3(40 \text{ amu}) + 2(31 \text{ amu}) + 8(16 \text{ amu}) = 310 \text{ amu}$$

Choice A is the answer.

3.6   THE MOLE

A **mole** is simply a particular number of things, like a dozen is any group of 12 things. One mole of any-thing contains 6.02×10^{23} entities. A mole of atoms is a collection of 6.02×10^{23} atoms; a mole of mol-ecules contains 6.02×10^{23} molecules, and so on. This number, 6.02×10^{23}, is called **Avogadro's number**, denoted by N_A (or N_0). What is so special about 6.02×10^{23}? The answer is based on the atomic mass unit, which is defined so that the mass of a carbon-12 atom is exactly 12 amu. *The number of carbon-12 atoms in a sample of mass of 12 grams is 6.02×10^{23}.* Avogadro's number is the link between atomic mass units and grams. For example, the periodic table lists the mass of sodium (Na, atomic number 11) as 23.0. This means that 1 atom of sodium has a mass of 23 atomic mass units, or that 1 *mole* of sodium atoms has a mass of 23 *grams*.

Since 1 mole of a substance has a mass in grams equal to the mass in amus of 1 formula unit of the sub-stance, we have the following formula:

$$\# \text{ moles} = \frac{\text{mass in grams}}{\text{molecular weight (MW)}}$$

Example 3-6:

a)   Which has the greater molecular weight: potassium dichromate ($K_2Cr_2O_7$) or lead azide $Pb(N_3)_2$?

b)   Which contains more formula units: a 1-mole sample of potassium dichromate or a 1-mole sample of lead azide?

Solution:

a)   The molecular weight of potassium dichromate is

$$2(39.1) + 2(52) + 7(16) = 294.2$$

and the molecular weight of lead azide is

$$207.2 + 6(14) = 291.2$$

Therefore, potassium dichromate has the greater molecular weight.

b)   Trick question. Both samples contain the same number of formula units, namely 1 mole of them. (Which weighs more: a pound of rocks or a pound of feathers?)

Example 3-7:   How many molecules of hydrazine, N_2H_4, are in a sample with a mass of 96 grams?

Solution: The molecular weight of N_2H_4 is $2(14) + 4(1) = 32$. This means that 1 mole of N_2H_4 has a mass of 32 grams. Therefore, a sample that has a mass of 96 grams contains 3 moles of molecules, because the formula above tells us that

$$n = \frac{96 \text{ g}}{32 \text{ g/mol}} = 3 \text{ moles}$$

3.7 PERCENTAGE COMPOSITION BY MASS

A molecule's molecular or empirical formula can be used to determine the molecule's percent mass composition. For example, let's find the mass composition of carbon, hydrogen, and nitrogen in $C_4H_4N_2$. Using the compound's empirical formula, C_2H_2N, will give us the same answer but the calculations will be easier because we'll have smaller numbers to work with. The empirical molecular weight is $2(12) + 2(1) + 14 = 40$, so each element's contribution to the total mass is

$$\%C = \frac{2(12)}{40} = \frac{12}{20} = \frac{60}{100} = 60\%, \quad \%H = \frac{2(1)}{40} = \frac{1}{20} = \frac{5}{100} = 5\%, \quad \%N = \frac{14}{40} = \frac{7}{20} = \frac{35}{100} = 35\%$$

We can also use information about the percentage composition to determine a compound's empirical formula. Suppose a substance is analyzed and found to consist, by mass, of 70 percent iron and 30 percent oxygen. To find the empirical formula for this compound, the trick is to start with 100 grams of the substance. We choose 100 grams since percentages are based on parts in 100. One hundred grams of this substance would then contain 70 g of Fe and 30 g of O. Now, how many *moles* of Fe and O are present in this 100-gram substance? Since the atomic weight of Fe is 55.8 and that of O is 16, we can use the formula given above in Section 3.6 and find

$$\# \text{ moles of Fe} = \frac{70 \text{ g}}{55.8 \text{ g/mol}} \approx \frac{70}{56} = \frac{5}{4} \quad \text{and} \quad \# \text{ moles of O} = \frac{30 \text{ g}}{16 \text{ g/mol}} = \frac{15}{8}$$

Because the empirical formula involves the ratio of the numbers of atoms, let's find the ratio of the amount of Fe to the amount of O:

$$\text{Ratio of Fe to O} = \frac{5/4 \text{ mol}}{15/8 \text{ mol}} = \frac{5}{4} \cdot \frac{8}{15} = \frac{2}{3}$$

Since the ratio of Fe to O is 2:3, the empirical formula of the substance is Fe_2O_3.

Example 3-8: What is the percent composition by mass of each element in sodium azide, NaN_3?

A) Sodium 25%; nitrogen 75%
B) Sodium 35%; nitrogen 65%
C) Sodium 55%; nitrogen 45%
D) Sodium 65%; nitrogen 35%

Solution: The molecular weight of this compound is $23 + 3(14) = 65$. Therefore, sodium's contribution to the total mass is

$$\%Na = \frac{23}{65} \approx \frac{1}{3} \approx 33\%$$

Without even calculating nitrogen's contribution, we already see that choice B is best.

Example 3-9: What is the percent composition by mass of carbon in glucose, $C_6H_{12}O_6$?

- A) 40%
- B) 50%
- C) 67%
- D) 75%

Solution: The empirical formula for this compound is CH_2O, so the empirical molecular weight is $12 + 2(1) + 16 = 30$. Therefore, carbon's contribution to the total mass is

$$\%C = \frac{12}{30} = 40\%$$

So choice A is the answer. We would have found the same answer using the molecular formula, but the numbers would have been messier:

$$\%C = \frac{6(12)}{6(12) + 12(1) + 6(16)} = \frac{72}{180} = 40\%$$

Example 3-10: What is the empirical formula of a compound that is, by mass, 90 percent carbon and 10 percent hydrogen?

- A) CH_2
- B) C_2H_3
- C) C_3H_4
- D) C_4H_5

Solution: A 100-gram sample of this compound would contain 90 g of C and 10 g of H. Since the atomic weight of C is 12 and that of H is 1, we have

$$\# \text{ moles of C} = \frac{90 \text{ g}}{12 \text{ g/mol}} = \frac{15}{2} \quad \text{and} \quad \# \text{ moles of H} = \frac{10 \text{ g}}{1 \text{ g/mol}} = 10$$

Therefore, the ratio of the amount of C to the amount of H is

$$\frac{15/2 \text{ mol}}{10 \text{ mol}} = \frac{3}{4}$$

Because the ratio of C to H is 3:4, the empirical formula of the compound is C_3H_4, and choice C is the answer.

Example 3-11: What is the percent, by mass of water, in the hydrate $MgCl_2 \cdot 5H_2O$?

- A) 27%
- B) 36%
- C) 49%
- D) 52%

3.7

Solution: The formula weight for this hydrate is $24.3 + 2(35.5) + 5[2(1) + 16] = 185.3$. Since water's total molecular weight in this compound is $5[2(1) + 16] = 90$, we see that water's contribution to the total mass is $\%H_2O = 90/185.3$, which is a little *less* than one half (50 percent). Therefore, the answer is C.

Example 3-12: In which of the following compounds is the mass percent of each of the constituent elements nearly identical?

    A)   NaCl
    B)   LiBr
    C)   HCl
    D) CaF_2

Solution: The question is asking us to identify the compound made up of equal amounts, by mass, of two elements. Looking at the given compounds, we see that

$$Na\ (23.0\ g/mol) \neq Cl\ (35.5\ g/mol)$$

$$Li\ (6.9\ g/mol) \neq Br\ (79.9\ g/mol)$$

$$H\ (1.0\ g/mol) \neq Cl\ (35.5\ g/mol)$$

$$Ca\ (40.1\ g/mol) \approx 2\ F\ (2\times19) = 38\ g/mol$$

Therefore, choice D is best.

3.8   CONCENTRATION

Molarity (*M*) expresses the concentration of a solution in terms of moles of solute per volume (in liters) of solution:

$$\text{Molarity}\ (M) = \frac{\#\ \text{moles of solute}}{\#\ \text{liters of solution}}$$

Concentration is denoted by enclosing the solute in brackets. For instance, "$[Na^+] = 1.0\ M$" indicates a solution in which the concentration is equivalent to 1 mole of sodium ions per liter of solution.

Mole fraction simply expresses the fraction of moles of a given substance (which we'll denote here by S) relative to the total moles in a solution:

$$\text{mole fraction of S} = X_S = \frac{\#\ \text{moles of substance S}}{\text{total}\ \#\ \text{moles in solution}}$$

Mole fraction is a useful way to express concentration when more than one solute is present, and is often used when discussing the composition of a mixture of gases.

3.9 CHEMICAL EQUATIONS AND STOICHIOMETRIC COEFFICIENTS

The equation

$$2\ Al + 6\ HCl \rightarrow 2\ AlCl_3 + 3\ H_2$$

describes the reaction of aluminum metal (Al) with hydrochloric acid (HCl) to produce aluminum chloride ($AlCl_3$) and hydrogen gas (H_2). The **reactants** are on the left side of the arrow, and the **products** are on the right side. A chemical equation is **balanced** if, for every element represented, the number of atoms on the left side is equal to the number of atoms on the right side. This illustrates the **Law of Conservation of Mass** (or of **Matter**), which says that the amount of matter (and thus mass) does not change in a chemical reaction. For a *balanced* reaction such as the one above, the coefficients (2, 6, 2, and 3) preceding each compound—which are known as **stoichiometric coefficients**—tell us in what proportion the reactants react and in what proportion the products are formed. For this reaction, 2 atoms of Al react with 6 molecules of HCl to form 2 molecules of $AlCl_3$ and 3 molecules of H_2. The equation also means that 2 *moles* of Al react with 6 *moles* of HCl to form 2 *moles* of $AlCl_3$ and 3 *moles* of H_2.

The stoichiometric coefficients give the ratios of the number of molecules (or moles) that apply to the combination of reactants and the formation of products. They do *not* give the ratios by mass.

Balancing Equations

Balancing most chemical equations is simply a matter of trial and error. It's a good idea to start with the most complex species in the reaction. For example, let's look at the reaction above:

$$Al + HCl \rightarrow AlCl_3 + H_2 \text{ (unbalanced)}$$

Start with the most complex molecule, $AlCl_3$. The total number of atoms, or moles of atoms, is calculated by multiplying the coefficient in front of a compound times the subscript within the formula. To get 3 atoms of Cl on the product side, we need to have 3 atoms of Cl on the reactant side; therefore, we put a 3 in front of the HCl:

$$Al + 3\ HCl \rightarrow AlCl_3 + H_2 \text{ (unbalanced)}$$

We've now balanced the Cl's, but the H's are still unbalanced. Since we have 3 H's on the left, we need 3 H's on the right to accomplish this, so we put a coefficient of 3/2 in front of the H_2:

$$Al + 3\ HCl \rightarrow AlCl_3 + 3/2\ H_2$$

Notice that we put a 3/2 (*not* a 3) in front of the H_2, because a hydrogen molecule contains 2 hydrogen atoms. All the atoms are now balanced—we see 1 Al, 3 H's, and 3 Cl's on each side. Because it's customary to write stoichiometric coefficients as whole numbers, we simply multiply through by 2 to get rid of the fraction and write

$$2\ Al + 6\ HCl \rightarrow 2\ AlCl_3 + 3\ H_2$$

Example 3-13: Balance each of these equations:

a) $NH_3 + O_2 \rightarrow NO + H_2O$
b) $CuCl_2 + NH_3 + H_2O \rightarrow Cu(OH)_2 + NH_4Cl$
c) $C_3H_8 + O_2 \rightarrow CO_2 + H_2O$
d) $C_8H_{18} + O_2 \rightarrow CO_2 + H_2O$

Solution:

a) $4\ NH_3 + 5\ O_2 \rightarrow 4\ NO + 6\ H_2O$
b) $CuCl_2 + 2\ NH_3 + 2\ H_2O \rightarrow Cu(OH)_2 + 2\ NH_4Cl$
c) $C_3H_8 + 5\ O_2 \rightarrow 3\ CO_2 + 4\ H_2O$
d) $2\ C_8H_{18} + 25\ O_2 \rightarrow 16\ CO_2 + 18\ H_2O$

3.10 STOICHIOMETRIC RELATIONSHIPS IN BALANCED REACTIONS

Once the equation for a chemical reaction is balanced, the stoichiometric coefficients tell us the relative amounts of the reactant species that combine and the relative amounts of the product species that are formed. For example, recall that the reaction

$$2\ Al + 6\ HCl \rightarrow 2\ AlCl_3 + 3\ H_2$$

tells us that 2 moles of Al react with 6 moles of HCl to form 2 moles of $AlCl_3$ and 3 moles of H_2.

Example 3-14: If 108 grams of aluminum metal are consumed, how many grams of hydrogen gas will be produced?

Solution: Because the stoichiometric coefficients give the ratios of the number of moles that apply to the combination of reactants and the formation of products—not the ratios by mass—we first need to determine how many *moles* of Al react. Since the molecular weight of Al is 27, we know that 27 grams of Al is equivalent to 1 mole. Therefore, 108 grams of Al is 4 moles. Now we use the stoichiometry of the balanced equation: for every 2 moles of Al that react, 3 moles of H_2 are produced. So, if 4 moles of Al react, we'll get 6 moles of H_2. Finally, we convert the number of moles of H_2 produced to grams. The molecular weight of H_2 is $2(1) = 2$. This means that 1 mole of H_2 has a mass of 2 grams. Therefore, 6 moles of H_2 will have a mass of $6(2\ g) = 12$ grams.

Example 3-15: How many grams of HCl are required to produce 534 grams of aluminum chloride?

Solution: First, we'll convert the desired mass of $AlCl_3$ into moles. The molecular weight of $AlCl_3$ is $27 + 3(35.5) = 133.5$. This means that 1 mole of $AlCl_3$ has a mass of 133.5 grams. Therefore, 534 grams of $AlCl_3$ is equivalent to $534/133.5 = 4$ moles. Next, we use the stoichiometry of the balanced equation. For every 2 moles of $AlCl_3$ that are produced, 6 moles of HCl are consumed. So, if we want to produce 4 moles of $AlCl_3$, we'll need 12 moles of HCl. Finally, we convert the number of moles of HCl consumed to grams. The molecular weight of HCl is $1 + 35.5 = 36.5$. This means that 1 mole of HCl has a mass of 36.5 grams. Therefore, 12 moles of HCl will have a mass of $12(36.5\ g) = 438$ grams.

Example 3-16: Consider the following reaction:

$$CS_2 + 3\,O_2 \rightarrow CO_2 + 2\,SO_2$$

How much carbon disulfide must be used to produce 64 grams of SO_2?

A) 38 g
B) 57 g
C) 76 g
D) 114 g

Solution: Since the molecular weight of SO_2 is 32.1 + 2(16) = 64, we know that 64 grams of SO_2 is equivalent to 1 mole. From the stoichiometry of the balanced equation, we see that for every 1 mole of CS_2 that reacts, 2 moles of SO_2 are produced. Therefore, to produce just 1 mole of SO_2, we need 1/2 mole of CS_2. The molecular weight of CS_2 is 12 + 2(32.1) ≈ 76, so 1/2 mole of CS_2 has a mass of 38 grams. The answer is A.

3.11 THE LIMITING REAGENT

Let's look again at the reaction of aluminum with hydrochloric acid:

$$2\,Al + 6\,HCl \rightarrow 2\,AlCl_3 + 3\,H_2$$

Suppose that this reaction starts with 4 moles of Al and 18 moles of HCl. We have enough HCl to make 6 moles of $AlCl_3$ and 9 moles of H_2. *However,* there's only enough Al to make 4 moles of $AlCl_3$ and 6 moles of H_2. There isn't enough aluminum metal (Al) to make use of all the available HCl. As the reaction proceeds, we'll run out of aluminum. This means that aluminum is the **limiting reagent** here, because we run out of this reactant *first*, so it limits how much product the reaction can produce.

Now suppose that the reaction begins with 4 moles of Al and 9 moles of HCl. There's enough Al metal to produce 4 moles of $AlCl_3$ and 6 moles of H_2. But there's only enough HCl to make 3 moles of $AlCl_3$ and 4.5 moles of H_2. There isn't enough HCl to make use of all the available aluminum metal. As the reaction proceeds, we'll find that all the HCl is consumed before the Al is consumed. In this situation, HCl is the limiting reagent. Notice that we had more moles of HCl than we had of Al and the initial mass of the HCl was greater than the initial mass of Al. Nevertheless, the limiting reagent in this case was the HCl. The limiting reagent is the reactant that is consumed first, not necessarily the reactant that's initially present in the smallest amount.

Example 3-17: Consider the following reaction:

$$2\ ZnS + 3\ O_2 \rightarrow 2\ ZnO + 2\ SO_2$$

If 97.5 grams of zinc sulfide undergoes this reaction with 32 grams of oxygen gas, what will be the limiting reagent?

A) ZnS
B) O_2
C) ZnO
D) SO_2

Solution: Since the molecular weight of ZnS is $65.4 + 32.1 = 97.5$ and the molecular weight of O_2 is $2(16)$ = 32, this reaction begins with 1 mole of ZnS and 1 mole of O_2. From the stoichiometry of the balanced equation, we see that 1 mole of ZnS would react completely with $\dfrac{3}{2}$ = 1.5 moles of O_2. Because we have only 1 mole of O_2, the O_2 will be consumed first; it is the limiting reagent, and the answer is B. Note that choice C and D can be eliminated immediately, because a limiting reagent is always a reactant.

3.12   SOME NOTATION USED IN CHEMICAL EQUATIONS

In addition to specifying what atoms or molecules are involved in a chemical reaction, an equation may contain additional information. One type of additional information that can be written right into the equation specifies the **phases** of the atoms or molecules in the reaction; that is, is the substance a solid, liquid, or gas? Another common condition is that a substance may be dissolved in water when the reaction proceeds. In this case, we'd say the substance is in aqueous solution. These four "states" are abbreviated and written in parentheses as follows:

Solid	(s)
Liquid	(l)
Gas	(g)
Aqueous	(aq)

These immediately follow the chemical symbol for the reactant or product in the equation. For example, the reaction of sodium metal with water, which produces sodium hydroxide and hydrogen gas, could be written like this:

$$2\ Na(s) + 2\ H_2O(l) \xrightarrow{\Delta} 2\ NaOH(aq) + H_2(g)$$

In some cases, the reactants are heated to produce the desired reaction. To indicate this, we write a "Δ"—or the word "heat"—above (or below) the reaction arrow. For example, heating potassium nitrate produces potassium nitrite and oxygen gas:

$$2\ KNO_3(s) \xrightarrow{\Delta} 2\ KNO_2(aq) + O_2(g)$$

Some reactions proceed more rapidly in the presence of a **catalyst**, which is a substance that increases the rate of a reaction without being consumed. For example, in the industrial production of sulfuric acid, an intermediate step is the reaction of sulfur dioxide and oxygen to produce sulfur trioxide. Not only are the reactants heated, but they are combined in the presence of vanadium pentoxide, V_2O_5. We indicate the presence of a catalyst by writing it below the arrow in the equation:

$$2\ SO_2 + O_2 \underset{V_2O_5}{\overset{\Delta}{\rightarrow}} 2\ SO_3$$

3.13 OXIDATION STATES

An atom's **oxidation state** (or **oxidation number**) is meant to indicate how the atom's "ownership" of its valence electrons changes when it forms a compound. For example, consider the formula unit NaCl. The sodium atom will transfer its valence electron to the chlorine atom, so the sodium's "ownership" of its valence electron has certainly changed. To indicate this, we'd say that the oxidation state of sodium is now +1 (or 1 *less* electron than it started with). On the other hand, chlorine accepts ownership of that 1 electron, so its oxidation state is −1 (that is, 1 *more* electron than it started with). Giving up ownership results in a more positive oxidation state; accepting ownership results in a more negative oxidation state.

This example of NaCl is rather special (and easy) since the compound is **ionic**, and we consider ionic compounds to involve the complete transfer of electrons. But what about a non-ionic (that is, a **covalent**) compound? *The oxidation state of an atom is the "charge" it would have if the compound were ionic.* Here's another way of saying this: the oxidation state of an atom in a molecule is the charge it would have if all the shared electrons were completely transferred to the more electronegative element. Note that for covalent compounds, this is not a real charge, just a bookkeeping trick.

The following list gives the rules for assigning oxidation states to the atoms in a molecule. If following one rule in the list causes the violation of another rule, the rule that is higher in the list takes precedence.

Rules for Assigning Oxidation States
1) The oxidation state of any element in its standard state is 0.
2) The sum of the oxidation states of the atoms in a neutral molecule must always be 0, and the sum of the oxidation states of the atoms in an ion must always equal the ion's charge.
3) Group 1 metals have a +1 oxidation state, and Group 2 metals have a +2 oxidation state.
4) Fluorine has a −1 oxidation state.

3.13

5) Hydrogen has a +1 oxidation state when bonded to something more electronegative than carbon, a –1 oxidation state when bonded to an atom less electronegative than carbon, and a 0 oxidation state when bonded to carbon.
6) Oxygen has a –2 oxidation state.
7) The rest of the halogens have a –1 oxidation state, and the atoms of the oxygen family have a –2 oxidation state.

It's worth noting a common exception to Rule 6: In peroxides (such as H_2O_2 or Na_2O_2), oxygen is in a –1 oxidation state.

As we will discuss later, the order of electronegativities of some elements can be remembered with the mnemonic FONClBrISCH (pronounced "fawn-cull-brish"). This lists the elements in order from the most electronegative (F) to the least electronegative (H). Hence, bonds from H to anything before C in FONClBrISCH will give hydrogen a +1 oxidation state, and bonds from H to anything *not* found in the list will give H a –1 oxidation state.

Let's find the oxidation number of manganese in $KMnO_4$. By Rule 3, K is +1, and by Rule 6, O is –2. Therefore, the oxidation state of Mn must be +7 in order for the sum of all the oxidation numbers in this electrically-neutral molecule to be zero (the unbreakable Rule 2).

Like many other elements, transition metals can assume different oxidation states, depending on the compound they're in. (Note, however, that a metal will never assume a negative oxidation state!) For example, iron has an oxidation number of +2 in $FeCl_2$ but an oxidation number of +3 in $FeCl_3$. The oxidation number of a transition metal is given as a Roman numeral in the name of the compound. Therefore, $FeCl_2$ is iron(II) chloride, and $FeCl_3$ is iron(III) chloride.

Example 3-18: Determine the oxidation state of the atoms in each of the following molecules:

a) NO_3^-
b) HNO_2
c) O_2
d) SF_4
e) Fe_3O_4

Solution:

a) By Rule 6, the oxidation state of O is –2; therefore, by Rule 2, the oxidation state of N must be +5
b) By Rule 5, the oxidation state of H is +1, and by Rule 6, O has an oxidation state of –2. Therefore, by Rule 2, N must have an oxidation state of +3 in this molecule.
c) By Rule 1 (which is higher in the list than Rule 5 and thus takes precedence), each O atom in O_2 has an oxidation state of 0.
d) By Rule 4, F has an oxidation state of –1. So, by Rule 2, S has an oxidation state of +4.
e) By Rule 6, O has an oxidation state of –2. So, by Rule 2, Fe has an oxidation state of +8/3. (Notice that oxidation states do not have to be whole numbers.)

3.13

Chapter 4
Atomic Structure and Periodic Trends

1 H 1.0																	2 He 4.0
3 Li 6.9	4 Be 9.0											5 B 10.8	6 C 12.0	7 N 14.0	8 O 16.0	9 F 19.0	10 Ne 20.2
11 Na 23.0	12 Mg 24.3											13 Al 27.0	14 Si 28.1	15 P 31.0	16 S 32.1	17 Cl 35.5	18 Ar 39.9
19 K 39.1	20 Ca 40.1	21 Sc 45.0	22 Ti 47.9	23 V 50.9	24 Cr 52.0	25 Mn 54.9	26 Fe 55.8	27 Co 58.9	28 Ni 58.7	29 Cu 63.5	30 Zn 65.4	31 Ga 69.7	32 Ge 72.6	33 As 74.9	34 Se 79.0	35 Br 79.9	36 Kr 83.8
37 Rb 85.5	38 Sr 87.6	39 Y 88.9	40 Zr 91.2	41 Nb 92.9	42 Mo 95.9	43 Tc (98)	44 Ru 101.1	45 Rh 102.9	46 Pd 106.4	47 Ag 107.9	48 Cd 112.4	49 In 114.8	50 Sn 118.7	51 Sb 121.8	52 Te 127.6	53 I 126.9	54 Xe 131.3
55 Cs 132.9	56 Ba 137.3	57 *La 138.9	72 Hf 178.5	73 Ta 180.9	74 W 183.9	75 Re 186.2	76 Os 190.2	77 Ir 192.2	78 Pt 195.1	79 Au 197.0	80 Hg 200.6	81 Tl 204.4	82 Pb 207.2	83 Bi 209.0	84 Po (209)	85 At (210)	86 Rn (222)
87 Fr (223)	88 Ra 226.0	89 †Ac 227.0	104 Rf (261)	105 Db (262)	106 Sg (266)	107 Bh (264)	108 Hs (277)	109 Mt (268)	110 Ds (281)	111 Rg (272)	112 Cn (285)	113 Uut (286)	114 Fl (289)	115 Uup (288)	116 Lv (293)	117 Uus (294)	118 Uuo (294)

*Lanthanide Series:

58 Ce 140.1	59 Pr 140.9	60 Nd 144.2	61 Pm (145)	62 Sm 150.4	63 Eu 152.0	64 Gd 157.3	65 Tb 158.9	66 Dy 162.5	67 Ho 164.9	68 Er 167.3	69 Tm 168.9	70 Yb 173.0	71 Lu 175.0

†Actinide Series:

90 Th 232.0	91 Pa (231)	92 U 238.0	93 Np (237)	94 Pu (244)	95 Am (243)	96 Cm (247)	97 Bk (247)	98 Cf (251)	99 Es (252)	100 Fm (257)	101 Md (258)	102 No (259)	103 Lr (260)

Periodic Table of the Elements

4.1 ATOMS

The smallest unit of any element is one **atom** of the element. All atoms have a central **nucleus**, which contains **protons** and **neutrons**, known collectively as **nucleons**. Each proton has an electric charge of +1 elementary unit; neutrons have no charge. Outside the nucleus, an atom contains electrons, and each **electron** has a charge of −1 elementary unit.

In every neutral atom, the number of electrons outside the nucleus is equal to the number of protons inside the nucleus. The electrons are held in the atom by the electrical attraction of the positively charged nucleus.

The number of protons in the nucleus of an atom is called its **atomic number**, Z. The atomic number of an atom uniquely determines what element the atom is, and Z may be shown explicitly by a subscript before the symbol of the element. For example, every beryllium atom contains exactly four protons, and we can write this as $_4$Be.

A proton and a neutron each have a mass slightly more than one atomic mass unit (1 amu $= 1.66 \times 10^{-27}$ kg), and an electron has a mass that's only about 0.05 percent the mass of either a proton or a neutron. So, virtually all the mass of an atom is due to the mass of the nucleus.

The number of protons plus the number of neutrons in the nucleus of an atom gives the atom's **mass number**, A. If we let N stand for the number of neutrons, then $A = Z + N$.

In designating a particular atom of an element, we refer to its mass number. One way to do this is to write A as a superscript. For example, if a beryllium atom contains 5 neutrons, then its mass number is $4 + 5 = 9$, and we would write this as $_4^9$Be or simply as ^{9}Be. Another way is simply to write the mass number after the name of the elements, with a hyphen; ^{9}Be is beryllium-9.

4.2 ISOTOPES

If two atoms of the same element differ in their numbers of neutrons, then they are called **isotopes**. The atoms shown below are two different isotopes of the element beryllium. The atom on the left has 4 protons and 3 neutrons, so its mass number is 7; it's ^{7}Be (or beryllium-7). The atom on the right has 4 protons and 5 neutrons, so it's ^{9}Be (beryllium-9).

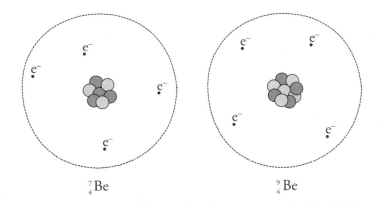

$^7_4$Be $^9_4$Be

(These figures are definitely not to scale. If they were, each dashed circle showing the "outer edge" of the atom would literally be about 1500 m—almost a mile across! The nucleus occupies only the *tiniest* fraction of an atom's volume, which is mostly empty space.) Notice that these atoms—like all isotopes of a given element—*have the same atomic number but different mass numbers.*

Example 4-1: An atom with 7 neutrons and a mass number of 12 is an isotope of what element?

A) Boron
B) Nitrogen
C) Magnesium
D) Potassium

Solution: If $A = 12$ and $N = 7$, then $Z = A - N = 12 - 7 = 5$. The element with an atomic number of 5 is boron. Therefore, choice A is the answer.

Atomic Weight

Elements exist naturally as a collection of their isotopes. The **atomic weight of an element** is a *weighted average* of the masses of its naturally occurring isotopes. For example, boron has two naturally occurring isotopes: boron-10, with an atomic mass of 10.013 amu, and boron-11, with an atomic mass of 11.009 amu. Since boron-10 accounts for 20 percent of all naturally occurring boron, and boron-11 accounts for the other 80 percent, the atomic weight of boron is

$$(20\%)(10.013 \text{ amu}) + (80\%)(11.009 \text{ amu}) = 10.810 \text{ amu}$$

and this is the value listed in the periodic table. (Recall that the atomic mass unit is defined so that the most abundant isotope of carbon, carbon-12, has a mass of precisely 12 amu.)

4.3 IONS

When a neutral atom gains or loses electrons, it becomes charged, and the resulting atom is called an **ion**. For each electron it gains, an atom acquires a charge of –1 unit, and for each electron it loses, an atom acquires a charge of +1 unit. A negatively charged ion is called an **anion**, while a positively charged ion is called a **cation**.

We designate how many electrons an atom has gained or lost by placing this number as a superscript after the chemical symbol for the element. For example, if a lithium atom loses 1 electron, it becomes the lithium cation Li^{1+}, or simply Li^+. If a phosphorus atom gains 3 electrons, it becomes the phosphorus anion P^{3-}, or phosphide.

Example 4-2: An atom contains 16 protons, 17 neutrons, and 18 electrons. Which of the following best indicates this ion?

A) $^{33}Cl^-$
B) $^{34}Cl^-$
C) $^{33}S^{2-}$
D) $^{34}S^{2-}$

Solution: Any nucleus that contains 16 protons is sulfur, so we can eliminate choices A and B immediately. Now, because $Z = 16$ and $N = 17$, the mass number, A, is $Z + N = 16 + 17 = 33$. Therefore, the answer is C.

Example 4-3: Of the following atoms/ions, which one contains the greatest number of neutrons?

A) $^{60}_{28}Ni$

B) $^{64}_{29}Cu^+$

C) $^{64}_{30}Zn$

D) $^{64}_{30}Zn^{2+}$

Solution: To find N, we just subtract Z (the subscript) from A (the superscript). The atom in choice A has $N = 60 - 28 = 32$; the ion in choice B has $N = 64 - 29 = 35$, and the atom or ion in both choices C and D have $N = 64 - 30 = 34$. Therefore, of the choices given, the ion in choice B contains the greatest number of neutrons.

4.4   NUCLEAR STABILITY AND RADIOACTIVITY

The protons and neutrons in a nucleus are held together by a force called the **strong nuclear force**. It's stronger than the electrical force between charged particles, since for all atoms besides hydrogen, the strong nuclear force must overcome the electrical repulsion between the protons. In fact, of the four fundamental forces of nature, the strong nuclear force is the most powerful even though it only works over extremely short distances, as seen in the nucleus.

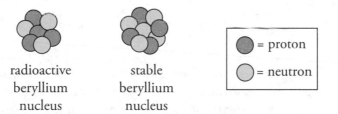

radioactive
beryllium
nucleus

stable
beryllium
nucleus

⬤ = proton
◯ = neutron

Unstable nuclei are said to be **radioactive**, and they undergo a transformation to make them more stable, altering the number and ratio of protons and neutrons or just lowering their energy. Such a process is called **radioactive decay**, and we'll look at three types: **alpha**, **beta** and **gamma**. The nucleus that undergoes radioactive decay is known as the **parent**, and the resulting more stable nucleus is known as the **daughter.**

Alpha Decay

When a large nucleus wants to become more stable by reducing the number of protons and neutrons, it emits an alpha particle. An **alpha particle**, denoted by $_2^4\alpha$, consists of 2 protons and 2 neutrons:

alpha particle

This is equivalent to a helium-4 nucleus, so an alpha particle can also be denoted by $_2^4$He. Alpha decay reduces the parent's atomic number by 2 and the mass number by 4. For example, polonium-210 is an α-emitter. It undergoes alpha decay to form the stable nucleus lead-206:

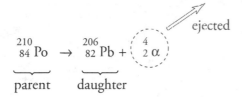

$$_{84}^{210}\text{Po} \rightarrow {}_{82}^{206}\text{Pb} + {}_{2}^{4}\alpha$$

parent   daughter

Although alpha particles are emitted with high energy from the parent nucleus, this energy is quickly lost as the particle travels through matter or air. As a result, the particles do not typically travel far, and can be stopped by the outer layers of human skin or a piece of paper.

Beta Decay

There are actually three types of beta decay: β^-, β^+, and electron capture. Each type of beta decay involves the conversion of a neutron into a proton (along with some other particles that are beyond the scope of the MCAT), or vice versa, through the action of the **weak nuclear force**.

Beta particles are more dangerous than alpha particles since they are significantly less massive. They therefore have more energy and a greater penetrating ability. However, they can be stopped by aluminum foil or a centimeter of plastic or glass.

β^- Decay

When an unstable nucleus contains too many neutrons, it may convert a neutron into a proton and an electron (also known as a β^- **particle**), which is ejected. The atomic number of the resulting daughter nucleus is 1 greater than the radioactive parent nucleus, but the mass number remains the same. The isotope carbon-14, the decay of which is the basis of radiocarbon dating of archaeological artifacts, is an example of a radioactive nucleus that undergoes β^- decay:

$$^{14}_{6}\text{C} \quad \rightarrow \quad ^{14}_{7}\text{N} \; + \; ^{0}_{-1}\beta \quad \text{ejected}$$

β^- decay is the most common type of beta decay, and when the MCAT mentions "beta decay" without any further qualification, it means β^- decay.

β^+ Decay (or Positron Emission)

When an unstable nucleus contains too few neutrons, it converts a proton into a neutron and a positron, which is ejected. This is known as β^+ **decay**. The positron is the electron's *antiparticle*; it's identical to an electron except its charge is positive. The atomic number of the resulting daughter nucleus is 1 less than the radioactive parent nucleus, but the mass number remains the same. The isotope fluorine-18, which can be used in medical diagnostic bone scans in the form Na^{18}F, is an example of a positron emitter:

$$^{18}_{9}\text{F} \quad \rightarrow \quad ^{18}_{8}\text{O} \; + \; ^{0}_{+1}\beta \quad \text{ejected}$$

Electron Capture

Another way for an unstable nucleus to increase its number of neutrons is to capture an electron from the closest electron shell (the $n = 1$ shell) and use it in the conversion of a proton into a neutron. Just like positron emission, **electron capture** causes the atomic number to be reduced by 1 while the mass number remains the same. The nucleus chromium-51 is an example of a radioactive nucleus that undergoes electron capture, becoming the stable nucleus vanadium-51:

$$\ce{^{51}_{24}Cr} + \ce{^{0}_{-1}e^-} \rightarrow \ce{^{51}_{23}V}$$

Gamma Decay

A nucleus in an excited energy state—which is usually the case after a nucleus has undergone alpha or any type of beta decay—can "relax" to its ground state by emitting energy in the form of one or more photons of electromagnetic radiation. These photons are called **gamma photons** (symbolized by γ) and have a very high frequency and energy. Gamma photons (or gamma rays) have neither mass nor charge, and can therefore penetrate matter most effectively. A few inches of lead or about a meter of concrete will stop most gamma rays. Their ejection from a radioactive atom changes neither the atomic number nor the mass number of the nucleus. For example, after silicon-31 undergoes β^- decay, the resulting daughter nucleus then undergoes gamma decay:

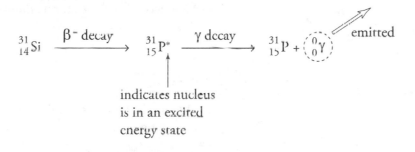

indicates nucleus
is in an excited
energy state

Notice that alpha and beta decay change the identity of the nucleus, but gamma decay does not. Gamma decay is simply an expulsion of energy.

Summary of Radioactive Decay

$N\downarrow\ Z\downarrow$	Alpha Decay	Decreases the number of neutrons *and* protons in large nucleus

Subtracts 4 from the mass number
Subtracts 2 from the atomic number

$$^{A}_{Z}X \xrightarrow{\ \alpha\ } {}^{A-4}_{Z-2}Y + {}^{4}_{2}\alpha$$

$N\downarrow\ Z\uparrow$	Beta$^-$ Decay	Decreases the number of neutrons, increases the number of protons

Adds 1 to the atomic number

$$^{A}_{Z}X \xrightarrow{\ \beta^-\ } {}^{A}_{Z+1}Y + {}^{0}_{-1}\beta$$

$N\uparrow\ Z\downarrow$	Positron Emission	Increases the number of neutrons, decreases the number of protons

Subtracts 1 from the atomic number

$$^{A}_{Z}X \xrightarrow{\ \beta^+\ } {}^{A}_{Z-1}Y + {}^{0}_{+1}\beta$$

$N\uparrow\ Z\downarrow$	Electron Capture	Increases the number of neutrons, decreases the number of protons

Subtracts 1 from the atomic number

$$^{A}_{Z}X + {}^{0}_{-1}e^- \xrightarrow{\ EC\ } {}^{A}_{Z-1}Y$$

	Gamma Decay	Brings an excited nucleus to a lower energy state

Doesn't change mass number or atomic number

$$^{A}_{Z}X^* \xrightarrow{\ \gamma\ } {}^{A}_{Z}X + {}^{0}_{0}\gamma$$

Example 4-4: Radioactive calcium-47, a known β^- emitter, is administered in the form of $^{47}CaCl_2$ by I.V. as a diagnostic tool to study calcium metabolism. What is the daughter nucleus of ^{47}Ca?

A) ^{46}K
B) ^{47}K
C) $^{47}Ca^+$
D) ^{47}Sc

Solution: Since β^- decay will always change the identity of an element, eliminate choice C. The β^- decay of ^{47}Ca is described by this nuclear reaction:

$$^{47}_{20}Ca \rightarrow {}^{47}_{21}Sc + {}^{0}_{-1}\beta$$

Therefore, the daughter nucleus is scandium-47, choice D.

Example 4-5: Americium-241 is used to provide intracavitary radiation for the treatment of malignancies. This radioisotope is known to undergo alpha decay. What is the daughter nucleus?

A) ^{237}Np
B) ^{241}Pu
C) ^{237}Bk
D) ^{243}Bk

Solution: Alpha decay will reduce the mass by 4, to 237, so eliminate choices B and D. It will reduce the nuclear charge by 2 from 95 to 93, so choose A. The α decay of ^{241}Am is described by this nuclear reaction:

$$^{241}_{95}Am \rightarrow ^{237}_{93}Np + ^{4}_{2}\alpha$$

Example 4-6: Vitamin B_{12} can be prepared with *radioactive* cobalt (^{58}Co), a known β^+ emitter, and administered orally as a diagnostic tool to test for defects in intestinal vitamin B_{12} absorption. What is the daughter nucleus of ^{58}Co?

A) ^{57}Fe
B) ^{58}Fe
C) ^{59}Co
D) ^{59}Ni

Solution: All types of β^+ decay leave the mass of the daughter and parent elements the same, thus the mass must be 58, making choice B the only option. The β^+ decay of ^{58}Co is described by this nuclear reaction:

$$^{58}_{27}Co \rightarrow ^{58}_{26}Fe + ^{0}_{+1}\beta$$

Example 4-7: A certain radioactive isotope is administered orally as a diagnostic tool to study pancreatic function and intestinal fat absorption. This radioisotope is known to undergo β^- decay, and the daughter nucleus is xenon-131. What is the parent radioisotope?

A) ^{131}Cs
B) ^{131}I
C) ^{132}I
D) ^{132}Xe

Solution: Eliminate choices C and D since the mass number should remain the same for all forms of β^- decay. The β^- decay that results in ^{131}Xe is described by this nuclear reaction:

$$^{131}_{53}I \rightarrow ^{131}_{54}Xe + ^{0}_{-1}\beta$$

Therefore, the parent nucleus is iodine-131, choice B.

Example 4-8: Which of these modes of radioactive decay causes a change in the mass number of the parent nucleus?

A) α
B) β^-
C) β^+
D) γ

Solution: Gamma decay causes no changes in the number of protons or neutrons, so we can eliminate choice D. Beta decay (β^-, β^+, and EC) changes both N and Z by 1, but always such that the change in the sum $N + Z$ (which is the mass number, A) is zero. Therefore, we can eliminate choices B and C. The answer is A.

Example 4-9: One of the naturally occurring radioactive series begins with radioactive ^{238}U. It undergoes a series of decays, one of which is: alpha, beta, beta, alpha, alpha, alpha, alpha, alpha, beta, beta, alpha, beta, alpha, beta. What is the final resulting nuclide of this series of decays?

A) ^{204}Pb
B) ^{204}Pt
C) ^{206}Pb
D) ^{206}Pt

Solution: Since there are so many individual decays, let's find the final daughter nucleus using a simple shortcut: For every alpha decay, we'll subtract 4 from the mass number (the superscript) and subtract 2 from the atomic number (the subscript); for every beta decay, we'll add 0 to the mass number and 1 to the atomic number. Since there are a total of 8 alpha-decays and 6 beta-decays, we get

$$^{238}_{92}\text{U} \xrightarrow{8\alpha} \begin{smallmatrix} 238 \ -8(4) \\ 92 \ -8(2) \end{smallmatrix} \xrightarrow[+6(1)]{6\beta^- \ +6(0)} = \ ^{206}_{82}\text{Pb}$$

Therefore, the final daughter nucleus is lead-206, choice C.

Half Life

Different radioactive nuclei decay at different rates. The **half-life**, which is denoted by $t_{1/2}$, of a radioactive substance is the time it takes for one-half of some sample of the substance to decay. Thus, the shorter the half-life, the faster the decay. The amount of a radioactive substance decreases exponentially with time, as illustrated in the following graph.

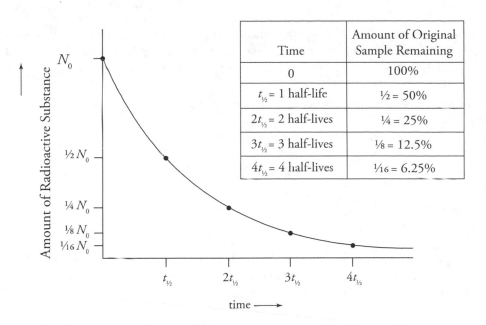

Time	Amount of Original Sample Remaining
0	100%
$t_{1/2}$ = 1 half-life	½ = 50%
$2t_{1/2}$ = 2 half-lives	¼ = 25%
$3t_{1/2}$ = 3 half-lives	⅛ = 12.5%
$4t_{1/2}$ = 4 half-lives	1/16 = 6.25%

For example, a radioactive sample with an initial mass of 80 grams and a half-life of 6 years will decay as follows:

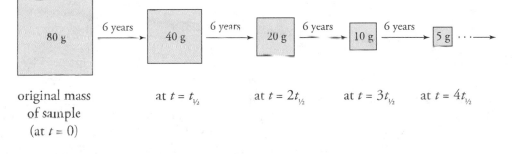

The equation for the exponential decay curve shown above is often written as $N = N_0 e^{-kt}$, but a simpler—and much more intuitive way—is

$$N = N_0(1/2)^{t/t_{1/2}}$$

where $t_{1/2}$ is the half-life. For example, when $t = 3t_{1/2}$, the number of radioactive nuclei remaining, N, is $N_0(1/2)^3 = 1/8\ N_0$, just what we expect. If the form $N_0 e^{-kt}$ is used, the value of k (known as the **decay constant**) is inversely proportional to the half-life: $k = (\ln 2)/t_{1/2}$. The shorter the half-life, the greater the decay constant, and the more rapidly the sample decays.

Example 4-10: Cesium-137 has a half-life of 30 years. How long will it take for only 0.3 g to remain from a sample that had an original mass of 2.4 g?

A) 60 years
B) 90 years
C) 120 years
D) 240 years

Solution: Since 0.3 grams is 1/8 of 2.4 grams, the question is asking how long it will take for the radio-isotope to decrease to 1/8 its original amount. We know that this requires 3 half-lives, since $1/2 \times 1/2 \times 1/2 = 1/8$. So, if each half-life is 30 years, then 3 half-lives will be $3(30) = 90$ years, choice B.

Example 4-11: Radiolabeled vitamin B_{12} containing radioactive cobalt-58 is administered to diagnose a defect in a patient's vitamin-B_{12} absorption. If ^{58}Co has a half-life of 72 days, approximately what percentage of the radioisotope will still remain in the patient a year later?

A) 3%
B) 5%
C) 8%
D) 10%

Solution: One year is approximately equal to 5 half-lives of this radioisotope, since $5 \times 72 = 360$ days = 1 year. After 5 half-lives, the amount of the radioisotope will drop to $(1/2)^5 = 1/32$ of the original amount administered. Because $1/32 = 3/100 = 3\%$, the best answer is choice A.

Example: 4-12 Iodinated oleic acid, containing radioactive iodine-131, is administered orally to study a patient's pancreatic function. If ^{131}I has a half-life of 8 days, how long after the procedure will the amount of ^{131}I remaining in the patient's body be reduced to 1/5 its initial value?

A) 19 days
B) 32 days
C) 40 days
D) 256 days

Solution: Although the fraction 1/5 is not a whole-number power of 1/2, we do know that it's between 1/4 and 1/8. If 1/4 of the sample were left, we'd know that 2 half-lives had elapsed, and if 1/8 of the sample were left, we'd know that 3 half-lives had elapsed. Therefore, because 1/5 is between 1/4 and 1/8, we know that the amount of time will be between 2 and 3 half-lives. Since each half-life is 8 days, this amount of time will be between $2(8) = 16$ days and $3(8) = 24$ days. Of the choices given, only choice A is in this range.

4.5   ATOMIC STRUCTURE

Emission Spectra

Imagine a glass tube filled with a small sample of an element in gaseous form. When electric current is passed through the tube, the gas begins to glow with a color characteristic of that particular element. If this light emitted by the gas is then passed through a prism—which will separate the light into its component wavelengths—the result is the element's **emission spectrum.**

An atom's emission spectrum gives an energetic "fingerprint" of that element because it consists of a unique sequence of *bright* lines that correspond to specific wavelengths and energies. The energies of the photons, or particles of light that are emitted, are related to their frequencies, *f*, and wavelengths, λ, by the equation

$$E_{photon} = hf = h\frac{c}{\lambda}$$

where *h* is a universal constant called **Planck's constant** (6.63×10^{-34} J·s) and *c* is the speed of light. For the following discussion, a general understanding of the electromagnetic spectrum will be useful. More detail on this topic can be found in Section 13.1 of the *MCAT Physics Review*.

The Bohr Model of the Atom

In 1913 the Danish physicist Niels Bohr realized that the model of atomic structure of his time was inconsistent with emission spectral data. In order to account for the limited numbers of lines that are observed in the emission spectra of elements, Bohr described a new model of the atom. In this model that would later take his name, he proposed that the electrons in an atom orbited the nucleus in circular paths, much as the planets orbit the sun in the solar system. Distance from the nucleus was related to the energy of the electrons; electrons with greater amounts of energy orbited the nucleus at greater distances. However, the electrons in the atom cannot assume any arbitrary energy, but have *quantized* energy states, and thereby only orbit at certain allowed distances from the nucleus.

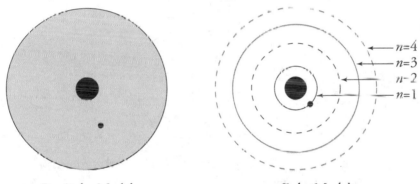

Pre-Bohr Model
Electrons assume arbitrary energies

Bohr Model
Electrons assume discrete energies

If an electron absorbs energy that's exactly equal to the difference in energy between its current level and that of an available higher lever, it "jumps" to that higher level. The electron can then "drop" to a lower energy level, emitting a photon with an energy exactly equal to the difference between the levels. This model predicted that elements would have line spectra instead of continuous spectra, as would be the case if transitions between all possible energies could be expected. An electron could only gain or lose very specific amounts of energy due to the quantized nature of the energy levels. Therefore, only photons with certain energies are observed. These specific energies corresponded to very specific wavelengths, as seen in the emission line spectra.

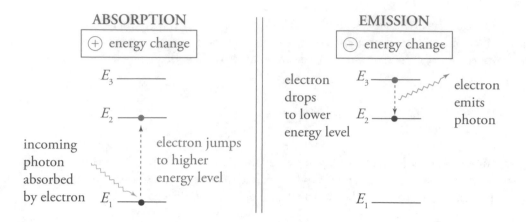

In the transition depicted below, an electron is initially in its **ground state** ($n = 1$), or its lowest possible energy level. When this electron absorbs a photon it jumps to a higher energy level, known as an **excited state** (in this case $n = 3$). Electrons excited to high energy don't always relax to the ground state in large jumps, rather they can relax in a series of smaller jumps, gradually coming back to the ground state. From this excited state the electron can relax in one of two ways, either dropping into the $n = 2$ level, or directly back to the $n = 1$ ground state. In the first scenario, we can expect to detect a photon with energy corresponding to the difference between $n = 3$ and $n = 2$. In the latter case we'd detect a more energetic photon of energy corresponding to the difference between $n = 3$ and $n = 1$.

Note: Distances between energy levels are not drawn to scale.

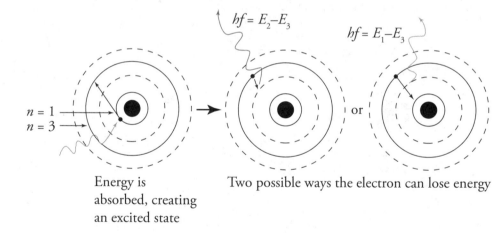

The energies of these discrete energy levels were given by Bohr in the following equation, which only accurately predicted the behavior of atoms or ions containing one electron, now known as Bohr atoms. The value n in this case represents the energy level of the electron.

$$E_n = \frac{(-2.178 \times 10^{-18}\,\text{J})}{n^2}$$

Since we can calculate the energies of the levels of a Bohr atom, we can predict the wavelengths of photons emitted or absorbed when electrons transition between any two energy levels. To do this we calculate the energy differences between discrete levels by subtracting the initial energy of the electron from the final energy of the electron. We can find the energies of the two possible emitted photons shown above as follows:

$$\Delta E_{3\rightarrow 2} = \frac{(-2.178\times 10^{-18}\,\text{J})}{(2)^2} - \frac{(-2.178\times 10^{-18}\,\text{J})}{(3)^2}$$

$$\Delta E_{3\rightarrow 2} = -3.025\times 10^{-19}\,\text{J}$$

$$\Delta E_{3\rightarrow 1} = \frac{(-2.178\times 10^{-18}\,\text{J})}{(1)^2} - \frac{(-2.178\times 10^{-18}\,\text{J})}{(3)^2}$$

$$\Delta E_{3\rightarrow 2} = -1.936\times 10^{-18}\,\text{J}$$

Note that both energies calculated above are negative, indicating that energy is being released by the electron as it falls from its excited state to a lower energy level. For electron transitions from the ground state to an excited state, the ΔE values will be positive, indicating energy is absorbed by the electron.

Once the energy is calculated, the wavelength of the photon can be found by employing the relation $\Delta E = h\dfrac{c}{\lambda}$. Not all electron transitions produce photons we can see with the naked eye, but all transitions in an atom will produce photons either in the ultraviolet, visible, or infrared region of the electromagnetic spectrum.

Example 4-13: Which of the following is NOT an example of a Bohr atom?

A)   H
B)   He⁺
C)   Li²⁺
D)   H⁺

Solution: A Bohr atom is one that contains only one electron. Since H⁺ has a positive charge from losing the one electron in the neutral atom thereby having no electrons at all, choice D is the answer.

Example 4-14: The first four electron energy levels of an atom are shown at the right, given in terms of electron volts. Which of the following gives the energy of a photon that could NOT be emitted by this atom?

A)   14 eV
B)   40 eV
C)   44 eV
D)   54 eV

———— $E_4 = -18$ eV

———— $E_3 = -32$ eV

———— $E_2 = -72$ eV

———— $E_1 = -288$ eV

Solution: The difference between E_4 and E_3 is 14 eV, so a photon of 14 eV would be emitted if an electron were to drop from level 4 to level 3; this eliminates choice A. Similarly, the difference between E_3 and E_2 is 40 eV, so choice B is eliminated, and the difference between E_4 and E_2 is 54 eV, so choice D is eliminated. The answer must be C; no two energy levels in this atom are separated by 44 eV.

Example 4-15: Consider two electron transitions. In the first case, an electron falls from $n = 4$ to $n = 2$, giving off a photon of light with a wavelength equal to 488 nm. In the second transition, an electron moves from $n = 3$ to $n = 4$. For this transition, we would expect that:

A) energy is emitted, and the wavelength of the corresponding photon will be shorter than the first transition.

B) energy is emitted, and the wavelength of the corresponding photon will be longer than the first transition.

C) energy is absorbed, and the wavelength of the corresponding photon will be shorter than the first transition.

D) energy is absorbed, and the wavelength of the corresponding photon will be longer than the first transition.

Solution: Since the electron is moving from a lower to higher energy level, we would expect that the atom absorbs energy (eliminating choices A and B). Since the electron transitions between energy levels that are closer together, the ΔE between levels is smaller. By the $\Delta E = h\dfrac{c}{\lambda}$ relationship, we know that energy and wavelength are inversely related. Therefore with a smaller energy change, the wavelength of the associated light will be longer. D is the correct answer.

The Quantum Model of the Atom

While one-electron atoms produce easily predicted atomic spectra, the Bohr model does not do a good job of predicting the atomic spectra of many-electron atoms. This shows that the Bohr model cannot describe the electron-electron interactions that exist in many-electron atoms. The quantum model of the atom was developed to account for these differences. Bohr's model suggested, and we still hold to be true, that electrons held by an atom can exist only at discrete energy levels—that is, electron energy levels are quantized. This quantization is described by a unique "address" for each electron, consisting of four quantum numbers designating the shell, subshell, orbital, and spin. While the details of quantum numbers are beyond the scope of the MCAT, it is still useful to understand the conceptual basis of the quantum model.

The Energy Shell

The energy shell (n) of an electron in the quantum model of the atom is analogous to the circular orbits in the Bohr model of the atom. An electron in a higher shell has a greater amount of energy and a greater average distance from the nucleus. For example, an electron in the 3rd shell ($n = 3$) has a higher energy than an electron in the 2nd shell (where $n = 2$), which has more energy than an electron in the 1st shell ($n = 1$).

The Energy Subshell

In the quantum model of the atom, however, we no longer describe the path of electrons around the nucleus as circular orbits, but focus on the probability of finding an electron somewhere in the atom. Loosely speaking, an **orbital** describes a three-dimensional region around the nucleus in which the electron is most likely to be found.

A subshell in an atom is comprised of one or more orbitals, and is denoted by a letter (*s, p, d,* or *f*) that describes the shape and energy of the orbital(s). The orbitals in the subshells get progressively more complex and higher in energy in the order listed above. Each energy shell has one or more subshells, and each higher energy shell contains one additional subshell. For example, the first energy shell contains the *s* subshell, while the second energy shell contains both the *s* and *p* subshell, etc.

4.5

The Orbital Orientation

Each subshell contains one or more orbitals of the same energy (also called degenerate orbitals), and these orbitals have different three-dimensional orientations in space. The number of orientations increases by two in each successive subshell. For example, the *s* subshell contains one orientation and the *p* subshell contains three orientations.

You should be able to recognize the shapes of the orbitals in the *s* and *p* subshells. Each *s* subshell has just one spherically symmetrical orbital.

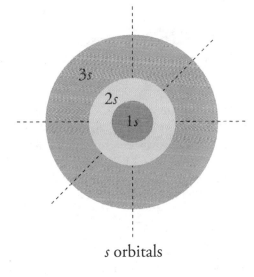

s orbitals

Each *p* subshell has three orbitals, each depicted as a dumbbell, with different spatial orientations.

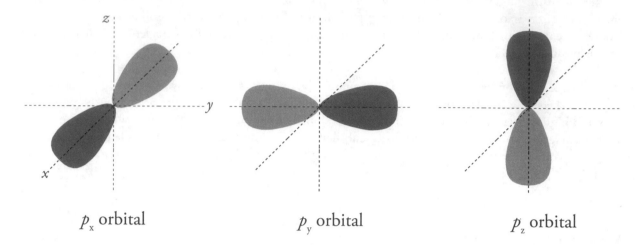

p_x orbital $\qquad$ p_y orbital $\qquad$ p_z orbital

The Electron Spin

Every electron has two possible spin states, which can be considered the electron's intrinsic magnetism. Because of this every orbital can accommodate a maximum of two electrons, one spin-up and one spin-down. If an orbital is full, we say that the electrons it holds are "spin-paired."

4.6 ELECTRON CONFIGURATIONS

Now that we've described the modern quantum model of the atom, let's see how this is represented as an electron configuration. There are three basic rules:

1) *Electrons occupy the lowest energy orbitals available.* (This is the **Aufbau principle**.) Electron subshells are filled in order of increasing energy. The periodic table is logically constructed to reflect this fact, and therefore one can easily determine shell filling for specific atoms based on where they appear on the table. We will detail this in the next section on "Blocks."

2) *Electrons in the same subshell occupy available orbitals singly, before pairing up.* (This is known as **Hund's rule**.)

3) *There can be no more than two electrons in any given orbital.* (This is the **Pauli exclusion principle**.)

For example, let's describe the locations for all the electrons in an oxygen atom, which contains eight electrons. Beginning with the first, lowest energy shell, there is only one subshell (*s*) and only one orientation in that subshell, and there can only be two electrons in that one orbital. Therefore, these two electrons fill the only orbital in the 1*s* subshell. We write this as $1s^2$, to indicate that there are two electrons in the 1*s* subshell.

We still have six electrons left, so let's move on to the second, next highest, energy shell. There are two subshells (*s* and *p*). Since the *s* subshell is lower in energy than the *p* subshell, the next two electrons go in the 2*s* subshell, that is, $2s^2$.

For the remaining four electrons, there would be three orientations of orbitals in the p subshell. According to Hund's rule, we place one spin up electron in each of these three orbitals. The eighth electron now pairs up with an electron in one of the $2p$ orbitals. So, the last four electrons go in the $2p$ subshell: $2p^4$ (or more explicitly, $2p_x^2 2p_y^1 2p_z^1$).

The complete electron configuration for oxygen can now be written like this:

$$\text{Oxygen} = 1s^2 2s^2 2p^4$$

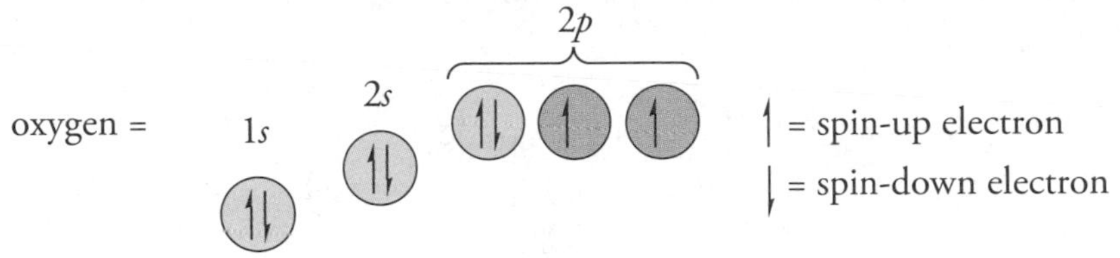

↑ = spin-up electron
↓ = spin-down electron

Here are the electron configurations for the first ten elements:

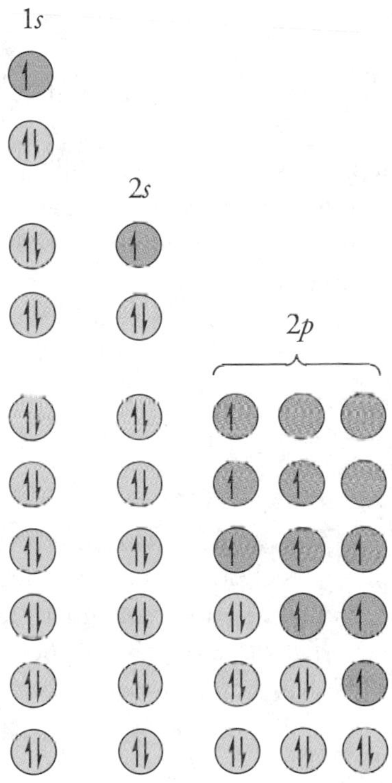

Example 4-16: What's the maximum number of electrons that can go into any s subshell? Any p subshell? Any d? Any f?

Solution: An s subshell has only one possible orbital orientation. Since only two electrons can fill any given orbital, an s subshell can hold no more than $1 \times 2 = 2$ electrons.

A p subshell has three possible orbital orientations (two more than an s subshell). Since again only two electrons can fill any given orbital, a p subshell can hold no more than $3 \times 2 = 6$ electrons.

A d subshell has five possible orbital orientations (two more than a p subshell). Since there are two electrons per orbital, a d subshell can hold no more than $5 \times 2 = 10$ electrons.

Finally, an f subshell has seven possible orbital orientations (two more than a d subshell). Since there are two electrons per orbital, an f subshell can hold no more than $7 \times 2 = 14$ electrons.

Example 4-17: Write down—and comment on—the electron configuration of argon (Ar, atomic number 18).

Solution: We have 18 electrons to successively place in the proper subshells, as follows:

$1s$:   2 electrons

$2s$:   2 electrons

$2p$:   6 electrons

$3s$:   2 electrons

$3p$:   6 electrons

Therefore,

$$[\text{Ar}] = 1s^2 2s^2 2p^6 3s^2 3p^6$$

Notice that $3s$ and $3p$ subshells have their full complement of electrons. In fact, the **noble gases** (those elements in the last column of the periodic table) all have their outer 8 electrons in filled subshells: 2 in the ns subshell plus 6 in the np. (The lone exception, of course, is helium; but its one and only subshell, the $1s$, is filled—with 2 electrons.) Because their 8 valence electrons are in filled subshells, we say that these atoms—Ne, Ar, Kr, Xe, and Rn—have a complete **octet**, which accounts for their remarkable chemical inactivity.

Diamagnetic and Paramagnetic Atoms

An atom that has all of its electrons spin-paired is referred to as **diamagnetic**. For example, helium, beryllium, and neon are diamagnetic. A diamagnetic atom must contain an even number of electrons and have all of its occupied subshells filled. Since all the electrons in a diamagnetic atom are spin-paired, the individual magnetic fields that they create cancel, leaving no net magnetic field. Such an atom will be *repelled* by an externally produced magnetic field.

4.6

If an atom's electrons are not all spin-paired, it is said to be **paramagnetic**. Paramagnetic atoms are *attracted* into externally produced magnetic fields.

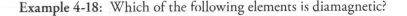

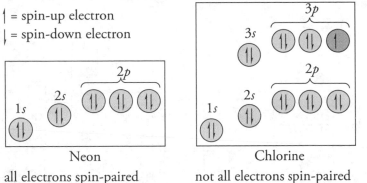

Neon

all electrons spin-paired
∴ diamagnetic
repelled from a magnetic field

Chlorine

not all electrons spin-paired
∴ paramagnetic
attracted into a magnetic field

Example 4-18: Which of the following elements is diamagnetic?

A) Sodium
B) Sulfur
C) Potassium
D) Calcium

Solution: First, a diamagnetic atom must contain an *even* number of electrons, because they all must be spin-*paired*. So, we can eliminate choices A and C, since sodium and potassium each contain an odd number of electrons (11 and 19, respectively). The electron configuration of sulfur is [Ne] $3s^2 3p^4$; by Hund's rule, the 4 electrons in the $3p$ subshell will look like this:

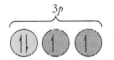

They're not all spin-paired, so sulfur is not diamagnetic. The answer must be D, calcium, because its configuration is [Ar] $4s^2$, and all of its electrons are spin-paired.

Blocks in the Periodic Table

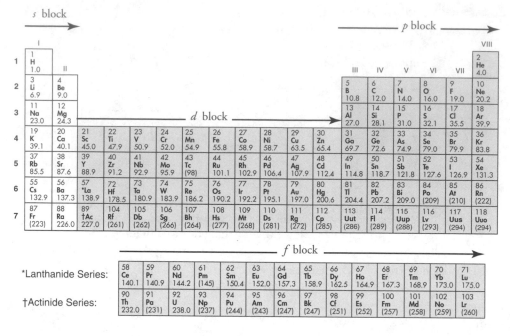

The periodic table can be divided into blocks, as shown above. The name of the block (s, p, d, or f) indicates the highest-energy subshell containing electrons in the ground-state of an atom within that block. For example, carbon is in the p block, and its electron configuration is $1s^2 2s^2 2p^2$; the highest-energy subshell that contains electrons (the $2p$) is a p subshell. In addition, each horizontal row in the periodic table is called a **period**, and each vertical column is called a **group** (or **family**). The bold numbers next to the rows on the left indicate the period number; for example, potassium (K, atomic number 19) is in Period 4.

How do we use this block diagram to write electron configurations? To illustrate, let's say we want to write the configuration for chlorine ($Z = 17$). To get to $Z = 17$, imagine starting at $Z = 1$ (hydrogen) and filling up the subshells as we move along through the rows to $Z = 17$. (Notice that helium has been moved over next to hydrogen for purposes of this block diagram.) We'll first have $1s^2$ for the 2 atoms in Period 1, s block ($Z = 1$ and $Z = 2$); the $2s^2$ for the next 2 atoms, which are in Period 2, s block ($Z = 3$ and $Z = 4$); then $2p^6$ for the next 6 atoms, which are in Period 2, p block ($Z = 5$ through $Z = 10$); the $3s^2$ for the next 2 atoms, which are in Period 3, s block ($Z = 11$ and $Z = 12$); then, finally, $3p^5$ for the atoms starting with aluminum, Al, in Period 3, p block and counting through to chlorine, Cl. So, we've gone through the rows and blocks from the beginning and stopped once we hit the atom we wanted, and along the way we obtained $1s^2 2s^2 2p^6 3s^2 3p^5$. This is the electron configuration of chlorine.

The noble gases are often used as starting points, because they are at the end of the rows and represent a shell being completely filled; all that's left is to count over in the next row until the desired atom is reached. We find the closest noble gas that has an atomic number less than that of the atom for which we want to find an electron configuration. In the case of chlorine ($Z = 17$), the closest noble gas with a smaller atomic number is neon ($Z = 10$). Starting with neon, we have 7 additional electrons to take care of. To get to $Z = 17$, we go through the 2 atoms in the s block of Period 3 ($3s^2$), then notice that Cl is the fifth element in the p block, giving us $3p^5$. Therefore, the electron configuration of chlorine is the same as that of neon plus $3s^2 3p^5$, which we can write like this: Cl = [Ne] $3s^2 3p^5$.

The simple counting through the rows and blocks works as long as you remember this simple rule: Whenever you're in the d block, *subtract 1 from the period number.* For example, the first row of the d block ($Z = 21$ through $Z = 30$) is in Period 4, but instead of saying that these elements have their outermost (or **valence**) electrons in the $4d$ subshell, we subtract 1 from the period number and say that these elements put their valence electrons in the $3d$ subshell.

In summary: The block in the table tells us in which subshell the outermost (valence) electrons of the atom will be. The period (row) gives the shell, n, as long as we remember the following fact about the atoms in the d block: electrons for an atom in the d block of Period n go into the subshell $(n-1)d$. For example, the electron configuration for scandium (Sc, atomic number 21) is $[Ar]4s^2 3d^1$. (Note: if you ever need to write the electron configuration for an element in the f block, the rule is: *In the f block, subtract 2 from the period number.*)

Example 4-19: Which of the following gives the electron configuration of an aluminum atom?

A) $1s^2 2s^2 2p^1$
B) $1s^2 2s^2 2p^2$
C) $1s^2 2s^2 2p^6 3s^2 3p^1$
D) $1s^2 2s^2 2p^6 3s^2 3p^2$

Solution: Since aluminum (Al) has atomic number 13, a neutral aluminum atom must have 13 electrons. This observation alone eliminates choices A, B, and D (which indicate a total of 5, 6, and 14 electrons, respectively), so the answer must be C.

Example 4-20: What is the maximum number of electrons that can be present in the $n = 3$ shell?

A) 6
B) 9
C) 12
D) 18

Solution: Every new energy level (n) adds a new subshell. That means that in the first energy level we have only the s subshell, while when $n = 2$ we have both s and p subshells, and when $n = 3$, there are s, p, and d subshells. Since there are 1, 3, and 5 s, p, and d orbitals, respectively, for a total of 9 orbitals, and since the maximum number of electrons in an orbital is 2, there can be a maximum of 18 electrons in the $n = 3$ shell.

Example 4-21: What's the electron configuration of a zirconium atom ($Z = 40$)?

A) $[Kr] 4d^4$
B) $[Kr] 5s^2 4d^2$
C) $[Kr] 5s^2 5p^2$
D) $[Kr] 5s^2 5d^2$

Solution: Zirconium (Zr) is in the d block of Period 5. After krypton (Kr, atomic number 36), we'll have $5s^2$ for the next 2 atoms in the Period 5, s block ($Z = 37$ and $Z = 38$). Then, remembering the rule that electrons for an atom in the d block of Period n go into the subshell $(n - 1)d$, we know that the last two electrons will go in the $4d$ (not the $5d$) subshell. Therefore, the answer is B.

Some Anomalous Electron Configurations

The process described above (reading across the periodic table, from top to bottom and left to right, using the blocks as a tool for the order of filling of subshells) to determine an atom's electron configuration works quite well for a large percentage of the elements, but there are a few atoms for which the anticipated electron configuration is not the actual configuration observed.

In a few instances, atoms can achieve a lower energy state (or a higher degree of stability) *by having a filled or half-filled, d subshell*. For example, consider chromium (Cr, $Z = 24$). On the basis of the block diagram, we'd expect its electron configuration to be [Ar] $4s^2 3d^4$. Recalling that a d subshell can hold a maximum of 10 electrons, it turns out that chromium achieves a more stable state by filling its d subshell with 5 electrons (*half-filled*) rather than leaving it with 4. This is accomplished by promoting one of its $4s$ electrons to the $3d$ subshell, yielding the electron configuration [Ar]$4s^1 3d^5$. As another example, copper (Cu, $Z = 29$) has an expected electron configuration of [Ar] $4s^2 3d^9$. However, a copper atom obtains a more stable, lower-energy state by promoting one of its $4s$ electrons into the $3d$ subshell, yielding [Ar] $4s^1 3d^{10}$ to give a *filled d* subshell.

Other atoms that display the same type of behavior with regard to their electron configuration as do chromium and copper include molybdenum (Mo, $Z = 42$, in the same family as chromium), as well as silver and gold (Ag and Au, $Z = 47$ and $Z = 79$, respectively, which are in the same family as copper).

Example 4-22: What is the electron configuration of an atom of silver?

Solution: As mentioned above, silver is one of the handful of elements with atoms that actually achieve greater overall stability by promoting one of its electrons into a higher subshell in order to make it filled. We'd expect the electron configuration for silver to be [Kr]$5s^2 4d^9$. But, by analogy with copper, we'd predict (correctly) that the actual configuration of silver is [Kr] $5s^1 4d^{10}$, where the atom obtains a more stable state by promoting one of its $5s$ electrons into the $4d$ subshell, to give a *filled d* subshell.

Electron Configurations of Ions

Recall that an ion is an atom that has acquired a nonzero electric charge. An atom with more electrons than protons is negatively charged and is called an anion; an atom with fewer electrons than protons is positively charged and is called a cation.

Atoms that gain electrons (anions) accommodate them in the first available orbital, the one with the lowest available energy. For example, fluorine (F, $Z = 9$) has the electron configuration $1s^2 2s^2 2p^5$. When a fluorine atom gains an electron to become the fluoride ion, F^-, the additional electron goes into the $2p$ subshell, giving the electron configuration $1s^2 2s^2 2p^6$, which is the same as the configuration of neon. For this reason, F^- and Ne are said to be **isoelectronic**.

In order to write the electron configuration of an ion for an element in the s or p blocks, we can use the blocks in the periodic table as follows. If an atom becomes an anion—that is, if it acquires one or more additional electrons—then we move to the *right* within the table by a number of squares equal to the number of electrons added in order to find the atom with the same configuration as the ion.

If an atom becomes a cation—that is, if it loses one or more electrons—then we move to the *left* within the table by a number of squares equal to the number of electrons lost in order to find the atom with the same configuration as the ion.

Example 4-23: What's the electron configuration of P^{3-}? Of Sr^+?

Solution: To find the configuration of P^{3-}, we locate phosphorus (P, $Z = 15$) in the periodic table and move 3 places to the *right* (because we have an anion with charge of $3-$); this lands us on argon (Ar, $Z = 18$). Therefore, the electron configuration of the anion P^{3-} is the same as that of argon: $1s^2 2s^2 2p^6 3s^2 3p^6$.

To find the configuration of Sr^+, we locate strontium (Sr, $Z = 38$) in the periodic table and move 1 place to the *left* (because we have a cation with charge $1+$), thus landing on rubidium (Rb, $Z = 37$). Therefore, the electron configuration of the anion Sr^+ is the same as that of rubidium: $[Kr]\,5s^1$.

Electrons that are removed (*ionized*) from an atom always come from the valence shell (the highest n level), and the highest energy orbital within that level. For example, an atom of lithium, Li ($1s^2 2s^1$), becomes Li^+ ($1s^2$) when it absorbs enough energy for an electron to escape. However, recall from our discussion above that **transition metals** (which are the elements in the d block) have both ns and $(n-1)d$ electrons. To form a cation, atoms will always lose their valence electrons first, and since $n > n-1$, transition metals lose s electrons *before* they lose d electrons. Only after *all* s electrons are lost do d electrons get ionized. For example, the electron configuration for the transition metal titanium (Ti, $Z = 22$) is $[Ar]\,4s^2 3d^2$. We might expect that the electron configuration of the ion Ti^+ to be $[Ar]\,4s^2 3d^1$ since the d electrons are slightly higher in energy. However, the *actual* configuration is $[Ar]\,4s^1 3d^2$, and the valence electrons (the ones from the highest n level) are ALWAYS lost first. Similarly, the electron configuration of Ti^{2+} is not $[Ar]\,4s^2$—it's actually $[Ar]\,3d^2$.

Example 4-24: Which one of the following ions has the same electron configuration as the noble gas argon?

A) Na^+
B) P^{2-}
C) Al^{3+}
D) Cl^-

Solution: Na^+ (choice A) has the same electron configuration as the noble gas *neon*, not argon, since one element to the left of Na is Ne. The ion P^{2-} has the same electron configuration as Cl, which is two elements to the right of P. Al^{3+}, like Na^+, has the same configuration as Ne. Of the choices given, only Cl^- (choice D) has the same configuration as Ar, since Ar is one element to the right of Cl.

Example 4-25: What's the electron configuration of Cu^+? Of Cu^{2+}? Of Fe^{3+}?

Solution: Copper (Cu, $Z = 29$) is a transition metal, so it will lose its valence s electrons before losing any d electrons. Recall the anomalous electron configuration of Cu (to give it a filled $3d$ subshell): $[Ar]\,4s^1 3d^{10}$. Therefore, the configuration of Cu^+ (the *cuprous* ion, Cu(I)) is $[Ar]\,3d^{10}$, and that of Cu^{2+} (the *cupric* ion, Cu(II)) is $[Ar]\,3d^9$. Since the electron configuration of iron (Fe, $Z = 26$) is $[Ar]\,4s^2 3d^6$, the configuration of Fe^{3+} (the *ferric* ion, Fe(III)) is $[Ar]\,3d^5$, since the transition metal atom Fe first loses both of its valence s electrons, then once they're ionized, one of its d electrons.

4.6

Excited State vs. Ground State

Assigning electron configurations as we've just discussed is aimed at constructing the *most probable* location of electrons, following the Aufbau principle. These configurations are the most probable because they are the lowest in energy, or as they are often termed, the ground state.

Any electron configuration of an atom that is *not* as we would assign it, provided it doesn't break any physical rules (no more than 2 e^- per orbital, no assigning non existent shells such as $2d$, etc....) is an excited state. The atom has absorbed energy, so the electrons now inhabit states we wouldn't predict as the most probable ones.

Example 4-26: Which of the following could be the electron configuration of an excited oxygen atom?

A) $1s^2 2s^2 2p^4$
B) $1s^2 2s^2 2p^5$
C) $1s^2 2s^2 2p^3 3s^1$
D) $1s^2 2s^2 2p^4 3s^1$

Solution: An oxygen atom contains 8 electrons; when excited, one (or more) of these electrons will jump to a higher energy level. Choice A is the configuration of a ground-state oxygen atom, and choices B and D show the placement of 9 electrons, not 8, so both may be eliminated. The answer must be C; one of the $2p$ electrons has jumped to the $3s$ subshell. (Note carefully that an excited atom is not an ion; electrons are not lost or gained; they simply jump to higher energy levels within the atom.

4.7 GROUPS OF THE PERIODIC TABLE AND THEIR CHARACTERISTICS

We will use the electron configurations of the atoms to predict their chemical properties, including their reactivity and bonding patterns with other atoms.

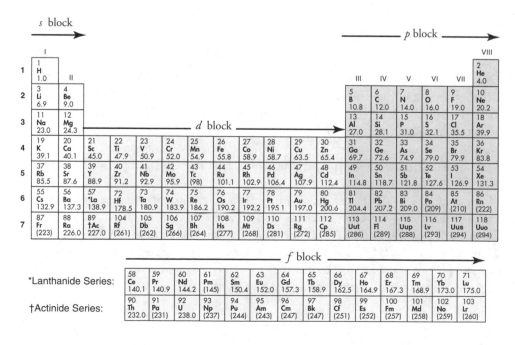

Recall that each horizontal row in the periodic table is called a **period**, and each vertical column is called a **group** (or **family**). Within any group in the periodic table, all of the elements have the same number of electrons in their outermost shell. For instance, the elements in Group II all have two electrons in their outermost shell. Electrons in an atom's outermost shell are called **valence** electrons, and it's the valence electrons that are primarily responsible for an atom's properties and chemical behavior.

Some groups (families) have special names.

Group	Name	Valence-Shell Configuration
Group I	*Alkali metals*	ns^1
Group II	*Alkaline earth metals*	ns^2
Group VII	*Halogens*	ns^2np^5
Group VIII	*Noble gases*	ns^2np^6
The *d* Block	*Transition metals*	
The *s* and *p* Blocks	*Representative elements*	
The *f* Block	*Rare earth metals*	

The valence-shell electron configuration determines the chemical reactivity of each group in the table. For example, in the noble gas family each element has eight electrons in its outermost shell (ns^2np^6). Such a closed-shell (fully-filled valence shell) configuration is called an octet and results in great stability (and therefore low reactivity) for an atom. For this reason, noble gases do not generally undergo chemical reactions, so most group VIII elements are inert. Helium is inert as well, but has a closed shell with a stable duet ($1s^2$) of electrons.

Other elements experience similar increases in stability upon reaching this stable octet electron configuration, and most chemical reactions can be regarded as the quest for atoms to achieve such closed-shell stability. The alkali metals and alkaline earth metals, for instance, possess one (ns^1) or two (ns^2) electrons in their valence shells, respectively, and behave as reducing agents (i.e., lose valence electrons) in redox reactions in order to obtain a stable octet, generally as an M^+ or M^{2+} cation.

Similarly, the halogens (ns^2np^5) require only a single electron to achieve a stable octet. To achieve this state in their elemental form, halogens naturally exist as diatomic molecules (e.g., F_2) where one electron from each atom is shared in a covalent bond. When combined with other elements, the halogens behave as powerful oxidizing agents (that is, gain electrons); they can become stable either as X^- anions or by sharing electrons with other nonmetals (more on bonding in Ch. 5).

Reactions between elements on opposite sides of the periodic table can be quite violent. This occurs due to the great degree of stability gained for both elements when the valence electrons are transferred from the metal to the nonmetal. The relative reactivities within these and all other groups can be further explained by the periodic trends detailed in the next section.

4.7

Example 4-27: Which of the following elements has a closed valence shell, but not an octet?

A) He
B) Ne
C) Br
D) Rn

Solution: Choice A, He, is the correct choice because He, along with H^- and Li^+, has a completed $n = 1$ shell with only 2 electrons, since the $n = 1$ shell can fit only 2 electrons.

Example 4-28: Which of the following could describe an ion with the same electron configuration as a noble gas?

A) An alkali metal that has gained an electron
B) A halogen that has lost an electron
C) A transition metal that has gained an electron
D) An alkaline earth metal that has lost two electrons

Solution: Choice A is wrong since it says "gained" rather than "lost." Choice B is incorrect since it says "lost" rather than "gained." Choice C is also incorrect, because no element in the *d* block could acquire a noble-gas configuration by gaining a single electron. The answer must be D. If an element in Group II loses two electrons, it can acquire a noble-gas electron configuration. (For example, Mg^{2+} has the same configuration as Ne, and Ca^{2+} has the same configuration as Ar.)

Example 4-29: Of the following, the element that possesses properties of both metals and nonmetals is:

A) Si
B) Al
C) Zn
D) Hg

Solution: Elements that possess qualities of both metals and nonmetals are called *metalloids*. These elements are shown below. Thus, choice A is the correct answer; the other choices are metals.

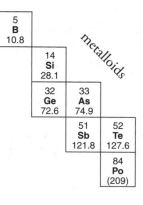

4.8 PERIODIC TRENDS

Shielding

Each filled shell between the nucleus and the valence electrons shields—or "protects"—the valence electrons from the full effect of the positively charged protons in the nucleus. This is called **nuclear shielding** or the **shielding effect**. As far as the valence electrons are concerned, the electrical pull by the protons in the nucleus is reduced by the negative charges of the electrons in the filled shells in between; the result is an effective reduction in the positive elementary charge, from Z to a smaller amount denoted by Z_{eff} (for *effective nuclear charge*).

Example 4-30: The electrons in a solitary He atom are under the influence of two forces, one attractive and one repulsive. What are these forces?

A) Electrostatic attraction between the electrons and the nuclear protons, and electrostatic repulsion between the electrons and nuclear neutrons.

B) Electrostatic attraction between the electrons and the nuclear protons, and electrostatic repulsion between the electrons.

C) Gravitational attraction between the electrons and the nuclear protons, and frictional repulsion between the electrons.

D) Gravitational attraction between the electrons and the entire nucleus, and frictional repulsion between the electrons.

Solution: Compared to the magnitude of electrostatic forces in an atom, gravitational forces between the electrons and nucleons of an atom are negligible, so choices C and D are eliminated. Furthermore, neutrons have no charge and thus do not participate in electrostatic forces, so choice A is eliminated. Remember that opposite charges attract and like charges repel. The best choice is B.

Atomic and Ionic Radius

With progression across any period in the table, the number of protons increases, and hence their total pull on the outermost electrons increases, too. New shells are initiated only at the beginning of a period. So, as we go across a period, electrons are being added, but new shells are not; therefore, the valence electrons are more and more tightly bound to the atom because they feel a greater effective nuclear charge. Therefore, as we move from left to right across a period, **atomic radius** *decreases*.

However, with progression down a group, as new shells are added with each period, the valence electrons experience increased shielding. The valence electrons are less tightly bound since they feel a smaller effective nuclear charge. Therefore, as we go down a group, atomic radius *increases* due to the increased shielding.

If we form an ion, the radius will decrease as electrons are removed (because the ones that are left are drawn in more closely to the nucleus), and the radius will increase as electrons are added. So, in terms of radius, we have $X^+ < X < X^-$; that is, cation radius < neutral-atom radius < anion radius.

Ionization Energy

Because the atom's positively charged nucleus is attracted to the electrons in the atom, it takes energy to remove an electron. The amount of energy necessary to remove the least tightly bound electron from an isolated atom is called the atom's (**first**) **ionization energy** (often abbreviated **IE** or IE_1). As we move from left to right across a period, or up a group, the ionization energy *increases* since the valence electrons are more tightly bound. The ionization energy of any atom with a noble-gas configuration will always be very large. (For example, the ionization energy of neon is 4 times greater than that of lithium.) The **second ionization energy** (IE_2) of an atom, X, is the energy required to remove the least tightly bound electron from the cation X^+. Note that IE_2 will always be greater than IE_1.

4.8

Electron Affinity

The energy associated with the addition of an electron to an isolated atom is known as the atom's **electron affinity** (often abbreviated **EA**). If energy is *released* when the electron is added, the usual convention is to say that the electron affinity is negative; if energy is *required* in order to add the electron, the electron affinity is positive. The halogens have large negative electron affinity values, since the addition of an electron would give them the much desired octet configuration. So they readily accept an electron to become an anion; the increase in stability causes energy to be released. On the other hand, the noble gases and alkaline earth metals have positive electron affinities, because the added electron begins to fill a new level or sublevel and destabilizes the electron configuration. Therefore, anions of these atoms are unstable. Electron affinities typically become more negative as we move to the right across a row or up a group (noble gases excepted), but there are anomalies in this trend.

Electronegativity

Electronegativity is a measure of an atom's ability to pull electrons to itself when it forms a covalent bond; the greater this tendency to attract electrons, the greater the atom's electronegativity. Electronegativity generally behaves as does ionization energy; that is, as we move from left to right across a period, electronegativity increases. As we go down a group, electronegativity decreases. You should know the order of electronegativity for the nine most electronegative elements:

$$F > O > N > Cl > Br > I > S > C \approx H$$

not accurate

Acidity

Acidity is a measure of how well a compound donates protons, accepts electrons, or lowers pH in a chemical system. A binary acid has the structure HX, and can dissociate in water in the following manner: $HX \rightarrow H^+ + X^-$. Stronger acids have resulting X^- anions that are likely to separate from H^+ because they are stable once they do. With respect to the *horizontal* periodic trend for acidity, the more electronegative the element is (X^-) the more stable the anion will be. Therefore acidity increases from left to right across a period. However, the *vertical* trend for acidity depends on the size of the anion. The larger the anion, the more the negative charge can be delocalized and stabilized. Therefore, acidity increases down a group or family in the periodic table.

Summary of Periodic Trends

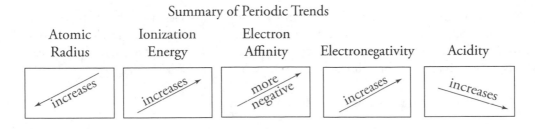

Example 4-31: Compared to calcium, beryllium is expected to have:

A) greater electronegativity and ionization energy.
B) smaller electronegativity and ionization energy.
C) greater electronegativity and smaller ionization energy.
D) smaller electronegativity and larger ionization energy

Solution: Beryllium and calcium are in the same group, but beryllium is higher in the column. We therefore expect beryllium to have greater ionization energy and a greater electronegativity than calcium (choice A), since both of these periodic trends tend to increase as we go up within a group.

Example 4-32: Which of the following will have a greater value for phosphorus than for magnesium?

I.   Atomic radius
II.   Ionization energy
III. Electronegativity

A) I only
B) I and II only
C) II and III only
D) I, II, and III

Solution: Magnesium and phosphorus are in the same period (row), but phosphorus is farther to the right. We therefore expect phosphorus to have a smaller atomic radius, making Roman numeral I false. This allows us to eliminate choices A, B, and D, leaving C as the correct answer. This is also consistent as we expect phosphorus to have a greater ionization energy and a greater electronegativity than magnesium, since both of these periodic trends tend to increase as we move to the right across a row. However, we expect the atomic radius of phosphorus to be smaller than that of magnesium, since atomic radii tend to *decrease* as we move to the right across a row. Therefore, the answer is C.

Example: 4-33 Of the following, which has the most negative electron affinity?

A) Barium
B) Bromine
C) Phosphorus
D) Chlorine

4.8

Solution: Barium is in Group II and therefore has a large positive electron affinity, so we can eliminate choice A immediately. Because electron affinity values tend to become more negative as we go to the right across a row or up within a column, we'd expect chlorine to have a more negative electron affinity than phosphorus or bromine. Therefore, choice D is the answer.

Example 4-34: Of the following, which has the smallest atomic radius?

A) Sodium
B) Oxygen
C) Calcium
D) Silicon

Solution: The atoms with the *smallest* atomic radius are those in the *upper right* portion of the periodic table, since atomic radius tends to increase as we move to the left or down a column. We can therefore eliminate choices A and C; these elements are in Groups I and II, respectively, at the far left end of the table. To decide between the remaining choices, we notice that oxygen is farther to the right *and* in a higher row than silicon, so we'd expect an oxygen atom to have a smaller radius than a silicon atom. Choice B is the best answer.

Example 4-35: Of the following, which is the strongest acid?

A) H_2O
B) H_2S
C) HCl
D) HBr

Solution: For binary acids, we expect acidity to increase with increasing stability of the conjugate base. When comparing anions in a period, those that are more electronegative are more stable. Since chloride is more electronegative than sulfide, choice B can be eliminated. In addition, when comparing anions in a family, those that are larger are more stable, so choices A and C can also be eliminated, making choice D the best answer.

4.8

- The nucleus contains protons and neutrons. Their sum corresponds to the mass number (A).

- The number of protons corresponds to the atomic number (Z).

- An overabundance of either protons or neutrons can result in unstable nuclei, which decay via the emission of various particles.

- For nuclear decay reactions, the sum of all mass and atomic numbers in the products must equal the same sum of these numbers in the reactants.

- The rate of nuclear decay is governed by a species' half-life.

- Electrons exist in discrete energy levels within an atom. Emission spectra are obtained from energy emitted as excited electrons fall from one level to another.

- The periodic table is organized into blocks based on the architecture of electron orbitals. Therefore, valence electron configurations can be determined based on an element's location in the table.

- In their ground state, electrons occupy the lowest energy orbitals available, and occupy subshell orbitals singly before pairing.

- Atoms and ions are most stable when they have an octet of electrons in their outer shell.

- The d subshell is always backfilled: for an atom in the d block of period n, the d subshell will have a principle quantum number of $n - 1$.

- A half filled (d^5) or filled (d^{10}) d subshell is exceptionally stable.

- Transition metals ionize from their valence s subshell before their d subshell.

- Atomic radius increases to the left and down the periodic table; for charged species, cations < neutral atom < anions for a given element; for isoelectronic ions, the species with more protons will have the smaller radius.

- Ionization energy, electron affinity, and electronegativity increase up and to the right on the periodic table, while acidity increases to the right and down the periodic table.

- The relative electronegativities of common atoms in decreasing order are F O N Cl Br I S C $\approx$ H.

CHAPTER 4 FREESTANDING PRACTICE QUESTIONS

1. When an atom of plutonium-239 is bombarded with an alpha particle, this element along with one free neutron is created:

   A) Californium-240
   B) Californium-241
   C) Curium-242
   D) Curium-243

2. Which of the following represents the correct ground state electronic configuration for ferrous ion, Fe^{2+}?

   A) $[Ar]\ 4s^2 3d^6$
   B) $[Ar]\ 4s^2 3d^4$
   C) $[Ar]\ 3d^6$
   D) $[Ar]\ 4s^2 3d^2$

3. Which atom has three unpaired electrons in its valence energy level?

   A) Li
   B) Be
   C) C
   D) N

4. Which of the following elements would be most strongly attracted to a magnetic field?

   A) Mg
   B) Ca
   C) Cr
   D) Zn

5. Which of the following colors would appear as a bright band in an emission spectrum of a yellow sodium vapor lamp?

   A) Yellow, indicating a lesser wavelength than ultraviolet light
   B) Yellow, indicating a greater wavelength than ultraviolet light
   C) Blue, indicating a lesser wavelength than ultraviolet light
   D) Blue, indicating a greater wavelength than ultraviolet light

6. Which of the following atoms/ions has electrons in the subshell of highest energy?

   A) Cl^-
   B) Ca^{2+}
   C) Cr^+
   D) As

7. Of the following metallic elements, which has the lowest second ionization energy?

   A) Na
   B) K
   C) Mg
   D) Ca

8. Which of the following has the smallest atomic or ionic radius?

   A) Cl^-
   B) Ar
   C) K^+
   D) Ca^{2+}

9. Metallic character results from an element's ability to lose electrons. On the periodic table it is expected that metallic character increases:

   A) from left to right, because the decrease in electronegativity would make it easier to lose electrons.
   B) from left to right, because the decrease in atomic radius would result in more stable positive ions.
   C) from right to left, because the decrease in ionization energy would make it easier to lose electrons.
   D) from right to left, because the decrease in electron affinity would result in more stable positive ions.

CHAPTER 4 PRACTICE PASSAGE

Atoms are the building blocks of molecules and they consist of electrons surrounding a nucleus composed of neutrons and protons. The identity of an atom depends on how many protons it contains. The stability and/or reactivity of an atom often depends on how many neutrons and electrons it contains.

Nucleons themselves are composed of elementary particles known as quarks. Quarks are held together by the *strong force* to generate composite particles referred to as *hadrons*. This strong force, sometimes called the *nuclear force*, is also responsible for holding protons and neutrons together in the nucleus and overcomes other forces that may be present. *Baryons*, which are hadrons containing three quarks, form a charged nucleon when two up quarks and one down quark combine and uncharged nucleons when one up quark combines with two down quarks. *Mesons*, which are the other family of hadrons, are unstable particles composed of one quark and one antiquark.

1. An atom contains 29 hadrons comprised of two down quarks and one up quark and 28 hadrons comprised of two up quarks and one down quark. Which one of the following is the identity of the atom?

   A) Iron-57
   B) Nickel-57
   C) Copper-57
   D) Nickel-58

2. An excited electron drops down to its ground state and in the process a photon of light with a wavelength of 525 nm is emitted. Which of the following types of electromagnetic radiation could the photon be?

   A) Infrared
   B) Visible light
   C) X-ray
   D) Cannot be determined from the information given

3. A scientist in a laboratory observes a nucleon composed of three quarks with charges of $+2/3$ e, $-1/3$ e, and $-1/3$ e respectively. Which of the following best describes the nucleon?

   A) The particle is a neutron and it contains two down quarks.
   B) The particle is a proton and it contains two down quarks.
   C) The particle is a neutron and it contains one down quark.
   D) The particle is a proton and it contains one down quark.

4. The first, second, and third ionization energies for strontium are 549.5 kJ/mol, 1064.2 kJ/mol, and 4138 kJ/mol respectively. Why is the third ionization energy so much higher than the first two ionization energies?

   A) The third electron is being removed from a completely full subshell.
   B) The third electron has a larger mass than the first two electrons being removed.
   C) The third electron being removed is less attracted to the nucleus than the first two electrons.
   D) The third electron is at a higher energy level than the first two electrons.

5. Particles with opposite charges attract one another and particles with like charges repel. How can protons, which are positively charged, coexist in the nucleus?

   A) The neutrons in the nucleus prevent the protons from touching one another.
   B) The nuclear force is stronger than the repulsive forces between protons.
   C) Hadrons do not experience forces with one another.
   D) The surrounding cloud of electrons generates an opposing force.

SOLUTIONS TO CHAPTER 4 FREESTANDING PRACTICE QUESTIONS

1. **C** The process described is transmutation, and the new nucleus can be determined by writing a balanced nuclear equation. The preliminary equation to balance is this:

    $$^{239}_{94}\text{Pu} + {}^{4}_{2}\alpha \rightarrow {}^{1}_{0}\text{n} + {}^{A}_{Z}?$$

    where the question mark stands for the new element formed. Balancing mass number gives $239 + 4 = 1 + A$, where $A = 242$; balancing the atomic number gives $94 + 2 = 0 + Z$, where $Z = 96$. Therefore, element number 96 is curium (eliminate choices A and B), and the appropriate isotope has a mass number of 242.

2. **C** When answering electron configuration questions, the first step is to eliminate all answer choices that do not display the correct number of electrons. In this case, ferrous ion possesses six electrons beyond those represented by [Ar] (eight for elemental iron minus two to generate the +2 cation). Thus, choices A and D can be eliminated. To choose between B and C, recall that when transition metals ionize, it is the outermost and therefore least tightly held electrons that are removed first. In this case, the $4s$ electrons are further from the nucleus and are less tightly held ($n = 4$ represents a greater radial distance from the nucleus than $n = 3$). Thus they are the first to be removed.

3. **D** Since Li has only one valence electron and Be has only two, neither choices A nor B can be correct. To choose between C and D, note that the valence configuration of C is $2s^2 2p^2$. Thus the $2s$ electrons are paired leaving only two unpaired p electrons. Nitrogen has a valence configuration of $2s^2 2p^3$, and by Hund's rule, the three p electrons will singly occupy the p_x, p_y, and p_z levels rather than pairing up to avoid electron repulsion.

4. **C** Diamagnetic atoms are repelled by magnetic fields and paramagnetic atoms are attracted to magnetic fields. Paramagnetic atoms have unpaired electrons in their valence orbitals. Mg and Ca are in the same group and have the same valence configuration, so both cannot be the right answer. Zn is at the end of the d block and has a valence shell with all of its electrons paired. Cr only has four electrons in its $3d$ subshell, resulting in four unpaired electron orbitals. Cr is the only choice that is paramagnetic and would be attracted to a magnetic field.

5. **B** All visible light has a greater wavelength than ultraviolet, eliminating choices A and C. The sodium lamp glows yellow and would therefore emit a yellow band on a dark background. If the question asked where dark bands would have been in an absorption spectrum, several lines would be seen in regions other than yellow since those colors are absorbed.

6. **D** Electron energy level is determined by the first two quantum numbers. Given $\text{Cl}^- = [\text{Kr}]$, $\text{Ca}^{2+} = [\text{Ar}]$, $\text{Cr}^+ = [\text{Ar}]\, 3d^5$, and $\text{As} = [\text{Ar}]\, 4s^2 3d^{10} 4p^3$, arsenic contains electrons in the highest energy subshell, $4p$.

7.   **D**   After their first ionizations, Na^+ and K^+ both have octet electron configurations, so a second ionization to remove another electron would require a very high amount of energy. This eliminates choices A and B. Ionization energy decreases down a group, due to increased nuclear shielding, so it is easier to remove electrons from Ca than Mg, making choice D the answer.

8.   **D**   All four answer choices have the same number of electrons and the same electron configuration. Ca^{2+} has the most protons pulling on these electrons, so it will be the smallest.

9.   **C**   Choice A is eliminated because electronegativity increases from left to right on the periodic table. Choice B is eliminated because the stability of positive ions increases as you go up and to the left on the periodic table. Finally, choice D is eliminated since electron affinity is the energy released upon gaining an electron and does not relate to the stability of a positive ion. Choice C is the correct answer because ionization energy, or the energy required to remove an electron, decreases from right to left due to a decrease in effective nuclear charge.

SOLUTIONS TO CHAPTER 4 PRACTICE PASSAGE

1.   **B**   A hadron with two up quarks and one down quark is a charged nucleon or proton. Because the atom has 28 of these protons, it must be nickel, eliminating choices A and C. Furthermore, a hadron with two down quarks and one up quark is a neutron. The atom has 29 of these, so the atomic mass must be $28 + 29 = 57$, eliminating choice D.

2.   **B**   Visible light has a wavelength range of 450-700 nm. The photon falls in this range, so visible light must have been emitted.

3.   **A**   The charges of the three quarks add up to 0, so the nucleon must be an uncharged neutron, eliminating choices B and D. The passage states that uncharged nucleons have two down quarks, eliminating choice C.

4.   **A**   All electrons in an atom have the same mass, eliminating choice B. To remove three electrons from Sr, the first two electrons are removed from the $5s$ subshell and the third electron is removed from the $4p$ subshell, eliminating choice D. Since the third electron is at a lower energy level, it experiences less shielding and would be more attracted to the nucleus than the first two electrons removed, eliminating choice C. The third electron comes from the completely full $4p$ subshell and is much more difficult to remove, making choice A the best answer.

5.   **B**   The passage describes the nuclear force as being responsible for holding the nucleons in the nucleus together and that it "overcomes other forces that may be present." Therefore, choice B is the best answer because it explains how protons are held together in close proximity despite having the same charge. The passage provides us with no indication that neutrons are preventing protons from touching one another, and particles need not physically touch in order to experience repulsion, eliminating choice A. The passage does describe how hadrons are held together by the strong force, eliminating choice C. The electron cloud surrounding the nucleus experiences an attractive force between the positive protons and the negative electrons. It is unlikely that this could generate an opposing force to prevent the repulsion of like-charged nucleons, eliminating choice D.

Chapter 5
Bonding and
Intermolecular Forces

The physical properties of a substance are determined at the molecular level, and the chemistry of molecules is dominated by the reactivity of covalent and ionic bonds. An understanding of the fundamentals of bonding can provide the intuitive grasp necessary to answer a wide range of questions in both general and organic chemistry. This chapter will briefly outline some basic principles, that when mastered, will help lay a strong foundation for many chemistry concepts you will encounter on the MCAT.

5.1 LEWIS DOT STRUCTURES

Each dot in the picture below represents one of fluorine's valence electrons. Fluorine is a halogen, with a general valence-shell configuration of ns^2np^5, so there are $2 + 5 = 7$ electrons in its valence shell. We simply place the dots around the symbol for the element, one on each side, and, if there are more than 4 valence electrons, we just start pairing them up. So, for fluorine, we'd have:

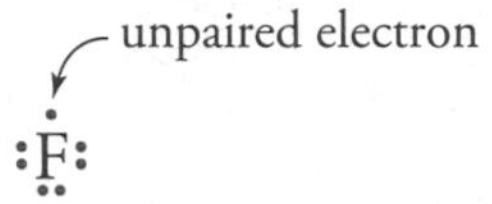

unpaired electron

:F:

This is known as a **Lewis dot symbol**. Here are some others:

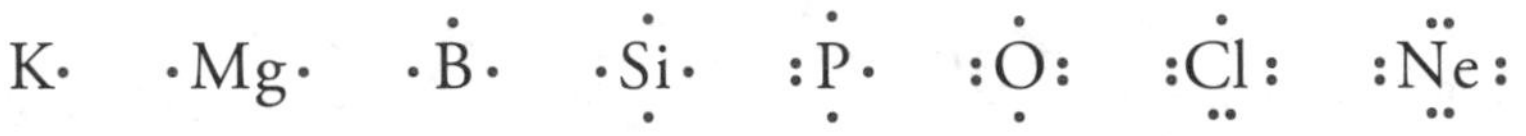

K·   ·Mg·   ·B·   ·Si·   :P·   :O: :Cl: :Ne:

(*Note*: Electrons in *d* subshells are not considered valence electrons for transition metals since valence electrons are in the highest *n* level.)

Example 5-1: Consider this Lewis dot symbol:

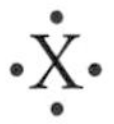

·X·

Among the following, X could represent:

A) carbon.
B) nitrogen.
C) sulfur.
D) argon.

Solution: Since there are four dots in the Lewis symbol, X will be an element in Group 4 of the periodic table. Of the choices given, only carbon (choice A) is in Group 4.

Lewis dot structures are one type of model we use to represent what compounds look like at the molecular level. Since it's the valence electrons that are responsible for creating bonds in molecules, a Lewis dot structure that accounts for the number and location of all valence electrons gives us a sense of how molecules are held together and helps us understand their reactivity.

To create a Lewis dot structure for a molecule, we begin to pair up electrons from two separate atoms since two electrons are required to form a single bond. By sharing a pair of electrons to form a bond, each atom may acquire an octet configuration, thereby stabilizing both atoms. For example, each of the fluorine atoms below can donate its unpaired valence electron to form a bond and give the molecule F_2. The shared electrons are attracted by the nuclei of *both* atoms in the bond, which hold the atoms together.

2 e^-s between atoms = single bond

:F· ·F: $\Longrightarrow$:F:F: $\Longrightarrow$ F—F

lone-pairs = nonbonding electrons
(unshared pairs of valence electrons)

Note that in addition to the **single bond** (a bond formed from two electrons) between the fluorine atoms, each fluorine atom has three pairs of electrons that are not part of a bond. They help satisfy the octets of the F atoms and are known as "lone pairs" of electrons. We'll see in a bit how these lone pairs are important for determining physical properties of compounds, so don't forget to write these out too.

We can also use Lewis dot structures to show atoms that form multiple bonds—**double bonds** use four electrons while **triple bonds** require six. Here are a couple of examples:

:Ö· ·Ö: $\Longrightarrow$:Ö:Ö: $\Longrightarrow$:Ö::Ö: $\Longrightarrow$ Ö=Ö

H· ·C· ·N: $\Longrightarrow$ H:C· ·N: $\Longrightarrow$ H:C::N:

$\Downarrow$

H—C≡N:

Formal Charge

The last Lewis dot structure shown above for the molecule consisting of 1 atom each of hydrogen, carbon, and nitrogen was drawn with C as the central atom. However, it could have been drawn with N as the central atom, and we could have still achieved closed-shell configurations for all the atoms:

H· ·N: ·C· $\Longrightarrow$ H:N::C: $\Longrightarrow$ H—N≡C: (?)

The problem is this doesn't give the correct structure for this molecule. The nitrogen atom is not actually bonded to the hydrogen. A helpful way to evaluate a proposed Lewis structure is to calculate the **formal charge** of each atom in the structure. These formal charges won't give the actual charges on the atoms; they'll simply tell us if the atoms are sharing their valence electrons in the "best" way possible, which will happen when the formal charges are all zero (or at least as small as possible). The formula for calculating the formal charge of an atom in a covalent compound is:

$$\text{Formal charge (FC)} = V - \frac{1}{2}B - L$$

where V is the number of valence electrons, B is the number of bonding electrons, and L is the number of lone-paired (non-bonding) electrons. We'll show the calculations of the formal charges for each atom in both Lewis structures:

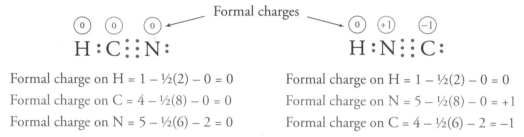

Formal charge on H = $1 - \frac{1}{2}(2) - 0 = 0$

Formal charge on C = $4 - \frac{1}{2}(8) - 0 = 0$

Formal charge on N = $5 - \frac{1}{2}(6) - 2 = 0$

Formal charge on H = $1 - \frac{1}{2}(2) - 0 = 0$

Formal charge on N = $5 - \frac{1}{2}(8) - 0 = +1$

Formal charge on C = $4 - \frac{1}{2}(6) - 2 = -1$

The best Lewis structures have an octet of electrons and a formal charge of zero on all the atoms. (Sometimes, this simply isn't possible, and then the best structure is the one that *minimizes* the magnitudes of the formal charges.) The fact that the HCN structure has formal charges of zero for all the atoms, but the HNC structure does not, tells us right away that the HCN structure is the better one. For dot structures that must contain formal charges on one or more atoms, the best structures have negative formal charges on the more electronegative element.

Example 5-2: What's the formal charge on each atom in phosgene, $COCl_2$?

Solution:

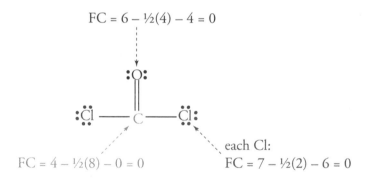

FC = $6 - \frac{1}{2}(4) - 4 = 0$

FC = $4 - \frac{1}{2}(8) - 0 = 0$

each Cl:
FC = $7 - \frac{1}{2}(2) - 6 = 0$

Example 5-3: Which of the following is the best Lewis structure for CH_2O?

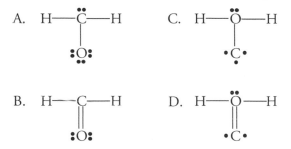

Solution: When faced with a question like this on the MCAT (and they're rather common), the first thing you should do is simply count the electrons. The correct structure for the molecule CH_2O must account for $4 + 2(1) + 6 = 12$ valence electrons. The structure in choice A has 14 and the structure in choice C has 11. Answer choices B and D both have 12 valence electrons. However, in choice D, oxygen is surrounded by 10 total electrons. This is not possible because oxygen, like all elements in the second row of the periodic table, cannot violate the octet rule and exceed 8 valence electrons. Choice B, then, with 12 valence electrons and the least electronegative atom as the central atom, is the best choice.

Resonance

Recall that Lewis dot structures are a model that we use to help us understand where the valence electrons are in a molecule. All models, being simplifications of reality, have limitations, and Lewis dot structures are no exception. Sometimes it is impossible for one structure to accurately represent the reality of a molecule's electron distribution. To account for this complexity, we need two or more structures, called **resonance structures**, to accurately depict the bonding in a molecule. These structures are often needed when there are double or triple bonds in molecules along with one or more lone pairs of electrons.

Let's draw the Lewis structure for sulfur dioxide.

formal charges ⋯⋯▶ (–1) (+1) (0)

We could also draw the structure like this:

(0) (+1) (–1) ◀⋯⋯ formal charges

In either case, there's one S—O single bond and one S=O double bond. This would imply that the double-bonded O would be closer to the S atom than the single-bonded O (see Section 5.2, Bond Length and Bond Dissociation Energy). Experiment, however, reveals that the bond lengths are the same. Therefore, to describe this molecule, we say that it's an "average" (or, technically, a **resonance hybrid**) of the equivalent Lewis structures shown:

We can also symbolize the resonance hybrid with a single picture, like this:

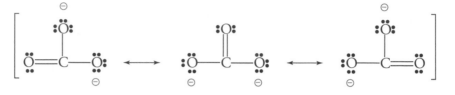

The dotted lines in the structure above indicate some double bond character for both S—O bonds, more of a "bond and a half." A molecule may be a resonance hybrid of more than two equivalent Lewis structures; for example, consider the carbonate ion, CO_3^{2-}:

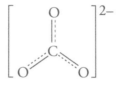

or, more simply,

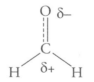

In addition, a molecule may have two or more non-equivalent resonance structures, and the resonance hybrid is then a weighted average of them, as shown with formaldehyde below:

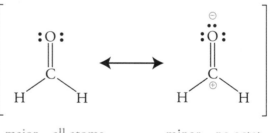

major—all atoms have octets and no formal charge

minor—no octet on C, atoms have formal charge

resonance hybrid

Example 5-4: Resonance structures are two or more structures where:

A) only atoms may move around.
B) only bonding electrons may move around.
C) only nonbonding electrons may move around.
D) only nonbonding electrons, and double and triple bonds may move around.

Solution: Choice D is the correct answer. (This definition is particularly important in organic chemistry.)

5.2 BOND LENGTH AND BOND DISSOCIATION ENERGY

While the term *bond length* makes good intuitive sense (the distance between two nuclei that are bonded to one another), **bond dissociation energy (BDE)** is not quite as intuitive. Bond dissociation energy is the energy required to break a bond *homolytically*. In **homolytic bond cleavage**, one electron of the bond being broken goes to each fragment of the molecule. In this process two radicals form. This is *not* the same thing as **heterolytic bond cleavage** (also known as *dissociation*). In heterolytic bond cleavage, both electrons of the electron pair that make up the bond end up on the same atom; this forms both a cation and an anion.

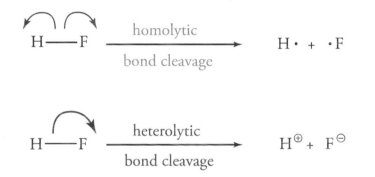

These two processes are very different and hence have very different energies associated with them. Here, we will only consider homolytic bond dissociation energies.

When one examines the relationship between bond length and bond dissociation energy for a series of similar bonds, an important trend emerges: For similar bonds, *the higher the bond order, the shorter and stronger the bond*. Bond order is defined as the number of bonds between adjacent atoms, so a single bond has a bond order of 1 while a triple bond has a bond order of 3. The following table, which lists the bond dissociation energies (BDE, in kcal/mol) and the bond lengths (*r*, in angstroms, where 1 Å = 10^{-10} m) for carbon-carbon and carbon-oxygen bonds, illustrates this trend:

	C—C	C=C	C≡C	C—O	C=O	C≡O
BDE	83	144	200	86	191	256
r (in Å)	1.54	1.34	1.20	1.43	1.20	1.13

An important caveat arises because of the varying atomic radii: *bond length/BDE comparisons should only be made for similar bonds*. Thus, carbon-carbon bonds should be compared only to other carbon-carbon bonds; carbon-oxygen bonds should be compared only to other carbon-oxygen bonds, and so on.

Recall the shapes of atomic orbitals: *s* orbitals are spherical about the atomic nucleus, while *p* orbitals are elongated "dumbbell"-shaped about the atomic nucleus.

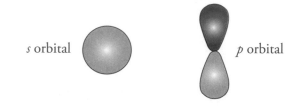

s orbital   *p* orbital

When comparing the same type of bonds, the greater the *s* character in the hybrid orbitals, the shorter the bond (because *s*-orbitals are closer to the nucleus than *p*-orbitals). A greater percentage of *p* character in the hybrid orbital also leads to a more directional hybrid orbital that is farther from the nucleus and thus a longer bond (see section 5.5 for all the details on hybridization). In addition, when comparing the same types of bonds, *the longer the bond, the weaker it is; the shorter the bond, the stronger it is*. In the following diagram, compare all the C—C bonds and all the C—H bonds:

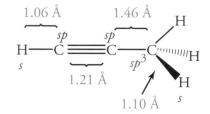

Bond	Bond length	Bond	Bond length
C—C (*sp* – *sp*)	1.21 Å	C–H (*sp* – *s*)	1.06 Å
C—C (*sp* – *sp³*)	1.46 Å	C–H (*sp³* – *s*)	1.10 Å

5.3   TYPES OF BONDS

Covalent Bonds

A **covalent bond** is formed between atoms when each contributes one or more of its unpaired valence electrons. The electrons are *shared* by both atoms to help complete both octets. There are minor variations in how the electrons are shared, however, so there are several classes of covalent bonds.

Polarity of Covalent Bonds

Recall that electronegativity refers to an atom's ability to attract another atom's valence electrons when it forms a bond. Electronegativity, in other words, is a measure of how much an atom will "hog" the electrons that it's sharing with another atom.

Consider the Lewis dot structures of hydrogen fluoride and fluorine:

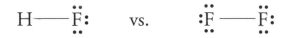

Fluorine is more electronegative than hydrogen (remember the order of electronegativity?), so the electron density will be greater near the fluorine than near the hydrogen in HF. That means that the H—F molecule is partially negative (denoted by δ^-) on the fluorine side and partially positive (denoted by δ^+) on the hydrogen side. We refer to this as **polarity** and say that the molecule has a **dipole moment**. A bond is **polar** if the electron density between the two nuclei is uneven. This occurs if there is a difference in electronegativity of the bonding atoms, and the greater the difference, the more uneven the electron density and the greater the dipole moment.

A bond is **nonpolar** if the electron density between the two nuclei is even. This occurs when there is little to no difference in electronegativity between the bonded atoms, generally when two atoms of the same element are bonded to each other, as we see in F_2.

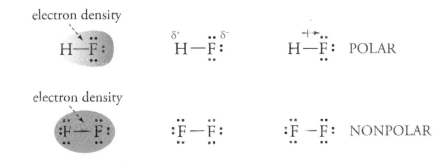

Coordinate Covalent Bonds

Sometimes, one atom will donate *both* of the shared electrons in a bond. That is called a **coordinate covalent bond**. For example, the nitrogen atom in NH_3 donates both electrons in its lone pair to form a bond to the boron atom in the molecule BF_3 to give the coordinate covalent compound F_3BNH_3:

coordinate covalent bond

5.3

Since the NH_3 molecule donates a pair of electrons, it is known as a **Lewis base.** A Lewis Base can act as a ligand, or a nucleophile (nucleus loving), and so all three terms are synonymous. Since the BF_3 molecule accepts a pair of electrons, it's known as a **Lewis acid** or **electrophile** (electron loving). When a coordinate covalent bond breaks, the electrons that come from the ligand will leave *with* that ligand.

Example 5-5: Identify the Lewis acid and the Lewis base in the following reaction, which forms a coordination complex:

$$4\ NH_3 + Zn^{2+} \rightarrow Zn(NH_3)_4{}^{2+}$$

Solution: Each of the NH_3 molecules donates its lone pair to the zinc atom, thus forming four coordinate covalent bonds. Since the zinc ion accepts these electron pairs, it's the Lewis acid; since each ammonia molecule donates an electron pair, they are Lewis bases (or ligands):

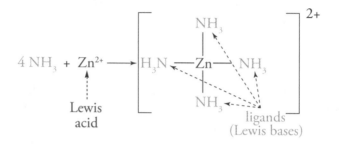

Example 5-6: Which one of the following anions *cannot* behave as a Lewis base/ligand?

A) F^-
B) OH^-
C) $NO_3{}^-$
D) $BH_4{}^-$

Solution: A Lewis base/ligand is a molecule or ion that donates a pair of nonbonding electrons. So, in order to even be a candidate Lewis base/ligand, a molecule must have a pair of nonbonding electrons in the first place. The ion in choice D does not have any nonbonding electrons.

Example 5-7: Carbon atoms with nonbonding electrons are excellent Lewis bases/ligands. Therefore, which of the following molecules is *not* a potential Lewis base/ligand?

A) CO_2
B) CO
C) CN^-
D) $CH_3{}^-$

Solution: The Lewis structures for the given molecules/ions arc as follows:

$$O{=}C{=}O \qquad :C{\equiv}O: \qquad :C{\equiv}N:^{\ominus} \qquad :CH_3^{\ominus}$$

Therefore, choice A (carbon dioxide) is not a good ligand and is the correct answer here.

Ionic Bonds

While sharing valence electrons is one way atoms can achieve the stable octet configuration, the octet may also be obtained by gaining or losing electrons. For example, a sodium atom will give its valence electron to an atom of chlorine. This results in a sodium cation (Na^+) and a chloride anion (Cl^-), which form sodium chloride. They're held together by the electrostatic attraction between a cation and anion; this is an **ionic bond**.

$$Na \quad \cdot \ddot{\underset{\cdot\cdot}{Cl}} : \quad \Longrightarrow \quad Na^{\oplus} \quad : \ddot{\underset{\cdot\cdot}{Cl}} :^{\ominus}$$

For an ionic bond to form between a metal and a non-metal, there has to be a big difference in electronegativity between the two elements. Generally speaking, the strength of the bond is proportional to the charges on the ions, and it decreases as the ions get farther apart, or as the ionic radii increase. We can use this to estimate the relative strength of ionic systems. For example, consider MgS and NaCl. For MgS, the magnesium ion has a +2 charge and sulfide ion has a –2 charge, while for NaCl, the charges are +1 for sodium and –1 for chloride. Therefore, the MgS "bond" is expected to be about four times stronger than the NaCl "bond," assuming the sizes of the ions are very nearly the same.

Example 5-8: Which of the following is most likely an ionic compound?

A) NO
B) HI
C) ClF
D) KBr

Solution: A diatomic compound is ionic if the electronegativities of the atoms are very different. Of the atoms listed in the choices, those in choice D have the greatest electronegativity difference (K is an alkali metal, and Br is a halogen); K will give up its lone valence electron to Br, forming an ionic bond.

5.4   VSEPR THEORY

The shapes of simple molecules are predicted by **valence shell electron-pair repulsion (VSEPR) theory**. There's one rule: Since electrons repel one another, electron pairs, whether bonding or nonbonding, attempt to move as far apart as possible.

For example, the bonding electrons in beryllium hydride, BeH_2, repel one another and attempt to move as far apart as possible. In this molecule, two pairs of electrons point in opposite directions:

$$180°$$
$$H — Be — H$$

The angle between the bonds is 180°. A molecule with this shape is said to be linear.

5.4

As the BeH_2 example shows, the total number of electron groups on the central atom of a molecule determines its bond angles and *orbital geometry*. Electron groups are defined as any type of bond (single, double, triple) and lone pairs of electrons. Double and triple bonds count only as one electron group, even though they involve two and three pairs of electrons, respectively. To illustrate, the number of electron groups and orbital geometries of the central atom are shown for some example molecules:

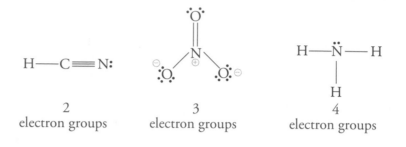

2	3	4
electron groups	electron groups	electron groups

The shape of a molecule (also referred to as the **molecular geometry**) is also a function of the location of the nuclei of its constituent atoms. Therefore, when lone electron pairs are present on the central atom of a molecule, as in NH_3 above, the shape is not the same as the orbital geometry. The table below shows how the presence of lone pairs determines the shape of a molecule:

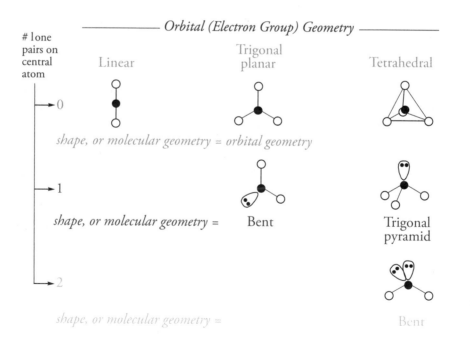

Example 5-9: Determine the orbital geometry and predict the shape of each of the following molecules or ions:

a) H_2O
b) SO_2
c) NH_4^+
d) PCl_3
e) CO_3^{2-}

Solution:

a)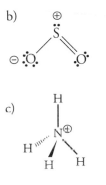

orbital geometry: *tetrahedral*
shape: *bent*

b)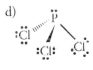

orbital geometry: *trigonal planar*
shape: *bent*

c)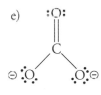

orbital geometry: *tetrahedral*
shape: *tetrahedral*

d)

orbital geometry: *tetrahedral*
shape: *trigonal pyramid*

e)

orbital geometry: *trigonal planar*
shape: *trigonal planar*

5.5 HYBRIDIZATION

In order to rationalize observed chemical and structural trends, chemists developed the concept of orbital hybridization. In this model, one imagines a mathematical combination of atomic orbitals centered on the same atom to produce a set of composite, **hybrid** orbitals. For example, consider an s and a p orbital on an atom.

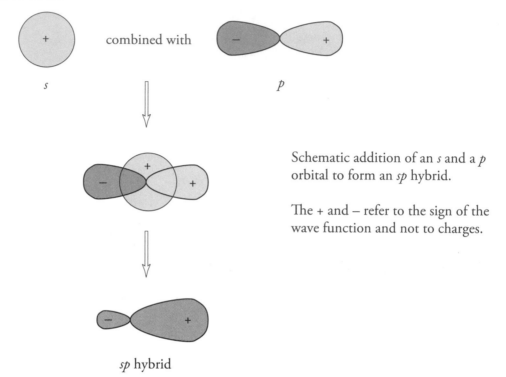

Schematic addition of an s and a p orbital to form an sp hybrid.

The + and – refer to the sign of the wave function and not to charges.

Notice that the new orbital is highly directional; this allows for better overlap when bonding.

There will be two such sp hybrid orbitals formed because two orbitals (the s and the p) were originally combined; that is, the total number of orbitals is conserved in the formation of hybrid orbitals. For this reason, the number of hybrid orbitals on a given atom of hybridization sp^x is $1 + x$ (1 for the s, x for the p's), where x may be either 1, 2, or 3.

The percentages of the s character and p character in a given sp^x hybrid orbital are listed below:

sp^x hybrid orbital	s character	p character
sp	50%	50%
sp^2	33%	67%
sp^3	25%	75%

To determine the hybridization for most atoms in simple molecules, add the number of attached atoms to the number of non-bonding electron pairs (localized) and use the brief table below (which also gives the ideal bond angles and orbital geometry). The number of attached atoms plus the number of lone pairs is equal to the number of orbitals combined to make the new hybridized orbitals.

Electron Groups (# atoms + # lone pairs)	Hybridization	Bond Angles (ideal)	Orbital Geometry
2	sp	180°	linear
3	sp^2	120°	trigonal planar
4	sp^3	109.5°	tetrahedral

sp hybridization:

sp hybridized oxygen
(1 attached atom + 1 lone pair)

sp hybridized nitrogen
(1 attached atom + 1 lone pair)

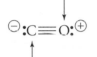

sp hybridized carbon
(1 attached atom + 1 lone pair)

sp hybridized carbon
(2 attached atoms + 0 lone pairs)

sp² hybridization:

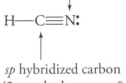

sp² hybridized carbon
(3 attached atoms + 0 lone pairs)

sp² hybridized nitrogen
(2 attached atoms + 1 lone pair)

sp³ hybridization:

sp³ hybridized carbon
(4 attached atoms + 0 lone pairs)

sp³ hybridized nitrogen
(3 attached atoms + 1 lone pair)

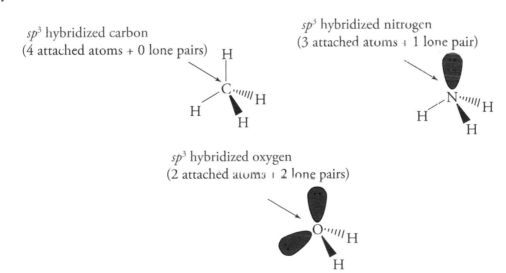

sp³ hybridized oxygen
(2 attached atoms + 2 lone pairs)

Example 5-10: Determine the hybridization of the central atom in each of the following molecules or ions from the previous example:

a) H_2O
b) SO_2
c) NH_4^+
d) PCl_3
e) CO_3^{2-}

Solution:

a) Hybridization of O is sp^3.
b) Hybridization of S is sp^2.
c) Hybridization of N is sp^3.
d) Hybridization of P is sp^3.
e) Hybridization of C is sp^2.

Sigma (σ) Bonds

A **σ bond** consists of two electrons that are localized between two nuclei. It is formed by the end-to-end overlap of one hybridized orbital (or an s orbital in the case of hydrogen) from each of the two atoms participating in the bond. Below, we show the σ bonds in ethane, C_2H_6:

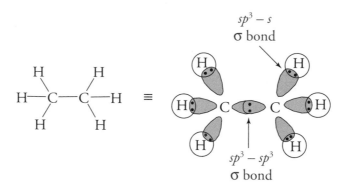

Remember that an sp^3 carbon atom has 4 sp^3 hybrid orbitals, which are derived from one s orbital and three p orbitals.

Example 5-11: Label the hybridization of the orbitals comprising the σ bonds in the molecules shown below:

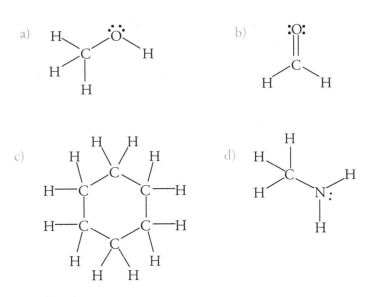

a)

b)

c)

d)

Solution:

a)   Bonds to H are sp^3-s σ bonds. The C—O bond is an sp^3-sp^3 σ bond.
b)   The bonds to H are sp^2-s σ bonds. The C=O bond contains an sp^2-sp^2 σ bond. (It's also composed of a π bond, which we'll discuss in the next section.)
c)   All C—C bonds are sp^3-sp^3 σ bonds, while all C—H bonds are sp^3-s σ bonds.
d)   All bonds to H are sp^3-s σ bonds. The C—N bond is an sp^3-sp^3 σ bond.

Pi (π) Bonds

A π **bond** is composed of two electrons that are localized to the region that lies on opposite sides of the plane formed by the two bonded nuclei and immediately adjacent atoms, not directly between the two nuclei as with a σ bond. A π bond is formed by the proper, parallel, side-to-side alignment of two unhybridized p orbitals on adjacent atoms. (An sp^2 hybridized atom has three sp^2 orbitals—which come from one s and two p orbitals—plus one p orbital that remains unhybridized.) Below, we show the π bonds in ethene, C_2H_4:

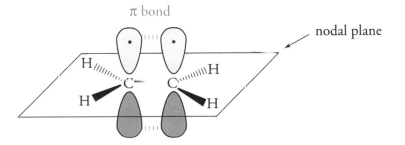

In any multiple bond, *there is only one σ bond; the remainder are π bonds.* Therefore:

a single bond: composed of 1 σ bond
a double bond: composed of 1 σ bond and 1 π bond
a triple bond: composed of 1 σ bond and 2 π bonds

Example 5-12: Count the number of σ bonds and π bonds in each of the following molecules. (Don't forget to count all of the C–H σ bonds!)

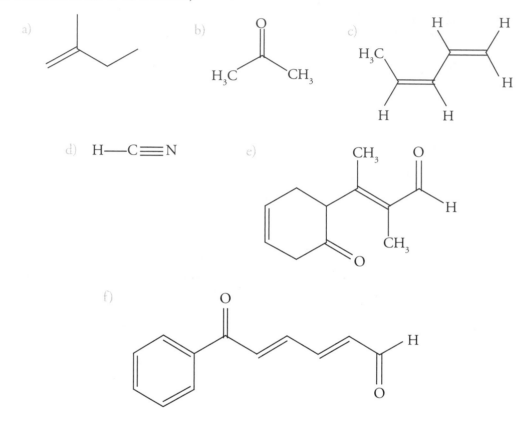

d) H—C≡N

Solution:

a) 14 σ, 1 π
b) 9 σ, 1 π
c) 12 σ, 2 π
d) 2 σ, 2 π
e) 27 σ, 4 π
f) 24 σ, 7 π

5.6 MOLECULAR POLARITY

A molecule as a whole may also be polar or nonpolar. If a molecule contains no polar bonds, it cannot be polar. In addition, if a molecule contains two or more symmetrically oriented polar bonds, the bond dipoles effectively cancel each other out, evenly distributing the electron density over the entire molecule. However, if the polar bonds in a molecule are not symmetrically oriented around the central atom (generally, though not always due to the presence of a lone pair of electrons on the central atom), the individual bond dipoles will not cancel. Therefore, there will be an uneven distribution of electron density over the entire molecule, and this results in a polar molecule.

Example 5-13: For each of the molecules N_2, OCS, and CCl_4, describe the polarity of each bond and of the molecule as a whole.

5.6

Solution:

- The N≡N bond is nonpolar (since it's a bond between two identical atoms), and since this *is* the molecule, it's nonpolar, too; no dipole moment.
- For the molecule O=C=S, each bond is polar, since it connects two different atoms of unequal electronegativities. Furthermore, the O=C bond is more polar that then C=S bond, because the difference between the electronegativities of O and C is greater than the difference between the electronegativities of C and S. Therefore, the molecule as a whole is polar (that is, it has a dipole moment):

$$O\!\!=\!\!C\!\!=\!\!S \implies O\!\!=\!\!C\!\!=\!\!S$$

polar bonds   polar molecule

- For the molecule CCl_4, each bond is polar, since it connects two different atoms of unequal electronegativities. However, the bonds are symmetrically arranged around the central C atom, leaving the molecule as a whole nonpolar, with no dipole moment:

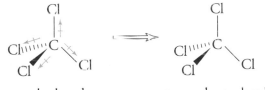

polar bonds   non-polar molecule

5.7 INTERMOLECULAR FORCES

Liquids and solids are held together by intermolecular forces, such as dipole-dipole forces and London dispersion forces. **Intermolecular forces** are the relatively weak interactions that take place between neutral molecules.

Polar molecules are attracted to ions, producing **ion-dipole** forces. **Dipole-dipole forces** are the attractions between the positive end of one polar molecule and the negative end of another polar molecule. (Hydrogen bonding [which we will look at more closely below] is the strongest dipole-dipole force.) A permanent dipole in one molecule may induce a dipole in a neighboring nonpolar molecule, producing a momentary **dipole-induced dipole force**.

Finally, an instantaneous dipole in a nonpolar molecule may induce a dipole in a neighboring nonpolar molecule. The resulting attractions are known as **London dispersion forces**, which are very weak and transient interactions between the instantaneous dipoles in nonpolar molecules. They are the weakest of all intermolecular interactions, and they're the "default" force; all an atom or molecule needs to experience them is electrons. In addition, as the size (molecular weight) of the molecule increases, so does its number of electrons, which increases its polarizability. As a result, the partial charges of the induced dipoles get larger, so the strength of the dispersion forces increases.

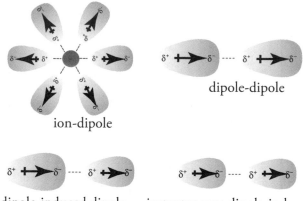

ion-dipole

dipole-dipole

dipole-induced dipole

instantaneous dipole-induced dipole
(London dispersion force)

Despite being weak, all intermolecular forces, including London dispersion forces, can have a profound impact on the physical properties of a particular molecule. Specifically, substances with stronger intermolecular forces will exhibit greater melting points, greater boiling points, greater viscosities, and lower vapor pressures (more on this below) than similar compounds with weaker intermolecular forces. For example, many substances that experience only dispersion forces, like fluorine (F_2) and chlorine (Cl_2), exist as gases under standard conditions (1 atm and 25°C). However, bromine (Br_2) is a liquid and iodine (I_2) is a solid because the strength of the dispersion forces increase as atomic size increases.

A final note: Dipole forces, hydrogen bonding, and London forces are *all* collectively known as **van der Waals forces**. However, you may sometimes see the term "van der Waals forces" used to mean only London dispersion forces.

Hydrogen Bonding

Hydrogen bonding is the strongest type of intermolecular force between neutral molecules. In order for a hydrogen bond to form, two very specific criteria must be fulfilled: 1) a molecule must have a covalent bond between H and either N, O, or F, and 2) another molecule must have a lone pair of electrons on an N, O, or F atom. A very common example of a substance that experiences hydrogen bonding is water:

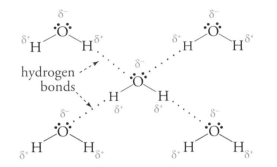

5.7

One of the consequences of hydrogen bonding is the high boiling points of compounds such as NH_3, H_2O, and HF. The boiling points of these hydrogen-containing compounds are higher than those of the hydrogen-containing compounds of other elements from Groups V, VI, and VII (the groups where N, O, and F reside). For example, the boiling point of H_2S is approximately –50°C, while that of H_2O is (of course) 100°C.

Example 5-14: Identify the mixture of compounds that *cannot* experience hydrogen bonding with each other:

A) NH_3 / H_2O
B) H_2O / HF
C)   HF / CO_2
D) H_2S / HCl

Solution: Hydrogen bonding occurs when an H covalently bonded to an F, O, or N electrostatically interacts with another F, O, or N (which doesn't need to have an H). Therefore, choices A, B, and C can all experience hydrogen bonding. Choice D, however, cannot, and this is the answer.

Vapor Pressure

One of the physical properties determined by the strength of the intermolecular forces of a substance is its vapor pressure. **Vapor pressure** is the pressure exerted by the gaseous phase of a liquid that evaporated from the exposed surface of the liquid. The weaker a substance's intermolecular forces, the higher its vapor pressure and the more easily it evaporates. For example, if we compare diethyl ether ($H_5C_2OC_2H_5$) and water, we notice that while water undergoes hydrogen bonding, diethyl ether does not, so despite its greater molecular mass, diethyl ether will vaporize more easily and have a higher vapor pressure than water. Easily vaporized liquids—liquids with *high* vapor pressures—like diethyl ether are said to be **volatile.**

While a substance's vapor pressure is determined in part by its intermolecular forces, vapor pressure is also temperature dependent and increases with the temperature of the substance. Increasing the average kinetic energy of the particles (which is proportional to temperature), allows them to overcome the intermolecular forces holding them together and increases the proportion of particles that can move into the gas phase. As a result, the vapor pressure of a substance is indirectly related to its boiling point, a topic we'll discuss in more detail in Chapter 7.

Example 5-15: An understanding of intermolecular forces is of critical importance because they govern so many physical properties of a substance. The property *least* likely to be influenced by intermolecular force strength is:

A)   color.
B)   melting point.
C)   solubility.
D)   vapor pressure.

Solution: Any physical property that involves separating molecules from one another will very much depend upon the strength of intermolecular forces. Molecules are spread out during melting (choice B), dissolving (choice C), and evaporation (choice D). Choice A is therefore the best choice here.

5.8   TYPES OF SOLIDS

Ionic Solids

An **ionic solid** is held together by the electrostatic attraction between cations and anions in a lattice structure. The bonds that hold all the ions together in the crystal lattice are the same as the bonds that hold each pair of ions together. Ionic bonds are strong, and most ionic substances (like NaCl and other salts) are solid at room temperature. As discussed previously, the strength of the bonds is primarily dependent on the magnitudes of the ion charges, and to a lesser extent, the size of the ions. The greater the charge, the stronger the force of attraction between the ions. The smaller the ions, the more they are attracted to each other.

Network Solids

In a **network solid**, atoms are connected in a **lattice** of covalent bonds, meaning that all interactions between atoms are covalent bonds. Like in an ionic solid, in a network solid the *inter*molecular forces are identical to the *intra*molecular forces. You can think of a network solid as one big molecule; in a network solid there are only intramolecular forces. As a result, network solids are very strong, and tend to be very hard solids at room temperature. Diamond (one of the allotropes of carbon) and quartz (a form of silica, SiO_2) are examples of network solids.

Metallic Solids

A sample of metal can be thought of as a covalently bound lattice of nuclei and their inner shell electrons, surrounded by a "sea" or "cloud" of electrons. At least one valence electron per atom is not bound to any one particular atom and is free to move throughout the lattice. These freely roaming valence electrons are called **conduction electrons**. As a result, metals are excellent conductors of electricity and heat, and are malleable and ductile. Metallic bonds vary widely in strength, but almost all metals are solids at room temperature.

Molecular Solids

The particles at the lattice points of a crystal of a molecular solid are molecules. These molecules are held together by one of three types of *inter*molecular interactions—hydrogen bonds, dipole-dipole forces, or London dispersion forces. Since these forces are *significantly* weaker than ionic, network, or metallic bonds, molecular compounds typically have much lower melting and boiling points than the other types of solids above. Molecular solids are often liquids or gases at room temperature, and are more likely to be solids as the strength of their intermolecular forces increase.

5.8

Example 5-16: Of the following, which one will have the lowest melting point?

A) MgO
B) CH_4
C) Cr
D) HF

Solution: Almost all ionic compounds are solids at room temperature. Therefore, choice A is eliminated. Similarly, all metals except for mercury (Hg) are solids at room temperature, so eliminate choice C. Both answers B and D will be molecular solids. Hydrogen fluoride is able to hydrogen bond and will therefore have stronger intermolecular interactions than the nonpolar methane. Since choice B has the weakest intermolecular forces (London dispersion), it will be easiest to melt.

- The best Lewis dot or resonance structures have 1) octets around all atoms, 2) minimized formal charge, and 3) negative charges on more electronegative elements.

- Covalent bonds form between elements with similar electronegativities (two nonmetals).

- Nonpolar bonding means equal electron sharing; polar bonding means unequal electron sharing, and electron density is higher around the more electronegative element.

- Coordinate covalent bonds form between a Lewis base (e^- pair donor) and a Lewis acid (e^- pair acceptor); electrons are shared.

- Ionic bonds form between elements with large differences in electronegativity (metals + nonmetals), and the strength of that bond depends on the charge and the size of the ions. Larger charges and smaller ions make the strongest ionic bonds.

- VSEPR theory predicts the shape of molecules; angles between electron groups around the central atom are maximized for greatest stability.

- The hybridization of an atom is dependent on the number of electron groups on the atom (two e^- groups = sp, three e^- groups = sp^2, four e^- groups = sp^3).

- Sigma (σ) bonds generally form through the end-on-end overlap of hybrid orbitals; pi (π) bonds form through the side-to-side overlap of unhybridized p orbitals.

- If bond dipoles are symmetrically oriented in a molecule, the molecule as a whole is nonpolar; if the dipoles are asymmetrical, the molecule will be polar.

- Intermolecular forces are cohesive, and determine the physical properties (melting and boiling points, solubility, vapor pressure, etc.) of a compound based on relative strengths.

- While all molecules have London dispersion forces, they are the predominant intermolecular force that holds nonpolar molecules together. Dipole-dipole forces are the predominant intermolecular force that holds polar molecules together.

- Molecules with an H—F, H—O, or H—N bond and an N, O, or F with a lone electron pair can hydrogen bond.

CHAPTER 5 FREESTANDING PRACTICE QUESTIONS

1. Which of these molecules has the strongest dipole moment?

   A) PBr_3O
   B) PF_5
   C) CCl_4
   D) SF_6

2. A pure sample of which of the following ions/molecules will participate in intermolecular hydrogen bonding?

   I. CH_3CO_2H
   II. CO_2
   III. H_2S

   A) I only
   B) III only
   C) I and II
   D) I and III

3. Which of the following best describes the intramolecular bonding present within a cyanide ion (CN^-)?

   A) Ionic bonding
   B) Covalent bonding
   C) Van der Waals forces
   D) Induced dipole

4. All of the following would be categorized as having tetrahedral orbital geometry EXCEPT:

   A) NH_3
   B) NH_4^+
   C) CO_2
   D) CH_4

5. Rank the following from highest to lowest boiling point:

   I. H_2SO_4
   II. NH_3
   III. CO_2
   IV. H_2O

   A) I > IV > II > III
   B) II > I > IV > III
   C) I > III > IV > II
   D) IV > III > I > II

6. Which of the following most specifically accounts for neon's ability to form a solid at 1 atm and 25 K?

   A) Gravitational forces
   B) Electrostatic forces
   C) London dispersion forces
   D) Strong nuclear forces

7. In the following reaction, which of the following most accurately describes the type of bond formed?

   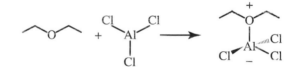

   A) Covalent
   B) Electrostatic
   C) Metallic
   D) Coordinate covalent

CHAPTER 5 PRACTICE PASSAGE

Molecules are not rigid, unchanging structures. Their atoms are in constant motion even relative to each other, ceaselessly oscillating around their average bond lengths and bond angles. For instance, in non-linear triatomic molecules there are three possible modes of vibration. There is the symmetric stretch in which both bonds in the molecule lengthen and contract in unison. In the asymmetric stretch, one bond lengthens while the other contracts. Finally, there is the bend in which the bond angle alternately widens and narrows.

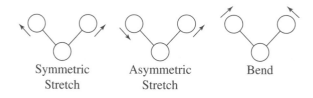

| Symmetric | Asymmetric | Bend |
| Stretch | Stretch | |

Figure 1 Vibrations of a Triatomic Molecule

More generally, each atom in a molecule is capable of moving in three distinct directions, often represented by x, y and z. In a molecule with N atoms, there will be $3N$ possible atomic movements. However, if all the atoms in a molecule move in the same direction, translational movement and not vibration will result. Likewise, there are some combinations of atomic motions that result in rotation of the molecule and not vibration. Taking this into account, in a molecule containing N atoms there will be $3N - 6$ normal modes of vibration in non-linear molecules and $3N - 5$ normal modes of vibration in linear molecules.

If we make the rough approximation that atoms in a molecule are harmonic oscillators, then the energy of their vibration is given by:

$$E = \left(v + \frac{1}{2}\right)\left(\frac{h}{2\pi}\right)\sqrt{\frac{k}{u}} \text{ for } v = 0,1,2,...$$

where v is the quantum vibrational number, h is Planck's constant, k is the force constant of the bond which increases with bond strength, and u is the reduced mass of the molecule. Changes in the vibrational quantum state are associated with energies similar to infrared photons. Thus, IR spectroscopy is the study of the energetics of a molecule's vibrational quantum states. However, only those normal modes of vibration that induce a change in the dipole moment of a molecule can be excited with IR light.

Table 1 Bond Energies of Select Diatomic Elements

Molecule	Bond Energy (kJ/mol)
H_2	436
N_2	946
O_2	497
F_2	155

1. Which of the following molecules has nine normal modes of vibration?

A) NI_3
B) CH_4
C) PF_5
D) SCl_6

2. A change in which of the following combinations of molecular movement can never produce a peak in an IR spectrum?

A) Translation and rotation
B) Stretching and bending
C) Vibration and translation
D) Rotation and bending

3. Assuming their reduced masses are the same, which molecule will have the highest energy of vibration in the $v = 0$ state?

A) N_2
B) O_2
C) F_2
D) Cannot be determined from the information given.

4. All of the following molecules will display absorption peaks in an IR spectrum EXCEPT

A) $HClO_4$
B) SO_3
C) CO
D) O_2

5. In VSEPR theory, T-shaped is a sub-class of the trigonal bipyramidal geometric family in which the central atom has exactly three atoms bound to it and two lone pairs of electrons. Which of the following molecules is T-shaped?

A) SF_4
B) NH_3
C) $BrCl_3$
D) FO_3^-

6. For a diatomic molecule, the reduced mass is given by $u = (m_1 \times m_2) / (m_1 + m_2)$ where m_1 and m_2 are the atomic weights of the two bonded atoms. What will be the ratio of the ground state vibration energies of D_2 to H_2 assuming the force constant k is the same for both?

A) 0.5
B) 0.7
C) 1.4
D) 2.0

7. Nitrate is best described by a resonance average of three structures:

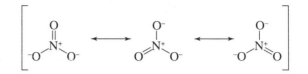

What best describes the peaks in an IR spectrum that result from the three N—O bond stretches?

A) One peak at the double bond N=O stretch frequency and two peaks at the single bond N—O stretch frequency
B) One peak at the double bond N=O stretch frequency and one peak at the single bond N—O stretch frequency
C) One peak at the double bond N=O stretch frequency and one peak between the single N—O and double bond N=O stretch frequencies
D) One peak between the single N—O and double bond N=O stretch frequencies

SOLUTIONS TO CHAPTER 5 FREESTANDING PRACTICE QUESTIONS

1. **A** A bond has a dipole moment when the two atoms involved in the bond differ in electronegativity. However, an entire molecule can only have a dipole if it contains bond dipoles and is asymmetrical. Choice A is tetrahedral and not all four substituents are the same. Therefore, it is asymmetrical and has a small negative dipole in the direction of the most electronegative substituent, oxygen. The remaining choices are trigonal bipyramidal, tetrahedral, and octahedral respectively. All have identical substituents, are symmetrical, and have no net dipole moment.

2. **A** In order to participate in intermolecular hydrogen bonding, a molecule must be able to act as both a hydrogen bond donor and acceptor. In order to act as a hydrogen bond donor, a molecule must possess a hydrogen (H) atom covalently bound to a nitrogen (N), oxygen (O), or fluorine (F) atom. In order to act as a hydrogen bond acceptor, a molecule must have an oxygen, nitrogen, or fluorine atom with an unshared pair of electrons. CH_3CO_2H meets both of these requirements, and is therefore a valid choice. CO_2 does not possess any hydrogen atoms and is therefore an invalid option. While H_2S may seem like an enticing choice, sulfur is not sufficiently electronegative to produce hydrogen bonding when covalently bound to hydrogen atoms.

3. **B** Van der Waals forces and induced dipoles are both examples of intermolecular forces, not intramolecular bonding, therefore choices C and D can be eliminated. The disparity in electronegativities between the carbon (C) and nitrogen (N) atoms in cyanide is not sufficient enough to produce ionic bonding, therefore choice B, covalent bonding, is the best answer.

$$\ddot{N}\!\!\equiv\!\!\overset{\ominus}{C}\!:$$

4. **C** The central atom, N, possesses three bonding electron groups and one lone pair of electrons. NH_3 therefore has tetrahedral orbital geometry.

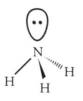

The central atom, N, possesses four bonding electron groups and zero lone pairs. NH_4^+ therefore has tetrahedral geometry.

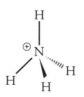

The central atom, C, possesses two bonding electron groups and zero lone pairs. Recall that double bonds count as a single electron group. CO_2 therefore has linear geometry.

$$\ddot{O} = C = \ddot{O}$$

The central atom, C, possesses four bonding electron groups and zero lone pairs. CH_4 therefore has tetrahedral geometry.

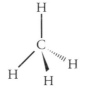

5. A   When answering ranking questions, it is best to determine the extremes and eliminate answer choices. Of the four molecules, only H_2O and H_2SO_4 are liquids at room temperature, and therefore would have higher boiling points than the two gases. Both experience strong hydrogen bonding, but the H_2SO_4 molecule is substantially larger, and, aside from this, has more sites to accept H-bonds from surrounding molecules. Therefore, H_2SO_4 should have the highest boiling point, eliminating answer choices B and D. Both NH_3 and CO_2 are gases at room temperature. However, NH_3 experiences hydrogen bonding, and therefore its boiling point would be higher than CO_2, eliminating choice C and making choice A the correct answer.

6. C   For neon to form a solid, there must be intermolecular forces holding the atoms or molecules in relatively fixed positions. Gravitational force is given by $F = G\frac{m_1 m_2}{r^2}$. With the constant G on the order of 10^{-11} and the mass of neon on the order of 10^{-26}, this force is negligible and choice A is eliminated. Electrostatic force is given by $F = k\frac{q_1 q_2}{r^2}$. Choice B is incorrect because neon is a neutral atom without any charge, so there are no significant electrostatic forces at play. Choice D is incorrect because strong nuclear forces act over a very small distance essentially limited to the size of the nucleus. Choice C is correct. Neon is a neutral molecule and has induced dipole-dipole interactions, also known as London dispersion forces. Because this is the weakest of the van der Waals forces, neon must be cooled down close to absolute zero before forming a solid.

7. D   This is an example of a Lewis acid-base reaction. In this type of reaction, one species accepts an electron pair from another species and a coordinate covalent bond is formed. One member of the bond donates *both* electrons in the bond. Whereas a coordinate covalent bond is a type of covalent interaction, the questions asks for the best answer, and coordinate covalent is more specific (eliminate choice A). Therefore, choice D is correct. An electrostatic bond is an ionic bond (eliminate choice B), and a metallic bond involves long-range delocalization of valence electrons, which is not the case in the product molecule (eliminate choice C).

SOLUTIONS TO CHAPTER 5 PRACTICE PASSAGE

1. **B** None of these molecules are linear. The passage states that the number of normal modes of vibration is $3N - 6$ for non-linear molecules. If there are nine normal modes of vibration, $3N - 6 = 9$, and $N = 5$. Only methane, choice B, has 5 atoms.

2. **A** From the passage, stretching and bending are types of vibration, while translation and rotation are not. All vibrations can potentially produce peaks in IR spectra, so choices B, C, and D are eliminated. Changes in translational and rotational movements alone do not show up in IR.

3. **A** If $v = 0$ and h and u are constant, the equation for vibration energy reduces as follows:

$$E = \left(v + \frac{1}{2}\right)\left(\frac{h}{2\pi}\right)\sqrt{\frac{k}{u}}$$

$$E \propto \sqrt{k}$$

The energy of the ground state is proportional to the square root of the force constant k. The passage states that k is larger for stronger bonds, and the bond in N_2 is strongest since it has the highest bond energy (see Table 1). N_2 must have the highest vibrational energy in the ground state.

4. **D** The passage states that only those normal modes of vibration that produce a change in the dipole moment of a molecule will absorb IR light. Since O_2 has no dipole, it will not have any peaks in an IR spectrum. Note that while the molecule SO_3 as a whole has no dipole, its individual bonds do have detectable dipoles.

5. **C** As the question states, T-shaped molecules have trigonal bipyramidal orbital geometry because of its three bonded and two lone pairs of electrons around the central atom. SF_4 has four atoms bound so it cannot be T-shaped, eliminating choice A. Both FO_3^- and NH_3 have three atoms bound to their central atoms and one lone pair, so they have trigonal pyramidal molecular geometries, eliminating choices B and D. $BrCl_3$ has three atoms bound to it and two lone pairs, making choice C the correct answer.

6. **B** Deuterium (D) has one proton, one neutron, and an atomic mass of 2. For D_2, $u = (2 \times 2) / (2 + 2) = 1$. For H_2, $u = 1 \times 1 / (1 + 1) = 1/2$. Since v, h, and k are all constant in this comparison, the vibration energy equation in the passage reduces as follows:

$$E = \left(v + \frac{1}{2}\right)\left(\frac{h}{2\pi}\right)\sqrt{\frac{k}{u}}$$

$$E \propto \frac{1}{\sqrt{u}}$$

The ratio of this energy for D_2 to H_2 is:

$$\frac{E_{D_2}}{E_{H_2}} = \frac{\dfrac{1}{\sqrt{1}}}{\dfrac{1}{\sqrt{1/2}}} = \frac{1}{\sqrt{2}}$$

The quantity must be greater than 0.5 but less than 1, so only choice B is possible.

7. **D** A molecule essentially exists as an average of its resonance structures. No individual resonance structure exists in isolation. In nitrate there are three bonds of equal strength, containing about 33% N=O double bond character and about 67% N—O single bond character. Therefore, there will be only one stretch peak in the IR spectrum intermediate to the N—O and N=O stretches that accounts for all three of these bonds in nitrate.

Chapter 6
Thermodynamics

6.1 SYSTEM AND SURROUNDINGS

Why does anything happen? Why does a creek flow downhill, a volcano erupt, a chemical reaction proceed? It's all **thermodynamics**: the transformation of energy from one form to another. The laws of thermodynamics underlie any event in which energy is transformed.

The Zeroth Law of Thermodynamics

The Zeroth Law is often conceptually described as follows: If two systems are both in thermal equilibrium with a third system, then the two initial systems are in thermal equilibrium with one another.

Thus, the Zeroth Law establishes a definition of thermal equilibrium. When systems are in thermal equilibrium with one another, their temperatures must be the same. When bodies of different temperatures are brought into contact with one another, heat will flow from the body with the higher temperature into the body with lower temperature in order to achieve equilibrium at the same temperature value. This means that devices (thermometers) may be designed to achieve thermal equilibrium with their surroundings, and give a quantified, relative value of the temperature at this equilibrium.

In this way, the Zeroth Law defines what we call temperature, and is the logical basis for the subsequent thermodynamic laws that rely on it. It also establishes the link between heat and temperature. An important practical application of the Zeroth Law is calorimetry, which will be discussed in more detail in Chapter 7.

The First Law of Thermodynamics

The First Law states that *the total energy of the universe is constant*. Energy may be transformed from one form to another, but it cannot be created or destroyed.

An important result of the First Law is that an isolated system has a constant energy—no transformation of the energy is possible. When systems are in contact, however, energy is allowed to flow, and thermal equilibrium can be attained. In addition, the First Law also establishes that work can be put into a system to increase its overall energy. This may or may not occur with a corresponding change in temperature. The concept of work and its effects on physical thermodynamics can be examined more closely in the *MCAT Physics and Math Review*.

Conventions Used in Thermodynamics

In thermodynamics we have to designate a "starting line" and a "finish line" to be able to describe how energy flows in chemical reactions and physical changes. To do this we use three distinct designations to describe energy flow: the system, the surroundings, and the thermodynamic universe (or just universe).

The system is the thing we're looking at: a melting ice cube, a solid dissolving into water, a beating heart, anything we want to study. Everything else: the table the ice cube sits on and the surrounding air, the beaker that holds the solid and the water, the chest cavity holding the heart, is known collectively as the surroundings. The system and the surroundings taken together form the thermodynamic universe.

We need to define these terms so that we can assign a direction—and therefore a sign, either (+) or (–)—to energy flow. For chemistry (and for physics), we define everything in terms of what's happening to the *system*.

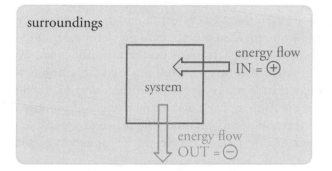

Consider energy flowing from the surroundings into the system, like the heat flowing from the table to the ice cube that's sitting on it. What is happening in the system? As energy flows in (here it's heat), the molecules in the system absorb it and start to jiggle faster. Eventually enough energy is absorbed to cause the ice to melt. Overall, the energy of the system *increased*, and we therefore give it a (+) sign. What about water when it freezes? Here energy (once again, heat) leaves the water (our system), and the water molecules' jiggling slows down. The energy of the system has *decreased*, and we therefore assign a (–) sign to energy flow. Finally, energy that flows into the system flows out of the surroundings, and energy that flows out of the system flows into the surroundings. Therefore, we can make these statements:

1) When energy flows into a system from the surroundings, the energy of the system increases and the energy of the surroundings decreases.
2) When energy flows out of a system into the surroundings, the energy of the system decreases and the energy of the surroundings increases.

Keep this duality in mind when dealing with energy.

6.2 ENTHALPY

Enthalpy is a measure of the heat energy that is released or absorbed when bonds are broken and formed during a reaction that's run at constant pressure. The symbol for enthalpy is *H*. Some general principles about enthalpy prevail over all reactions:

- When a bond is formed, energy is released. $\Delta H < 0$.
- Energy must be put into a bond in order to break it. $\Delta H > 0$.

In a chemical reaction, energy must be put into the reactants to break their bonds. Once the reactant bonds are broken, the atoms rearrange to form products. As the product bonds form, energy is released. The enthalpy of a reaction is given by the difference between the enthalpy of the products and the enthalpy of the reactants.

$$\Delta H = H_{products} - H_{reactants}$$

The enthalpy change, ΔH, is also known as the **heat of reaction**.

If the products of a chemical reaction have stronger bonds than the reactants, then more energy is released in the making of product bonds than was put in to break the reactant bonds. In this case, energy is released overall from the system, and the reaction is **exothermic**. The products are in a lower energy state than the reactants, and the change in enthalpy, ΔH, is negative, since heat flows out of the system. If the products of a chemical reaction have weaker bonds than the reactants, then more energy is put in during the breaking of reactant bonds than is released in the making of product bonds. In this case, energy is absorbed overall and the reaction is **endothermic**. The products are in a higher energy state than the reactants, and the change in enthalpy, ΔH, is positive, since heat had to be added to the system from the surroundings.

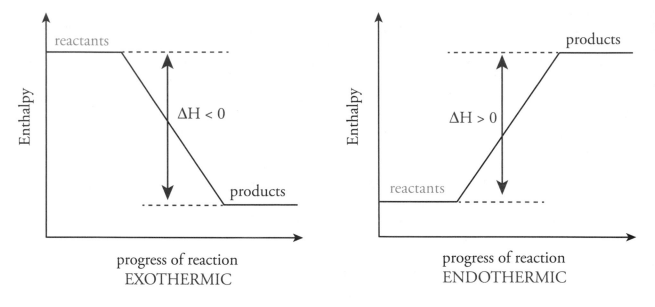

Example 6-1: The combustion of methanol is given by this reaction:

$$2\ CH_3OH(g) + 3\ O_2(g) \rightarrow 2\ CO_2(g) + 4\ H_2O(g), \qquad \Delta H = -1352\ kJ$$

a) How much heat is produced when 16 g of oxygen gas reacts with excess methanol?
b) Is the reaction exothermic or endothermic?
c) How many moles of carbon dioxide are produced when 676 kJ of heat is produced?

Solution:

a) The molecular weight of O_2 is $2(16) = 32$ g/mol, so 16 g represents one-half mole. If 1352 kJ of heat is released when 3 moles of O_2 react, then just $(1/6)(1352 \text{ kJ}) = 225$ kJ of heat will be released when one-half mole of O_2 reacts.

b) Because ΔH is negative, the reaction is exothermic. And since 6 moles of gaseous products are being formed from just 5 moles of gaseous reactants, the disorder (entropy) has increased.

c) The stoichiometry of the given balanced reaction tells us that 2 moles of CO_2 are produced when 1352 kJ of heat is produced. So, half as much CO_2 (that is, 1 mole) is produced when half as much heat, 676 kJ, is produced.

Example 6-2: Which one of the following processes does NOT contribute to the change in enthalpy, ΔH_{rxn}, of a chemical reaction?

A) Phase change
B) Formation of stronger intermolecular forces
C) Breaking covalent bonds
D) The presence of a heterogeneous catalyst

Solution: A catalyst lowers the activation energy, but does not affect an equilibrium constant, enthalpy, entropy, or free energy in any way. Choice D is the answer. The other choices do fall under the umbrella of enthalpy.

6.3 CALCULATION OF ΔH_{rxn}

The heat of reaction (ΔH_{rxn}) can be calculated in a number of ways. Each of these will lead to the same answer given accurate starting values. The three most important methods to be familiar with are the use of heats of formation (ΔH_f), Hess's law of heat summation, and the summation of individual bond enthalpies.

Standard Conditions

Essentially every process is affected by temperature and pressure, so scientists have a convention called **standard conditions** for which most constants, heats of formation, enthalpies, and so on are determined. Under standard conditions, the temperature is 298 K (25°C) and the pressure is 1 atm. All solids and liquids are assumed to be pure, and solutions are considered to be at a concentration of 1 M. Values that have been determined under standard conditions are designated by a ° superscript: $\Delta H°$, for example. Be careful not to confuse *standard conditions* with *standard temperature and pressure* (STP). STP is 0°C, while standard conditions means 25°C.

Heat of Formation

The **standard heat of formation**, ΔH°_{f}, is the amount of energy required to make one mole of a compound *from its constituent elements in their natural or standard state*, which is the way the element exists under standard conditions. The convention is to assign elements in their standard state forms a ΔH°_{f} of zero. For example, the ΔH°_{f} of C(*s*) (as graphite) is zero. Diatomic elements, such as O_2, H_2, Cl_2 and so on are also defined as zero, rather than their atomic forms (such as O, Cl, etc.), because the diatomic state is the *natural* state for these elements at standard conditions. For example, $\Delta H^{\circ}_{f} = 0$ for O_2, but for O, $\Delta H^{\circ}_{f} = 249$ kJ/mol at standard conditions, because it takes energy to break the O=O double bond.

When the ΔH°_{f} of a compound is positive, then an input of heat is required to make that compound from its constituent elements. When ΔH°_{f} is negative, making the compound from its elements gives off energy.

You can calculate the ΔH° of a reaction if you know the heats of formation of the reactants and products:

$$\Delta H^{\circ}_{rxn} = (\Sigma n \times \Delta H^{\circ}_{f,\, products}) - (\Sigma n \times \Delta H^{\circ}_{f,\, reactants})$$

In the above equation "*n*" denotes the stoichiometric coefficient applied to each species in a chemical reaction as written. ΔH°_{f} of a given compound is the heat needed to form one mole, and as such if two moles of a molecule are needed to balance a reaction one must double the corresponding ΔH°_{f} in the enthalpy equation. If only half a mole is required one must divide the ΔH°_{f} by 2.

Example 6-3: Which of the following substances does NOT have a heat of formation equal to zero at standard conditions?

    A) $F_2(g)$
    B) $Cl_2(g)$
    C) $Br_2(g)$
    D) $I_2(s)$

Solution: Heat of formation, ΔH°_{f}, is zero for a pure element in its natural phase at standard conditions. All of the choices are in their standard state, except for bromine, which is a liquid, not a gas, at standard conditions. The correct answer is C.

Example 6-4: What is ΔH° for the following reaction under standard conditions if the ΔH°_{f} of $CH_4(g) = -75$ kJ/mol, ΔH°_{f} of $CO_2(g) = -393$ kJ/mol, and ΔH°_{f} of $H_2O(l) = -286$ kJ/mol?

$$CH_4(g) + 2\, O_2(g) \rightarrow CO_2(g) + 2\, H_2O(l)$$

Solution: Using the equation for ΔH°_{rxn}, we find that

$$\Delta H^{\circ}_{rxn} = (\Delta H^{\circ}_{f} CO_2 + 2\, \Delta H^{\circ}_{f} H_2O) - (\Delta H^{\circ}_{f} CH_4 + 2\, \Delta H^{\circ}_{f} O_2)$$

$$= (-393 \text{ kJ/mol} + 2(-286) \text{ kJ/mol}) - (-75 \text{ kJ/mol} + 0 \text{ kJ/mol})$$

$$= -890 \text{ kJ/mol}$$

Hess's Law of Heat Summation

Hess's law states that if a reaction occurs in several steps, then the sum of the energies absorbed or given off in all the steps will be the same as that for the overall reaction. This is due to the fact that enthalpy is a state function, which means that changes are independent of the pathway of the reaction. Therefore, ΔH is independent of the pathway of the reaction.

For example, we can consider the combustion of carbon to form carbon monoxide to proceed by a two-step process:

1) $C(s) + O_2(g) \rightarrow CO_2(g)$ $\qquad \Delta H_1 = -394$ kJ
2) $CO_2(g) \rightarrow CO(g) + 1/2\ O_2(g)$ $\qquad \Delta H_2 = +283$ kJ

To get the overall reaction, we add the two steps:

$$C(s) +\ 1/2\ O_2(g) \rightarrow CO(g)$$

So, to find ΔH for the overall reaction, we just add the enthalpies of each of the steps:

$$\Delta H_{rxn} = \Delta H_1 + \Delta H_2 = -394\ \text{kJ} + 283\ \text{kJ} = -111\ \text{kJ}$$

It's important to remember the following two rules when using Hess's law:

1) *If a reaction is reversed, the sign of ΔH is reversed too.*
   For example, for the reaction $CO_2(g) \rightarrow C(s) + O_2(g)$, we'd have $\Delta H = +394$ kJ.

2) *If an equation is multiplied by a coefficient, then ΔH must be multiplied by that same value.*
   For example, for $1/2\ C(s) +\ 1/2\ O_2(g) \rightarrow 1/2\ CO_2(g)$, we'd have $\Delta H = -197$ kJ.

Summation of Average Bond Enthalpies

Enthalpy itself can be viewed as the energy stored in the chemical bonds of a compound. Bonds have characteristic enthalpies that denote how much energy is required to break them homolytically (often called the bond dissociation energy, or BDE; see Section 5.2).

As indicated at the start of this section, an important distinction should be made here in the difference in sign of ΔH for making a bond versus breaking a bond. One must, necessarily, infuse energy into a system to break a chemical bond. As such the ΔH for this process is positive; it is endothermic. On the other hand, creating a bond between two atoms must have a negative value of ΔH. It therefore gives off heat and is exothermic. If this weren't the case it would indicate that the bonded atoms were higher in energy than they were when unbound; such a bond would be unstable and immediately dissociate.

Therefore we have a very important relation that can help you on the MCAT:

> Energy is needed to break a bond.
>
> Energy is released in making a bond.

From this we come to the third method of determining ΔH_{rxn}. If a question provides a list of bond enthalpies, ΔH_{rxn} can be determined through the following equation:

$$\Delta H_{rxn} = \Sigma \text{ (BDE bonds broken)} - \Sigma \text{ (BDE bonds formed)}$$

One can see that if stronger bonds are being formed than those being broken, then ΔH_{rxn} will be negative. More energy is released than supplied and the reaction is exothermic. If the opposite is true and breaking strong bonds takes more energy than is regained through the making of weaker product bonds, then the reaction is endothermic.

Example 6-5: Given the table of average bond dissociation energies below, calculate ΔH_{rxn} for the combustion of methane given in Example 6-4.

Bond	Average Bond Dissociation Energy (kJ/mol)
C—H	413
O—H	467
C=O	799
C=N	615
H—Cl	427
O=O	495

A) 824 kJ/mol
B) 110 kJ/mol
C) −824 kJ/mol
D) −110 kJ/mol

Solution: First determine how many of each type of bond are broken in the reactants and formed in the products based on the stoichiometry of the balanced equation. Then using the bond dissociation energies we can calculate the enthalpy change:

$$\Delta H_{rxn} = \Sigma \text{ (BDE bonds broken)} - \Sigma \text{ (BDE bonds formed)}$$

$$\Delta H_{rxn} = (4(C-H) + 2(O=O)) - (2(C=O) + 4(O-H))$$

$$= (4(413) + 2(495)) - (2(799) + 4(467))$$

$$= -824 \text{ kJ/mol}$$

The correct answer is C. You may notice that the two methods of calculating the reaction enthalpy for the same reaction did not produce exactly the same answer. This is due to the fact that bond energies are reported as the average of many examples of that type of bond, whereas heats of formation are determined for each individual chemical compound. The exact energy of a bond will be dependent not only on the two atoms bonded together but also the chemical environment in which they reside. The average bond energy gives an approximation of the strength of an individual bond, and as such, the summation of bond energies give an approximation of ΔH_{rxn}.

6.4 ENTROPY

The Second Law of Thermodynamics

There are several different ways to state the **second law of thermodynamics**, each appropriate to the particular system under study, but they're all equivalent. One way to state this law is that the disorder of the universe increases in a spontaneous process. For this to make sense, let's examine what we mean by the term *spontaneous*. For example, water will spontaneously splash and flow down a waterfall, but it will not spontaneously collect itself at the bottom and flow up the cliff. A bouncing ball will come to rest, but a ball at rest will not suddenly start bouncing. If the ball is warm enough, it's got the energy to start moving, but heat—the disorganized, random kinetic energy of the constituent atoms—will not spontaneously organize itself and give the ball an overall kinetic energy to start it moving. From another perspective, heat will spontaneously flow from a plate of hot food to its cooler surroundings, but thermal energy in the cool surroundings will not spontaneously concentrate itself and flow into the food. None of these processes would violate the first law, but they do violate the second law.

Nature has a tendency to become increasingly disorganized, and another way to state the second law is that *all processes tend to run in a direction that leads to maximum disorder*. Think about spilling milk from a glass. Does the milk ever collect itself together and refill the glass? No, it spreads out randomly over the table and floor. In fact, it needed the glass in the first place just to have any shape at all. Likewise, think about the helium in a balloon: It expands to fill its container, and if we empty the balloon, the helium diffuses randomly throughout the room. The reverse doesn't happen. Helium atoms don't collect themselves from the atmosphere and move into a closed container. The natural tendency of *all* things is to increase their disorder.

We measure disorder or randomness as **entropy**. The greater the disorder of a system, the greater is its entropy. Entropy is represented by the symbol S, and the change in entropy during a reaction is represented by the symbol ΔS. The change in entropy is determined by the equation

$$\Delta S = S_{products} - S_{reactants}$$

If randomness increases—or order decreases—during the reaction, then ΔS is positive for the reaction. If randomness decreases—or order increases—then ΔS is negative. For example, let's look at the decomposition reaction for carbonic acid:

$$H_2CO_3 \rightleftharpoons H_2O + CO_2$$

In this case, one molecule breaks into two molecules, and disorder is increased. That is, the atoms are less organized in the water and carbon dioxide molecules than they are in the carbonic acid molecule. The entropy is increasing for the forward reaction. Let's look at the reverse process: If CO_2 and H_2O come together to form H_2CO_3, we've decreased entropy because the atoms in two molecules have become more organized by forming one molecule.

In general, entropy is predictable in many cases:

- Liquids have more entropy than solids.
- Gases have more entropy than solids or liquids.
- Particles in solution have more entropy than undissolved solids.
- Two moles of a substance have more entropy than one mole.
- The value of ΔS for a reverse reaction has the same magnitude as that of the forward reaction, but with opposite sign: $\Delta S_{reverse} = -\Delta S_{forward}$.

While the overall drive of nature is to increase entropy, reactions can occur in which entropy decreases, but we must either put in energy or gain energy from making more stable bonds. (We'll explore this further when we discuss Gibbs free energy.)

Example 6-6: Which of the following processes would have a negative ΔS?

A) The evaporation of a liquid.
B) The freezing of a liquid.
C) The melting of a solid.
D) The sublimation of a solid.

Solution: Only the change described in choice B involves a decrease in randomness—the molecules of a solid are more ordered and organized than those in a liquid. So this process would have a negative change in entropy.

Example 6-7: Of the following reactions, which would have the greatest positive entropy change?

A) $2 NO(g) + O_2(g) \rightarrow 2 NO_2(g)$
B) $2 HCl(aq) + Mg(s) \rightarrow MgCl_2(aq) + H_2(g)$
C) $2 H_2O(g) + Br_2(g) + SO_2(g) \rightarrow 2 HBr(g) + H_2SO_4(aq)$
D) $2 I^-(aq) + Cl_2(g) \rightarrow I_2(s) + 2 Cl^-(aq)$

Solution: The reactions in choices A, C, and D all describe processes involving a decrease in randomness, that is, an increase in order. However, the process in choice B has a highly ordered solid on the left, but a highly disordered gas on the right, so we'd expect this reaction to have a positive entropy change.

Example 6-8: For the endothermic reaction

$$2 CO_2(g) \rightarrow 2 CO(g) + O_2(g)$$

which of the following is true?

A) ΔH is positive, and ΔS is positive.
B) ΔH is positive, and ΔS is negative.
C) ΔH is negative, and ΔS is positive.
D) ΔH is negative, and ΔS is negative.

Solution: Since we're told that the reaction is endothermic, we know that ΔH is positive. This eliminates choices C and D. Now, what about ΔS? Has the disorder increased or decreased? On the reactant side, we have one type of gas molecule, while on the right we have two. The reaction increases the numbers of gas molecules, so this describes an increase in disorder. ΔS is positive, and the answer is A.

Example 6-9: A gas is observed to undergo condensation. Which of the following is true about the process?

A) ΔH is positive, and ΔS is positive.
B) ΔH is positive, and ΔS is negative.
C) ΔH is negative, and ΔS is positive.
D) ΔH is negative, and ΔS is negative.

Solution: Condensation is the phase change from gas to liquid, which *releases* heat (since the reverse process, vaporization, requires an input of heat). Therefore, ΔH is negative, and choices A and B are eliminated. Now, because the change from gas to liquid represents an increase in order—since gases are so highly disordered—this process will have a negative change in entropy. The answer is therefore D.

The Third Law of Thermodynamics

The Third Law defines absolute zero to be a state of zero-entropy. At absolute zero, thermal energy is absent and only the least energetic thermodynamic state is available to the system in question. If only one state is possible, then there is no randomness to the system and $S = 0$. In this way, the Third Law describes the least thermally energetic state, and therefore the lowest achievable temperature. Kelvin defined the temperature at this state as 0 on his temperature scale.

6.5 GIBBS FREE ENERGY

The magnitude of the change in **Gibbs free energy**, ΔG, is the energy that's available (free) to do useful work from a chemical reaction. The spontaneity of a reaction is determined by changes in enthalpy and in entropy, and G includes both of these quantities. Now we have a way to determine whether a given reaction will be spontaneous. In some cases—namely, when ΔH and ΔS have different signs—it's easy. For example, if ΔH is negative and ΔS is positive, then the reaction will certainly be spontaneous (because the products have less energy and more disorder than the reactants; there are two tendencies for a spontaneous reaction: to decrease enthalpy and/or to increase entropy). If ΔH is positive and ΔS is negative, then the reaction will certainly be nonspontaneous (because the products would have more energy and less disorder than the reactants).

But what happens when ΔH and ΔS have the *same* sign? Which factor—enthalpy or entropy—will dominate and determine the spontaneity of the reaction? The sign of the single quantity ΔG will dictate whether or not a process is spontaneous, and we calculate ΔG from this equation:

Change in Gibbs Free Energy
$$\Delta G = \Delta H - T\Delta S$$

where T is the absolute temperature (in kelvins). And now, we can then say this:

- $\Delta G < 0 \rightarrow$ spontaneous in the forward direction
- $\Delta G = 0 \rightarrow$ reaction is at equilibrium
- $\Delta G > 0 \rightarrow$ nonspontaneous in the forward direction

If ΔG for a reaction is positive, then the value of ΔG for the *reverse* reaction has the same magnitude but is negative. Therefore, the reverse reaction is spontaneous.

ΔG and Temperature

The equation for ΔG shows us that the entropy ($T\Delta S$) term depends directly on temperature. At low temperatures, the entropy doesn't have much influence on the free energy, and ΔH is the dominant factor in determining spontaneity. But as the temperature increases, the entropy term becomes more significant relative to ΔH and can dominate the value for ΔG. In general, the universe tends towards increasing disorder (positive ΔS) and stable bonds (negative ΔH), and a favorable combination of these will make a process spontaneous. The following chart summarizes the combinations of ΔH and ΔS that determine ΔG and spontaneity.

ΔH	ΔS	ΔG	Reaction is...?
–	+	–	spontaneous
+	+	– at sufficiently high T + at low T	spontaneous nonspontaneous
–	–	+ at high T – at sufficiently low T	nonspontaneous spontaneous
+	–	+	nonspontaneous

Important note: While values of ΔH are usually reported in terms of kJ, values of ΔS are usually given in terms of J. When using the equation $\Delta G = \Delta H - T\Delta S$, make sure that your ΔH and ΔS are expressed *both* in kJ or *both* in J.

Example 6-10: What must be true about a spontaneous, endothermic reaction?

A) ΔH is negative.
B) ΔG is positive.
C) ΔS is positive.
D) ΔS is negative.

Solution: Since the reaction is spontaneous, we know that ΔG is negative, and since we know the reaction is endothermic, we also know that ΔH is positive. The equation $\Delta G = \Delta H - T\Delta S$ then tells us that ΔS must be positive, choice C.

Example 6-11: If it's discovered that a certain nonspontaneous reaction becomes spontaneous if the temperature is lowered, then which of the following must be true?

A) ΔS is negative and ΔH is positive.
B) ΔS is negative and ΔH is negative.
C) ΔS is positive and ΔH is positive.
D) ΔS is positive and ΔH is negative.

Solution: Here's one (rather mathematical) approach. The nonspontaneous reaction has $\Delta G_1 = \Delta H - T_1\Delta S$, and the spontaneous reaction has $\Delta G_2 = \Delta H - T_2\Delta S$. Subtracting these equations, we find that $\Delta G_1 - \Delta G_2 = (T_2 - T_1)\Delta S$. Since $\Delta G_1 > 0$ and $\Delta G_2 < 0$, we know that the left-hand side is positive, so the right-hand side must be positive also. Because $T_2 < T_1$, the term $(T_2 - T_1)$ is negative. This implies that ΔS must be negative, and we eliminate choices C and D. Now let's figure out the sign of ΔH. From the equation $\Delta G_2 = \Delta H - T_2\Delta S$, we get $\Delta H = \Delta G_2 + T_2\Delta S$. Because ΔG_2 and $T_2\Delta S$ are both negative, so is ΔH, and the answer is B.

6.6 REACTION ENERGY DIAGRAMS

A chemical reaction can be graphed as it progresses in a reaction energy diagram. True to its name, a reaction energy diagram plots the free energy of the total reactions versus the conversion of reactants to products.

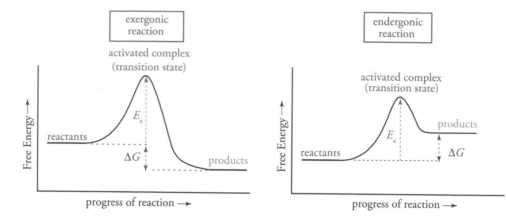

The ΔG of the overall reaction is the difference between the energy of the products and the energy of the reactants: $\Delta G_{rxn} = G_{products} - G_{reactants}$. When the value of $T\Delta S$ is very small, then ΔG can approximate ΔH, with the difference between the energy of products and reactants being very close to the heat of reaction, ΔH.

The activation energy, E_a, is the extra energy the reactants required to overcome the activation barrier, and determines the kinetics of the reaction. The higher the barrier, the slower the reaction proceeds towards equilibrium; the lower the barrier, the faster the reaction proceeds towards equilibrium. However, E_a does *not* determine the equilibrium, and an eternally slow reaction (very big E_a) can have a very favorable (large) K_{eq}. Many more details of both kinetics and equilibrium will be discussed in Chapters 9 and 10, respectively.

Kinetics vs. Thermodynamics

Just because a reaction is thermodynamically favorable (i.e., *spontaneous*), does not automatically mean that it will be taking place rapidly. **Do not confuse kinetics with thermodynamics** (this is something the MCAT will *try* to get you to do many times!). They are separate realms. *Thermodynamics predicts the spontaneity (and the equilibrium) of reactions, not their rates.* If you had a starting line and a finish line, thermodynamics tells you how far you will go, while kinetics tells you how quickly you will get there. A classic example to illustrate this is the formation of graphite from diamond. Graphite and diamond are two of the several different forms (**allotropes**) of carbon, and the value of $\Delta G°$ for the reaction $C_{(diamond)} \rightarrow C_{(graphite)}$ is about -2900 J/mol. Because $\Delta G°$ is negative, this reaction is spontaneous under standard conditions. But it's *extremely* slow. Even diamond heirlooms passed down through many generations are still in diamond form.

Reversibility

Reactions follow the principle of microscopic reversibility: The reverse reaction has the same magnitude for all thermodynamic values (ΔG, ΔH, and ΔS) but of the opposite sign, and the same reaction pathway, but in reverse. This means that the reaction energy diagram for the reverse reaction can be drawn by simply using the mirror image of the forward reaction. The incongruity you should notice is that E_a is different for the forward and reverse reactions. Coming from the products side towards the reactants, the energy barrier will be the difference between $G_{products}$ and the energy of the activated complex.

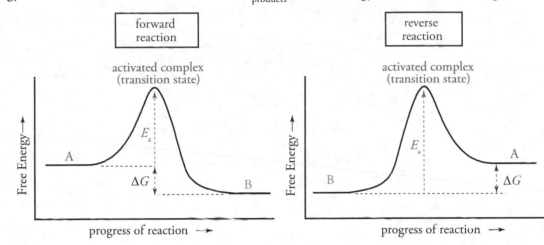

- The Zeroth Law of Thermodynamics states that energy will flow from a body at a higher temperature to a body at a lower temperature until both bodies have the same temperature.

- Energy flow into a system has a positive sign. Energy flow out of a system has a negative sign.

- The First Law of Thermodynamics states that energy cannot be created or destroyed.

- The internal energy of an object is proportional to its temperature.

- The Second Law of Thermodynamics states that all processes tend toward maximum disorder, or entropy (S).

- Enthalpy (H) is a measure of the energy stored in the bonds of molecules.

- Breaking bonds requires energy $(+\Delta H)$, while forming bonds releases energy $(-\Delta H)$.

- Standard conditions are 1 atm and 298 K, 1 M concentrations. Standard conditions are denoted by a superscript "$\circ$".

- An endothermic reaction has a $\Delta H > 0$. An exothermic reaction has a $\Delta H < 0$.

- $\Delta H_{reaction} = H_{products} - H_{reactants}$. This equation can also be applied to ΔG and ΔS.

- ΔG, the Gibbs free energy, is the amount of energy in a reaction available to do chemical work.

- For a reaction under any set of conditions, $\Delta G = \Delta H - T\Delta S$.

- If $\Delta G < 0$, the reaction is spontaneous in the forward direction. If $\Delta G > 0$, the reaction is nonspontaneous in the forward direction. If $\Delta G = 0$, the reaction is at equilibrium.

CHAPTER 6 FREESTANDING PRACTICE QUESTIONS

1. During the electrolysis of liquid water into hydrogen and oxygen gas at standard temperature and pressure, energy is:

A) absorbed during the breaking of H—H bonds and the reaction is spontaneous.
B) released during the formation of H—H bonds and the reaction is nonspontaneous.
C) absorbed during the formation of O=O bonds and the reaction is spontaneous.
D) released during the breaking of O—H bonds and the reaction is nonspontaneous.

2. What could make the following nonspontaneous endothermic reaction spontaneous?

$$2\ H_2O(l) \rightarrow 2\ H_2(g) + O_2(g)$$

A) Decreasing volume
B) Increasing temperature
C) Decreasing temperature
D) The reaction will always be nonspontaneous.

3. Which of the following should have the highest enthalpy of vaporization?

A) N_2
B) Br_2
C) Hg
D) Al

4. A 36 gram sample of water requires 93.4 kJ to sublime. What are the heats of fusion (ΔH_{fus}) and vaporization (ΔH_{vap}) for water?

A) $\Delta H_{fus} = -20$ kJ/mol, $\Delta H_{vap} = 66.7$ kJ/mol
B) $\Delta H_{fus} = 40.7$ kJ/mol, $\Delta H_{vap} = 6.0$ kJ/mol
C) $\Delta H_{fus} = 6.0$ kJ/mol, $\Delta H_{vap} = 40.7$ kJ/mol
D) $\Delta H_{fus} = 12.0$ kJ/mol, $\Delta H_{vap} = 81.4$ kJ/mol

5. Given the standard enthalpies of formation (ΔH_f°) at 298 K for the compounds below, all of the following reactions are exothermic EXCEPT:

Compound	ΔH_f° (kJ/mol)
$C_2H_5OH(l)$	−238.86
$CH_3CHO(l)$	−77.80
$CH_3COOH(l)$	−484.50
$H_2O(l)$	−285.83

A) $CH_3COOH(l) \rightarrow CH_3CHO(l) + \frac{1}{2} O_2(g)$
B) $C_2H_5OH(l) + \frac{1}{2} O_2(g) \rightarrow CH_3CHO(l) + H_2O(l)$
C) $CH_3CHO(l) + \frac{1}{2} O_2(g) \rightarrow CH_3COOH(l)$
D) $C_2H_5OH(l) + O_2(g) \rightarrow CH_3COOH(l) + H_2O(l)$

6. The citric acid cycle consists of reactions that break down acetate into carbon dioxide. Given that some steps are thermodynamically unfavorable, why does the cycle proceed in the forward direction overall?

A) The rate constant for the unfavorable reactions is very large.
B) The cycle contains exergonic reactions that drive the endergonic reactions forward.
C) The endothermically unfavorable reactions also have a negative entropy change.
D) The activation energies of the unfavorable reactions are lowered by catalysts.

CHAPTER 6 PRACTICE PASSAGE

The extent to which a salt dissolves in water can be quantified by its solubility product constant, (K_{sp}) which is defined, for a hypothetical salt X_aY_b, as shown in Equation 2. The greater the value of K_{sp}, the more soluble the compound. The K_{sp} of a salt is related to the free energy of dissolution by the equation $\Delta G^o_{diss} = -RT \ln(K_{sp})$. Table 1 lists the K_{sp} values for some insoluble salts.

$$X_aY_b(s) \rightleftharpoons a\,X^{b+}(aq) \ + \ b\,Y^{a-}(aq)$$

Equation 1

$$K_{sp} = [X^{b+}]^a\,[Y^{a-}]^b$$

Equation 2

Salt	K_{sp}
$PbCl_2$	1.2×10^{-5}
$MgCO_3$	6.8×10^{-6}
$BaSO_4$	1.1×10^{-10}
$AgCl$	5.4×10^{-13}

Table 1 K_{sp} values for select insoluble salts

When a solid completely dissolves, solute particles are separated and encapsulated by solvent molecules. This process requires several steps: 1) breaking all solute-solute interactions, 2) disrupting some solvent-solvent interactions, and 3) forming new solute-solvent interactions. The combination of these processes determines the overall enthalpy change for the dissolution, which can be either exothermic or endothermic regardless of the solubility of the salt. Table 2 shows the enthalpies of dissolution for several soluble salts.

Salt	ΔH_{diss} (kJ/mol)
LiCl	−37.03
KCH_3CO_2	−15.33
NaCl	3.87
NH_4NO_3	25.69
$KClO_4$	41.38

Table 2 Dissolution enthalpies for some soluble salts

As solids are low entropy materials, their dissolution entails an increase in entropy. The size of ΔS_{diss} is dependent on the organization of solvent molecules in the solvation sphere of the dissolved ions.

1. Which of the following species is isoelectronic with the silver ion in AgCl?

A) Rh^+
B) Pd
C) Cd^{2+}
D) In^-

2. Given that the dissolution of sodium chloride is endothermic and spontaneous below the saturation concentration, which of the following statements must be true?

A) Forming solute-solvent interactions requires energy, while breaking solute-solute and solvent-solvent interactions releases energy.
B) The increase in entropy must outweigh the endothermic process to create a negative Gibbs free energy.
C) Sodium chloride is only soluble at high temperatures.
D) All ionically-bound materials are substantially soluble in water.

3. Which one of the salts in Table 1 has the smallest value of ΔG^o_{diss}?

A) $PbCl_2$
B) $MgCO_3$
C) $BaSO_4$
D) $AgCl$

4. Which of the following is consistent with the differences in $\Delta H°_{diss}$ for NaCl and LiCl?

A) The electrostatic forces in solid LiCl are much stronger than in solid NaCl, while coordination of water is equivalent for both salts.

B) The electrostatic forces in the two solids are approximately equivalent, while water molecules coordinate much more effectively to Na^+ than Li^+.

C) The electrostatic forces in solid LiCl are weaker than in solid NaCl, while water cannot effectively coordinate to the very small Li^+ cation.

D) The electrostatic forces in solid NaCl are slightly weaker than in solid LiCl, while water far more efficiently coordinates Li^+ than Na^+.

5. The transfer of heat to or from a solution changes the temperature of the solution according to the equation $q = mc\Delta T$ where q is the heat transferred, m is the mass of solvent, and c is the specific heat of the solvent. If a 1 g sample of a salt was dissolved in 20 mL of water (specific heat = 4.18 J/g°C) in an insulated beaker and the temperature was found to decrease by 4°C, which of the following salts was used? Assume no phase change for the water.

A) LiCl
B) KCH_3CO_2
C) NH_4NO_3
D) NaCl

SOLUTIONS TO CHAPTER 6 FREESTANDING PRACTICE QUESTIONS

1. **B** Electrolysis requires energy. Water will not split into hydrogen and oxygen gas spontaneously at standard temperature and pressure which eliminates choices A and C. When bonds are broken, energy is absorbed (eliminates choice D). Energy is released when bonds are formed.

2. **B** Choice A is eliminated because decreasing volume would cause an increase in pressure, which would inhibit the transformation of a liquid to a gas. The question alludes that the process has a positive ΔH. Since the reaction involves changing two moles of liquid to three moles of gas, entropy increases so it will have a positive ΔS. Using the equation $\Delta G = \Delta H - T\Delta S$, a reaction with a positive ΔH and ΔS will be spontaneous only at high enough temperatures. Therefore, choices C and D can be eliminated, making choice B correct.

3. **D** Enthalpy of vaporization is the heat energy required per mole to change from the liquid to gas phase. N_2 is a gas at room temperature, Br_2 and Hg are both liquids at room temperature, and Al is a solid at room temperature. Therefore, it is expected that Al will have the highest enthalpy of vaporization, making choice D correct.

4. **C** Both fusion (melting) and vaporization (boiling) require energy and are endothermic, eliminating choice A. Comparing both processes, vaporization takes substantially more energy. During vaporization, intermolecular forces are essentially completely overcome, and gaseous molecules separate widely due to their increased kinetic energy. Choice B is therefore eliminated. A 36 gram sample of water is 2 moles, so the heat of sublimation of 1 mole is half of 93.4 kJ, or 46.7 kJ/mol. This eliminates choice D. Examining the fusion and vaporization of water and adding their enthalpies by Hess's law gives choice C as the correct answer:

$$H_2O(s) \rightarrow H_2O(l) \qquad \Delta H_{fus} = X \ (6.0 \text{ kJ/mol})$$

$$H_2O(l) \rightarrow H_2O(g) \qquad \Delta H_{vap} = Y \ (40.7 \text{ kJ/mol})$$

$$H_2O(s) \rightarrow H_2O(g) \qquad \Delta H_{vap} = X + Y = 46.7 \text{ kJ/mol}$$

5. **A** The change in enthalpy (ΔH) for a reaction is equal to the sum of ΔH_f° for products minus the sum of ΔH_f° for reactants: $\Delta H = \Sigma \ \Delta H_{f \ (products)} - \Sigma \ \Delta H_{f \ (reactants)}$. For choice A, the lone reduction reaction, $\Delta H = (-77.8 \text{ kJ/mol}) - (-484.50 \text{ kJ/mol})$. This is a positive value indicating that enthalpy is absorbed and the reaction is endothermic. Note that the heat of formation of diatomic oxygen gas or any element in its naturally occurring form is defined as 0. The other answer choices, which are all oxidation reactions, will yield a negative value indicating they are exothermic.

6.   B   The question is asking about thermodynamic principles, so answer choices A and D that involve kinetics can be eliminated. Reactions with a positive ΔH and a negative ΔS are never spontaneous according to $\Delta G = \Delta H - T\Delta S$, eliminating choice C. If the sum of all reactions is more exergonic ($-\Delta G$) than endergonic ($+\Delta G$), the net release of free energy will drive the cycle forward, making choice B the best answer.

SOLUTIONS TO CHAPTER 6 PRACTICE PASSAGE

1.   C   Isoelectronic species have the same electron configurations, and hence the same number of electrons. Ag^+ has 46 electrons, eliminating choices A and D because they have 44 and 50 electrons, respectively. The electron configuration of Ag^+ is [Kr] $4d^{10}$. The electron configuration of Pd is [Kr] $5s^2 3d^7$ (eliminate choice B). The electron configuration of Cd^{2+} is [Kr] $4d^{10}$, which is isoelectronic with Ag^+.

2.   B   Similar to bond formation, forming solute-solvent interactions is exothermic, meaning energy is released, not required; similarly breaking solute-solute or solvent-solvent interactions is endothermic (requires energy), like bond breaking (eliminate choice A). In addition, sodium chloride is soluble at room temperature (eliminate choice C). Salts are held together by ionic bonds, but Table 1 shows through the small K_{sp} values that not all of them are substantially soluble (eliminate choice D). For the dissolution of sodium chloride to be spontaneous, the increase in entropy must outweigh the endothermic process, yielding a negative Gibbs free energy.

3.   A   The important relationship between the standard state Gibbs free energy of dissolution and the solubility product constant is given in the passage:

$$\Delta G^\circ_{diss} = -RT \ln K_{sp}$$

Since the question asks for an extreme, first eliminate the two choices for K_{sp} in Table 1 that are the middle values (choices B and C). The ln function is similar to the log function, and can be thought of in the same way when judging relative magnitudes of ΔG°_{diss} in the equation above. For values of $K_{sp} > 1$, the ΔG° value will be negative, and for values of $K_{sp} < 1$, the ΔG° value will be positive. Therefore, the larger value of K_{sp} for $PbCl_2$ will give the smallest value for ΔG°.

4.   D   Effective dissolution involves the endothermic step of overcoming the electrostatic charges holding the solid salts together and the exothermic step of coordinating solvents to the separated ions. A negative value of ΔH°_{diss} likely indicates relatively weak electrostatic forces in the solid (small endothermic step), and effective solvation by water (large exothermic step). Table 2 shows that LiCl has a much more negative value of ΔH°_{diss} than NaCl. Choice A, stronger electrostatic forces in LiCl and no difference in solvation, would lead to a more negative ΔH°_{diss} for NaCl. Choice B would also result in a more negative value of ΔH°_{diss} for NaCl, as it indicates that electrostatics are equivalent while Na^+ has stronger interactions with water. Choice C is incorrect because a large negative value of ΔH°_{diss} would be difficult to achieve if water were unable to coordinate Li^+. Choice D includes a viable combination of slightly weaker attractive forces in NaCl but much better solvation for Li^+.

5. C   Since the question states that the temperature of the solution decreased, the salts with exo-thermic dissolution enthalpies (choices A and B) can be eliminated. Using the calorimetry equation given in the question stem ($q = mc\Delta T$), we can estimate:

$$20 \text{ g} \times \approx 4 \text{ J/g°C} \times 4°C = \approx 320 \text{ J} = \approx 0.32 \text{ kJ} = q$$

Since this heat is associated with 1 g of salt, in order to compare to the $\Delta H°_{diss}$ in Table 2, convert this energy to a per mole basis by multiplying by the molar mass of the salt.

For choice C (NH_4NO_3, MW = 80 g/mol), this yields:

$$\approx 0.3 \text{ kJ/1g } NH_4NO_3 \times 80 \text{ g } NH_4NO_3/\text{mol} = 24 \text{ kJ/mol}$$

which is close to the given 25.69 kJ/mol in the table. The comparable calculation for NaCl yields:

$$\approx 0.3 \text{ kJ/1g NaCl} \times \approx 60 \text{ g NaCl/mol} = 18 \text{ kJ/mol}$$

so choice D can be eliminated.

Chapter 7
Phases

7.1 PHYSICAL CHANGES

Matter can undergo physical changes as well as chemical changes. Melting, freezing, and boiling are all examples of physical changes. A key property of a physical change is that no *intra*molecular bonds are made or broken; a physical change affects only the *inter*molecular forces between molecules or atoms. For example, ice melting to become liquid water does not change the molecules of H_2O into something else. Melting reflects the disruption of the attractive interactions between the molecules.

Every type of matter experiences intermolecular forces such as dispersion forces, dipole interactions, and hydrogen bonding. All molecules have some degree of attraction towards each other (dispersion forces at least), and it's the intermolecular interactions that hold matter together as solids or liquids. The strength and the type of intermolecular forces depend on the identity of the atoms and molecules of a substance and vary greatly. For example, $NaCl(s)$, $H_2O(l)$ and $N_2(g)$ all have different kinds and strengths of intermolecular forces, and these differences give rise to their widely varying melting and boiling points.

Phase Transitions

Physical changes are closely related to temperature. What does temperature tell us about matter? Temperature is a measure of the amount of internal kinetic energy (the energy of motion) that molecules have. The average kinetic energy of the molecules of a substance directly affects its **state** or **phase**: whether it's a **solid, liquid,** or **gas.** Kinetic energy is also related to the degree of disorder, or **entropy.** In general, the higher the average kinetic energy of the molecules of a substance, the greater its entropy.

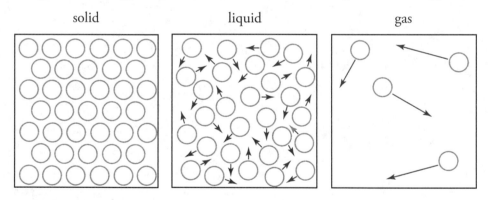

If we increase the temperature at a given pressure, a solid typically transforms into liquid and then into gas. What causes the phase transitions as the temperature increases? Phase changes are simply the result of breaking (or forming) intermolecular interactions. At low temperatures, matter tends to exist as a solid and is held together by intermolecular interactions. The molecules in a solid may jiggle a bit, but they're restricted to relatively fixed positions and form an orderly array, because the molecules don't have enough kinetic energy to overcome the intermolecular forces. Solids are the most ordered and least energetic of the phases. As a solid absorbs heat its temperature increases, meaning the average kinetic energy of the molecules increases. This causes the molecules to move around more, loosening the intermolecular interactions and increasing the entropy. When enough energy is absorbed for the molecules to move freely around one another, the solid melts and becomes liquid. At the molecular level, the molecules in a liquid are still in contact and interact with each other, but they have enough kinetic energy to escape fixed positions. Liquids have more internal kinetic energy and greater entropy than solids. If enough heat is absorbed by the liquid, the kinetic energy increases until the molecules have enough speed to escape intermolecular forces and vaporize into the gas phase. Molecules in the gas phase move freely of one another and experience very little, if any, intermolecular forces. Gases are the most energetic and least ordered of the phases.

To illustrate these phase transitions, let's follow ice through the transitions from solid to liquid to gas. Ice is composed of highly organized H_2O molecules held rigidly by hydrogen bonds. The molecules have limited motion. If we increase the temperature of the ice, the molecules will eventually absorb enough heat to move around, and the organized structure of the molecules will break down as fixed hydrogen bonds are replaced with hydrogen bonds in which the molecules are *not* in fixed positions. We observe the transition as ice melting into liquid water. If we continue to increase the temperature, the kinetic energy of the molecules eventually becomes great enough for the individual molecules to overcome all hydrogen bonding and move freely. This appears to us as vaporization, or boiling of the liquid into gas. At this point the H_2O molecules zip around randomly, forming a high-entropy, chaotic swarm. All the phase transitions are summarized here.

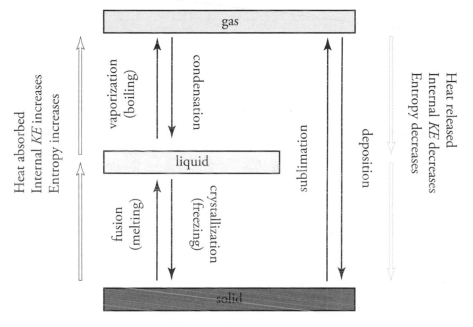

Example 7-1: Which of these phase changes releases heat energy?

A) Melting
B) Fusion
C) Condensation
D) Sublimation

Solution: Phase changes that bring molecules together (*condensation, freezing, deposition*) release heat, while phase changes that spread molecules out (*melting/fusion, vaporization, sublimation*) absorb heat. Choice C is the correct answer. (Note also that choices A and B are identical, so you know they have to be wrong no matter what.)

7.2 HEATS OF PHASE CHANGES

When matter undergoes a phase transition, energy is either absorbed or released. The amount of energy required to complete a transition is called the **heat of transition**, symbolized ΔH. For example, the amount of heat that must be absorbed to change a solid into liquid is called the **heat of fusion**, and the energy absorbed when a liquid changes to gas is the **heat of vaporization**. Each substance has a specific heat of transition for each phase change, and the magnitude is directly related to the strength and number of the intermolecular forces that substance experiences.

The amount of heat required to cause a change of phase depends on two things: the type of substance and the amount of substance. For example, the heat of fusion for H_2O is 6.0 kJ/mol. So, if we wanted to melt a 2 mol sample of ice (at 0°C), 12 kJ of heat would need to be supplied. The heat of vaporization for H_2O is about 41 kJ/mol, so vaporizing a 2 mol sample of liquid water (at 100°C) would require 82 kJ of heat. If that 2 mol sample of steam (at 100°C) condensed back to liquid, 82 kJ of heat would be released. In general, the amount of heat, q, accompanying a phase transition is given by

$$q = n \times \Delta H_{\text{phase change}}$$

where n is the number of moles of the substance. If ΔH and q are positive, heat is absorbed; if ΔH and q are negative, heat is released.

Example 7-2: The melting point of iron is 1530°C, and its heat of fusion is 64 cal/g. How much heat would be required to completely melt a 50 g chunk of iron at 1530°C?

Solution: Since the heat of transition is given in units of cal/g, we can simply multiply it by the given mass

$$q = m \times \Delta H_{\text{fusion}} = 50 \text{ g} \times 64 \text{ cal/g} = 3200 \text{ cal}$$

By the way, a **calorie** is, by definition, the amount of heat required to raise the temperature of 1 gram of water by 1°C. The SI unit of heat (and of all forms of energy) is the **joule**. Here's the conversion between joules and calories: 1 cal ≈ 4.2 J. (The popular term *calorie*—the one most of us are concerned with day to day when we eat—is actually a kilocalorie [10^3 cal] and is sometimes written as Calorie [with a capital C]).

Example 7-3: What happens when a container of liquid water (holding 100 moles of H_2O) at 0°C completely freezes? (Note: $\Delta H_{\text{fusion}} = 6$ kJ/mol, and $\Delta H_{\text{vap}} = 41$ kJ/mol.)

A) 600 kJ of heat is absorbed.
B) 600 kJ of heat is released.
C) 4100 kJ of heat is absorbed.
D) 4100 kJ of heat is released.

Solution: In order for ice to melt, it must absorb heat; therefore, the reverse process—water freezing into ice—must *release* heat. This eliminates choices A and C. The heat of transition from liquid to solid is $-\Delta H_{\text{fusion}}$, so in this case the heat of transition is $q = (100 \text{ mol})(-6 \text{ kJ/mol}) = -600$ kJ, so choice B is the answer.

7.3 CALORIMETRY

In between phase changes, matter can absorb or release energy without undergoing transition. We observe this as an increase or a decrease in the temperature of a substance. When a sample is undergoing a phase change, it absorbs or releases heat *without* a change in temperature, so when we talk about a temperature change, we are considering only cases where the phase doesn't change. One of the most important facts about physical changes of matter is this (and it will bear repeating):

> When a substance absorbs or releases heat, one of two things can happen: either its temperature changes *or* it will undergo a phase change *but not both at the same time.*

The amount of heat absorbed or released by a sample is proportional to its change in temperature. The constant of proportionality is called the substance's **heat capacity**, C, which is the product of its **specific heat**, c, and its mass, m; that is, $C = mc$. We can write the equation $q = C\Delta T$ in this more explicit form:

$$q = mc\Delta T$$

where

q = heat added to (or released by) a sample
m = mass of the sample
c = specific heat of the substance
ΔT = temperature change

A substance's specific heat is an *intrinsic* property of that substance and tells us how resistant it is to changing its temperature. For example, the specific heat of liquid water is 1 calorie per gram-°C. (This is actually the definition of a **calorie**: the amount of heat required to raise the temperature of 1 gram of water by 1°C.) The specific heat of copper, however, is much less: 0.09 cal/g-°C. So, if we had a 1 g sample of water and a 1 g sample of copper and each absorbed 10 calories of heat, the resulting changes in the temperatures would be

$$\Delta T_{water} = \frac{q}{mc_{water}} \qquad \Delta T_{copper} = \frac{q}{mc_{copper}}$$

$$= \frac{10\ \text{cal}}{(1\ \text{g})(1\frac{\text{cal}}{\text{g-°C}})} \qquad = \frac{10\ \text{cal}}{(1\ \text{g})(0.09\frac{\text{cal}}{\text{g-°C}})}$$

$$= 10°\text{C} \qquad\qquad = 111°\text{C}$$

That's a big difference! So, while it's true that the temperature change is proportional to the heat absorbed, it's *inversely* proportional to the substance's heat capacity. A substance like water, with a relatively high specific heat, will undergo a smaller change in temperature than a substance (like copper) with a lower specific heat.

A few notes:

1) The specific heat of a substance also depends upon phase. For example, the specific heat of ice is different from that of liquid water.
2) The SI unit for energy is the joule, not the calorie. You may see specific heats (and heat capacities) given in terms of joules rather than calories. Remember, the conversion between joules and calories is: 1 cal ≈ 4.2 J.
3) Specific heats may also be given in terms of kelvins rather than degrees Celsius; that is, you may see the specific heat of water, say, given as 4.2 J/g K rather than 4.2 J/g°C. However, since the size of a Celsius degree is the same as a Kelvin (that is, if two temperatures differ by 1°C, they also differ by 1K), the numerical value of the specific heat won't be any different if kelvins are used.

Example 7-4: The specific heat of tungsten is 0.03 cal/g-°C. If a 50-gram sample of tungsten absorbs 100 calories of heat, what will be the change in temperature of the sample?

Solution: From the equation $q = mc\Delta T$, we find that

$$\Delta T = \frac{q}{mc} = \frac{100 \text{ cal}}{(50 \text{ g})(0.03 \text{ cal/g°C})} = \frac{2}{3/100}°C = 67°C$$

Example 7-5: Equal amounts of heat are absorbed by 10 g solid samples of four different metals, aluminum, lead, tin, and iron. Of the four, which will exhibit the *smallest* change in temperature?

A) Aluminum (specific heat = 0.9 J/g-K)
B) Lead (specific heat = 0.13 J/g-K)
C) Tin (specific heat = 0.23 J/g-K)
D) Iron (specific heat = 0.45 J/g-K)

Solution: Since q and m are constant, ΔT is inversely proportional to c. So, the substance with the greatest specific heat will undergo the smallest change in temperature. Of the metals listed, aluminum (choice A) has the greatest specific heat.

Example 7-6: A researcher attempts to determine the specific heat of a substance by gradually heating a sample of it over time and measuring the temperature change. His first trial fails because it produces no significant change in temperature. Which changes to his experimental procedure would be most effective in producing a larger temperature change in his second trial?

A) Increasing the mass of the sample and increasing the heat input
B) Increasing the mass of the sample and decreasing the heat input
C) Decreasing the mass of the sample and increasing the heat input
D) Decreasing the mass of the sample and decreasing the heat input

Solution: Since $\Delta T = q/mc$, to increase ΔT, the researcher should increase q and decrease m. *(Intuitively, adding more heat to a smaller sample should result in a greater temperature increase.)* Therefore, the answer is C.

Example 7-7: Molecules that experience strong intermolecular forces tend to have high specific heats. Of the following molecules, which one is likely to have the highest specific heat?

A) CH_4
B) $(CH_3)_4Si$
C) CO
D) CH_3OH

Solution: We're looking for the molecule with the strongest intermolecular forces. Choices A and B are eliminated because these are nonpolar molecules that only experience weak London dispersion forces. Methanol (choice D) is a better choice than carbon monoxide (choice C), because methanol will experience hydrogen bonding while carbon monoxide experiences only weak dipole forces. Therefore, choice D is the answer.

7.4   PHASE TRANSITION DIAGRAM

Let's consider the complete range of phase changes from solid to liquid to gas. The process in this direction requires the input of heat. As heat is added to the solid, its temperature increases until it reaches its melting point. At that point, absorbed heat is used to change the phase to liquid, not to increase the temperature. Once the sample has been completely melted, additional heat again causes its temperature to rise, until the boiling point is reached. At that point, absorbed heat is used to change the phase to gas, not to increase the temperature. Once the sample has been completely vaporized, additional heat again causes its temperature to rise. We can summarize all this with a **phase transition diagram**, which plots the temperature of the sample versus the amount of heat absorbed. The figure below is a typical phase transition diagram.

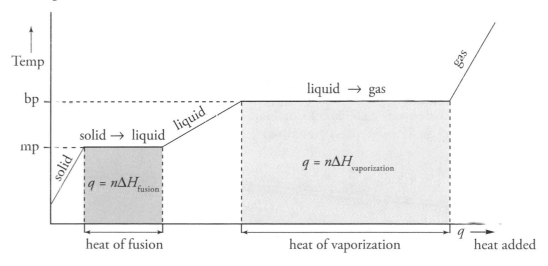

The horizontal axis represents the amount of heat added, and the vertical axis is the corresponding temperature of the substance. Notice the flat lines when the substance reaches its melting point (mp) and boiling point (bp). *During a phase transition, the temperature of the substance does not change.* Also, the greater the value for the heat of transition, the longer the flat line. A substance's heat of vaporization is always greater than its heat of fusion. The sloped lines show how the temperature changes (within a phase) as heat is added. Since $\Delta T = q/C$, the slopes of the non-flat lines are equal to $1/C$, the reciprocal of the substance's heat capacity in that phase.

Example 7-8: How much heat (in calories) is necessary to raise the temperature of 2 g of solid H_2O from 0°C to 85°C? (*Note:* Heat of fusion for water = 80 cal/g and the specific heat of water is 1 cal/g-°C.)

A) 85 cal
B) 165 cal
C) 170 cal
D) 330 cal

Solution: There are two steps here: (1) melt the ice at 0°C to liquid water at 0°C, and (2) heat the water from 0°C to 85°C.

$$\begin{aligned} q_{total} &= q_1 + q_2 \\ &= m\Delta H_{fusion} + mc_{water}\Delta T \\ &= (2 \text{ g})(80 \text{ cal/g}) + (2 \text{ g})(1 \text{ cal/g}°C)(85°C) \\ &= (160 \text{ cal}) + (170 \text{ cal}) \\ &= 330 \text{ cal} \end{aligned}$$

The correct answer is D.

Example 7-9: Given that each of the following solutions is at equilibrium with its environment, which solution should have the lowest temperature at 1 atm?

A) A solution that is 1% ice and 99% liquid water
B) A solution that is 50% ice and 50% liquid water
C) A solution that is 99% ice and 1% liquid water
D) All these solutions will have the same temperature

Solution: As long as there is any amount of ice and liquid water coexisting at equilibrium, the temperature must be 0°C at 1 atm. Therefore, D is the answer.

Phase Diagrams

The phase of a substance doesn't depend just on the temperature, it also depends on the pressure. For example, even at high temperatures, a substance can be squeezed into the liquid phase if the pressure is high enough, and at low temperature, a substance can enter the gas phase if that pressure is low enough. A substance's **phase diagram** shows how its phases are determined by temperature and pressure. The figure below is a generic example of a phase diagram.

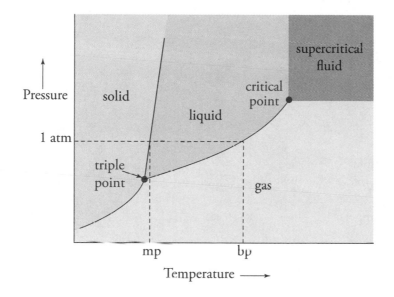

The boundary lines between phases represent points at which the two phases are in equilibrium. For example, a glass of liquid water at 0°C containing ice cubes is a two-phase system, and if its temperature and pressure were plotted in a phase diagram, it would be on the solid-liquid boundary line. Crossing a boundary line implies a phase transition. Notice that the solid phase is favored at low temperatures and high pressures, while the gas phase is favored at high temperatures and low pressures.

If we draw a horizontal line at the "1 atm" pressure level, the temperature at the point where this line crosses the solid-liquid boundary is the substance's **normal melting point**, and the temperature at the point where the line crosses the liquid-gas boundary is the **normal boiling point**.

The **triple point** is the temperature and pressure at which all three phases exist simultaneously in equilibrium.

The **critical point** marks the end of the liquid-gas boundary. Beyond this point, the substance displays properties of both a liquid (such as high density) and a gas (such as low viscosity). If a substance is in this state—where the liquid and gas phases are no longer distinct—it's called a **supercritical fluid**, and no amount of increased pressure can force the substance back into its liquid phase.

The Phase Diagram for Water

Water is the most common of a handful of substances that are denser in the liquid phase than in the solid phase. As a result, the solid-liquid boundary line in the phase diagram for water has a slightly *negative* slope, as opposed to the usual positive slope for most other substances. Compare these diagrams:

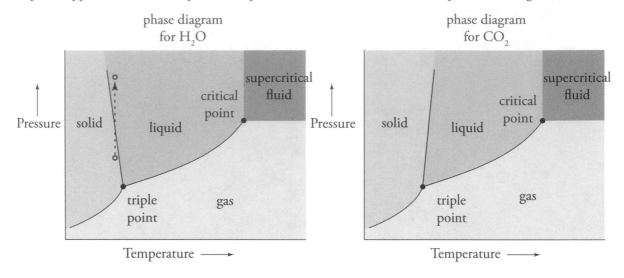

For H_2O, an increase in pressure at constant temperature can favor the *liquid* phase, not the solid phase as would be the case for most other substances (like CO_2, for example). You are probably already familiar with the following phenomenon: as the blade of an ice skate bearing all of the weight of the skater contacts the ice, the pressure increases, melting the ice under the blade and allowing the skate to glide over the liquid water. (The dashed arrow in the phase diagram for water above depicts this effect.) As the skater moves across the ice, each blade continually generates a thin layer of liquid water that refreezes as the blade passes. (This is also the reason why glaciers move.) The properties of CO_2 don't allow for skating because solid CO_2 will never turn to liquid when the pressure is increased. (And now you know why solid CO_2 is called *dry ice*!)

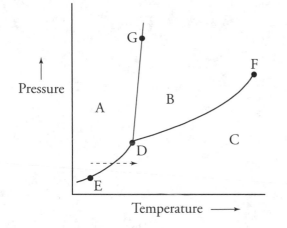

Example 7-10: In which region of the diagram above is the substance in the gas phase?

A)   A
B)   B
C)   C
D)   G

Solution: The gas phase is favored at high temperatures and low pressure, so we know that region C represents the gas phase.

Example 7-11: In which part of the diagram is gas in equilibrium with liquid?

A)   Along line ED
B)   Along line DG
C)   Along line DF
D)   In region B

Solution: The liquid phase is represented by region B and the gas phase by region C. Therefore, an equilibrium between liquid and gas phases is represented by a point on the boundary between regions B and C. This boundary is the "line" DF, choice C.

Example 7-12: The dashed arrow in the diagram indicates what type of phase transition?

A)   Evaporation
B)   Crystallization
C)   Deposition
D)   Sublimation

Solution: The arrow shows a substance in the solid phase (region A) moving directly to the gaseous phase (region C) without melting first. The phase transition from solid to gas is called sublimation, choice D.

- Changes in pressure and/or temperature of a substance can induce changes in phase.

- The three important phases are (in order of low-to-high entropy and low-to-high internal energy) solid, liquid, and gas.

- Specific heat (c) is an intrinsic property that defines how resistant a substance is to temperature change.

- The change in temperature associated with the input or extraction of heat when phase is uncharged is given by $q = mc\Delta T$, where c is the specific heat of a substance and m is the amount (either mass or moles, depending on c).

- Heat capacity (C) is given by $C = mc$, where m is the mass of the sample. Heat capacity is a proportionality constant that defines how much heat is required to change the temperature of a sample by 1°C.

- A substance cannot simultaneously undergo a phase change and a temperature change.

- The heat associated with a phase change is given by $q = n\Delta H_{phase\ change}$, where n is the number of moles of substance (or mass if ΔH is given in energy/mass).

- Lines on a phase diagram correspond to equilibria between phases and phase transitions. The intersection of all three lines on a phase diagram is known as the triple point, and represents equilibrium between all three phases.

- The phase diagram of water is unique in that its solid/liquid equilibrium line has a negative slope. This accounts for the fact that ice melts under increased pressure, and why the density of ice is less than that of liquid water.

CHAPTER 7 FREESTANDING PRACTICE QUESTIONS

1. Which of the following correctly describe(s) the physical properties of water?

    I.   The hydrogen bonds in water result in a lower boiling point than H_2S.
    II. Water has a high specific heat due to the hydrogen bonding between molecules.
    III. As pressure increases liquid water is favored over solid water.

A) II only
B) III only
C) II and III only
D) I, II and III

2. As a substance goes from the gas phase to the solid phase, heat is:

A) absorbed, internal energy decreases, and entropy decreases.
B) released, internal energy increases, and entropy decreases.
C) released, internal energy decreases, and entropy decreases.
D) released, internal energy decreases, and entropy increases.

3. In the following phase transition diagram, Substance X is in the solid phase during Segment A and in the gas phase during Segment C. What process is occurring during Segment B?

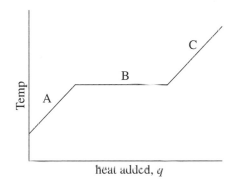

A) The substance is warming.
B) The substance is cooling.
C) Sublimation
D) Condensation

4. Denver is at a higher altitude than Los Angeles and therefore the atmospheric pressure is lower in Denver than in Los Angeles. Compared to Los Angeles, the melting point of water in Denver will be:

A) higher.
B) lower.
C) the same.
D) undetermined from the information given.

5. At 1 atm, deionized water can remain a liquid at temperatures down to –42°C. If a foreign body is added to the supercooled liquid, it will immediately turn into ice. Which of the following is true about this process?

A) The reaction is exothermic.
B) Tap water could also be supercooled to –42°C.
C) The transformation of a supercooled fluid to a solid is nonspontaneous.
D) Water's unique phase diagram allows it to be supercooled.

6. A pot containing 0.5 L of water at sea level is brought to 100°C. It is insulated around its sides to minimize heat loss to the environment, and heat is applied at the bottom of the container at a rate of 6 kJ/min over 3 minutes. What is the resulting temperature of the water? (ΔH_{vap} = 40.7 kJ/kg; $c(g)$ = 1.9 kJ/kg · °C; $c(l)$ = 4.2 kJ/kg · °C)

A) 115°C
B) 108°C
C) 104°C
D) 100°C

CHAPTER 7 PRACTICE PASSAGE

Lyophilization, or freeze drying, is a technique used to remove water from samples. Lyophilization uses sublimation to convert frozen, solid water directly to water vapor. This technique offers advantages over liquid-solvent removal techniques in that it can be performed at low temperatures, resulting in minimal damage to heat-sensitive samples.

A chamber containing the sample solution is attached to the lyophilizer, which freezes the sample at a temperature less than 0°C and then applies a vacuum, generally holding a pressure less than 0.006 atm. Under these conditions the frozen water sublimes and water vapor is pulled from the sample chamber into a condenser held at 50°C, where it is refrozen and held immobile.

The phase diagram for water is shown below, with its unique negatively sloped equilibrium line between the solid and liquid phase. At low pressures the solid phase of water is favored as long as any solute in the water is reasonably dilute. However, the freezing point of water decreases as the concentration of solute is increased. If concentrated enough, the sample can melt instead of sublime when pressure is decreased. In addition, volatile solvents often cannot be removed from the chamber by the condenser as their freezing point at low pressures is below −50°C. Volatile solvents remaining in the gaseous environment can compound the impurity of the remaining water, favoring the liquid phase even more.

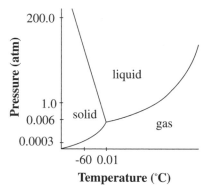

Figure 1 Phase diagram of water

1. The addition of which of the following substances is most likely to result in the melting of a sample during lyophilization?

   A) $(CH_3)_2CHOH$
   B) CH_3CH_2COOH
   C) $CH_3CH_2OCH_2CH_3$
   D) $CH_3(CH_2)_4OH$

2. If the temperature inside the chamber is 60°C, what pressure must the chamber be at in order for the sublimation reaction to be at equilibrium?

   A) 3×10^4 atm
   B) 3×10^3 atm
   C) 1 atm
   D) 125 atm

3. Lyophilization would most likely be employed industrially in which of the following separations?

   A) Salicylic acid dissolved in methanol
   B) An enzyme in aqueous solution
   C) NaCl in water
   D) A small molecular drug dissolved in dichloromethane

4. Sublimation of water inside the sample chamber causes the temperature of the chamber to:

   A) increase.
   B) decrease.
   C) stay the same.
   D) change in a manner dependent on the identity of the solvent.

5. The heat of sublimation of water is 46 kJ/mol. If heat is transferred to the sample by the environment at a rate of 0.1 kJ/min, approximately how long will it take to lyophilize 40 cm³ of frozen water (density = 0.91 g/mL) ?

   A) 7.7 hours
   B) 15.3 hours
   C) 77.0 hours
   D) 153.0 hours

SOLUTIONS TO CHAPTER 7 FREESTANDING PRACTICE QUESTIONS

1. **C** Since water experiences hydrogen bonding, more energy is required to boil water compared with SH_2, which leads to a higher boiling point, making Item I false and eliminating choice D. Since temperature is a measure of molecular motion, and hydrogen bonds bind molecules together, making this motion more difficult, hydrogen-bonded materials will require more energy to increase T and thus have high specific heats. Item II is true and choice B can be eliminated. The negative slope of the line between the solid and liquid phase on the phase diagram of water indicates that at higher pressures, liquid water is favored over solid, making Item III correct and C the best answer choice.

2. **C** As a substance undergoes deposition, it becomes a much more ordered substance, decreasing entropy (eliminate choice D). In addition, heat will be released (eliminate choice A) because the potential energy of the substance decreases (eliminate choice B).

3. **C** Substance X is changing from a solid to a gas during Segment B. This is an example of sublimation. Note that choices A and B cannot be correct answer choices because the temperature of Substance X remains constant during Segment B. Condensation occurs when a gas becomes a liquid, so choice D is eliminated.

4. **A** On a P vs. T phase diagram of water, the solid-liquid equilibrium line has a negative slope for water. Water's melting point increases with decreasing external pressure. Therefore, in Denver the melting point of water is higher than in Los Angeles.

5. **A** Upon nucleation with a foreign body, supercooled water will transition from liquid to solid phase. This phase transition (crystallization) requires heat to be released since intermolecular interactions are formed. Choice B is eliminated because tap water contains many dissolved particles that can serve as sites of nucleation. Choice C is incorrect because the supercooled fluids are only kinetically stabilized against freezing, and their transformation to a solid form is thermodynamically spontaneous. Since pressure remains constant, the negative sloped solid-liquid equilibrium line in water's phase diagram does not play a role in supercooling, eliminating Choice D.

6. **D** The addition of 6 kJ/min for three minutes imparts 18 kJ of heat to the sample. However, since the ΔH_{vap} of water is 40.7 kJ/mol, and 0.5 L is roughly 22 mol (1 L of $H_2O \approx 55$ mol), there is nowhere near enough heat provided to vaporize the entire sample. As such all the heat given to the sample is going toward vaporization and not toward increasing temperature. The temperature will remain constant at 100°C.

SOLUTIONS TO CHAPTER 7 PRACTICE PASSAGE

1. **C** The passage states that volatile chemicals cannot be used in samples subjected to lyophilization because they will hinder sublimation and favor the liquid phase through melting. This is because these compounds have a high vapor pressure and cannot be removed from the system by the condenser. Choices A, B, and D are all hydrogen donors and acceptors. Choice C, diethyl ether, can only act as a hydrogen bond acceptor. Therefore, it has the weakest intermolecular forces and is the most volatile.

2. **A** On a P vs. T diagram, sublimation equilibrium is indicated by the line separating the solid and vapor phases. On the graph in Figure 1, it is shown that at $-60°C$, the solid/gas line is at $P = 0.0003$ or 3×10^{-4} atm.

3. **B** Both dichloromethane and methanol are removed as liquids at reasonably low temperatures and have freezing points far lower than water. This eliminates choices A and D. The passage states that one of the major advantages to lyophilization is that it can be performed at low temperatures, and therefore preserve the activity of heat-sensitive samples. NaCl is a salt that is stable at high temperatures, whereas enzymes are proteins that denature at high temperatures. Therefore, lyophilization is best suited as a means to remove water from aqueous protein solutions.

4. **B** Sublimation is an endothermic reaction, requiring heat input. As this reaction removes heat from the surroundings, it lowers the temperature of the surroundings, in this case, the reaction chamber. This is very similar to sweat cooling the body as it evaporates off of the skin (also an endothermic process).

5. **B** 40 cm³ of ice is 36 g or 2 moles of water. The heat required to sublimate this sample is 46 kJ/mol(2 mol) = 92 kJ. If heat is transferred at 0.1 kJ/min, then 920 minutes are required. Dividing 920 min by 60 min/hour gives just over 15 hours. Overall:

$$Time = (40 cm^3) \left[\frac{0.91g}{mL} \right] \left[\frac{molH_2O}{18g} \right] \left[\frac{46kJ}{mol} \right] \left[\frac{min}{0.1kJ} \right] \left[\frac{hour}{60 \ min} \right]$$

$$Time \approx (40 cm^3) \left[\frac{0.9g}{mL} \right] \left[\frac{molH_2O}{18g} \right] \left[\frac{45kJ}{mol} \right] \left[\frac{min}{0.1kJ} \right] \left[\frac{hour}{60 \ min} \right]$$

$$Time \approx 15 \ hours$$

Chapter 8
Gases

8.1 GASES AND THE KINETIC-MOLECULAR THEORY

Unlike the condensed phases of matter (solids and liquids), **gases** have no fixed volume. A gas will fill all the available space in a container. Gases are *far* more compressible than solids or liquids, and their densities are very low (roughly 1 kg/m³ at standard temperature and pressure), about three to four orders of magnitude less than solids and liquids. But the most striking difference between a gas and a solid or liquid is that the molecules of a gas are free to move over large distances.

The most important properties of a gas are its **pressure**, **volume**, and **temperature**. How these macroscopic properties are related to each other can be derived from some basic assumptions concerning the *microscopic* behavior of gas molecules. These assumptions are the foundation of the **kinetic-molecular theory**.

Kinetic-molecular theory, a model for describing the behavior of gases, is based on the following assumptions:

1) The molecules of a gas are so small compared to the average spacing between them that the molecules themselves take up essentially no volume.

2) The molecules of a gas are in constant motion, moving in straight lines at constant speeds and in random directions between collisions. The collisions of the molecules with the walls of the container define the **pressure** of the gas (the average force exerted per unit area), and all collisions—molecules striking the walls and each other—are *elastic* (that is, the total kinetic energy is the same after the collision as it was before).

3) Since each molecule moves at a constant speed between collisions and the collisions are elastic, the molecules of a gas experience no intermolecular forces.

4) The molecules of a gas span a distribution of speeds, and the average kinetic energy of the molecules is directly proportional to the absolute temperature (the temperature in kelvins) of the sample: $KE_{avg} \propto T$.

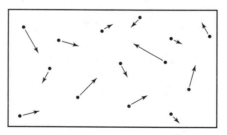

A gas that satisfies all these requirements is said to be an **ideal gas.** Most real gases behave like ideal gases under ordinary conditions, so the results that follow from the kinetic-molecular theory can be applied to real gases.

Units of Volume, Temperature, and Pressure

Volume

The SI unit for volume is the cubic meter (m³), but in chemistry, the **cubic centimeter** (**cm³** or **cc**) and **liter** (**L**) are commonly used. One cubic meter is equal to one thousand liters.

$$1 \text{ cm}^3 = 1 \text{ cc} = 1 \text{ mL} \quad \text{and} \quad 1 \text{ m}^3 = 1000 \text{ L}$$

Temperature

Temperature may be expressed in degrees Fahrenheit, degrees Celsius, or in kelvins (not degrees Kelvin). In scientific work, the Celsius scale is popular, where water freezes at 0°C and boils at 100°C (at standard atmospheric pressure). However, the "proper" unit for expressing temperatures is the kelvin (K), and this is the one we use when talking about gases (because of assumption #4 stated above for the kinetic-molecular theory). The relationship between kelvins and degrees Celsius is simple:

$$T \text{ (in K)} = T \text{ (in °C)} + 273.15$$

When dealing with gases, the best unit for expressing temperature is the kelvin (K). This is an absolute temperature scale whereby zero kelvin (0 K) defines a point of zero entropy (see Chapter 6) where molecular motion is at a minimum. From a practical perspective, this avoids the issue of calculations involving negative temperatures, so all of the gas laws equations on the MCAT require the use of absolute temperatures.

Pressure

Since pressure is defined as force per unit area, the SI unit for pressure is the **pascal** (abbreviated **Pa**), where $1 \text{ Pa} = 1 \text{ N/m}^2$. The unit is inconveniently small for normal calculations involving gases (for example, a nickel sitting on a table exerts about 140 Pa of pressure), so several alternative units for pressure are usually used.

At sea level, atmospheric pressure is about 101,300 pascals (or 101.3 kPa); this is 1 **atmosphere** (1 **atm**). Related to the atmosphere is the **torr**, where 1 atm = 760 torr. (Therefore, 1 torr is about the same as the pressure exerted by a nickel sitting on a table.) At 0°C, 1 torr is equal to 1 **mm Hg (millimeter of mercury)**, so we generally just take 1 atm to equal 760 mm Hg:

$$1 \text{ atm} = 760 \text{ torr} = 760 \text{ mm Hg} = 101.3 \text{ kPa}$$

Standard Temperature and Pressure

Standard Temperature and Pressure (STP) means a temperature of 0°C (273.15 K) and a pressure of 1 atm.

Example 8-1: A temperature of 273°C is equivalent to:

A) −100 K
B) 0 K
C) 100 K
D) 546 K

Solution: Choice A is eliminated, because negative values are not permitted when using the Kelvin temperature scale. Since $T \text{ (in K)} = T \text{ (in °C)} + 273$, we have

$$T \text{ (in K)} = 273 + 273 = 546 \text{ K}$$

Therefore, choice D is the answer.

Example 8-2: What would be the reading of a barometer (a device used to measure pressure) filled with a liquid of lower density than Hg if at that moment another nearby Hg barometer reads 752 mm Hg?

A) Less than 752 mm
B) 752 mm
C) Greater than 752 mm
D) It depends on the compressibility of the liquid.

Solution: In a mercury barometer, the atmospheric pressure pushes a column of Hg up a tube until the weight of the column of Hg balances the upward pressure of the atmosphere; one then reads the height of the suspended Hg column in millimeters. If a less dense liquid were used, then more liquid would have to get pushed up the column before it weighed enough to balance the atmospheric pressure. The liquid column would then have a greater strength, so choice C is the correct answer.

8.2   THE IDEAL GAS LAW

The volume, temperature, and pressure of an ideal gas are related by a simple equation called the **ideal gas law**. Most real gases under ordinary conditions act very much like ideal gases, so the ideal gas law applies to most gas behavior:

> **Ideal Gas Law**
>
> $$PV = nRT$$

where

P = the pressure of the gas in atmospheres
V = the volume of the container in liters
n = the number of moles of the gas
R = the universal gas constant, 0.0821 L-atm/K-mol
T = the absolute temperature of the gas (that is, T in kelvins)

Questions on gas behavior typically take one of two forms. The first type of question simply gives you some facts, and you use $PV = nRT$ to determine a missing variable. In the second type, "before" and "after" scenarios are presented for which you determine the effect of changing the volume, temperature, or pressure. In this case, you apply the ideal gas law twice, once for each scenario. We'll solve a typical example of each type of question.

1. If two moles of helium at 27°C fill a 3 L balloon, what is the pressure?

Take the ideal gas law, solve it for P, then plug in the numbers (and don't forget to convert the temperature in °C to kelvin!):

$$PV = nRT$$

$$P = \frac{nRT}{V}$$

$$P = \frac{(2 \text{ mol})(0.082 \text{ L-atm/K-mol})(300 \text{ K})}{3 \text{ L}}$$

$$P = 16 \text{ atm}$$

2. Argon, at a pressure of 2 atm, fills a 100 mL vial at a temperature of 0°C. What would the pressure of the argon be if we increase the volume to 500 mL, and the temperature is 100°C?

We're not told how much argon (the number of moles, n) is in the vial, but it doesn't matter since it doesn't change. Since R is also a constant, the ratio of PV/T, which is equal to nR, remains constant. Therefore,

$$\frac{P_1 V_1}{T_1} = \frac{P_2 V_2}{T_2} \quad \Rightarrow \quad P_2 = P_1 \frac{V_1}{V_2} \frac{T_2}{T_1}$$

$$P_2 = (2 \text{ atm}) \left(\frac{0.1 \text{ L}}{0.5 \text{ L}} \right) \left(\frac{373 \text{ K}}{273 \text{ K}} \right)$$

$$P_2 = 0.55 \text{ atm}$$

P-V-T Gas Laws in Systems Where n Is Constant

As we saw in answering Question 2 above, the amount of gas often remains the same, and the n drops out (we make this assumption in the equations that follow). Our work can be simplified even further if the pressure, temperature, or volume is also held constant. (And remember: when working with the gas laws, *temperature* always means *absolute temperature* [that is, T in kelvins].)

- If the pressure is constant, $V/T = k$ (where k is a constant). Therefore, the volume is proportional to the temperature: $V \propto T$

This is known as **Charles's law**. If the pressure is to remain constant, then a gas will expand when heated and contract when cooled. If the temperature of the gas is increased, the molecules will move faster, hitting the walls of the container with more force; in order to keep the pressure the same, the frequency of the collisions would need to be reduced. This is accomplished by expanding the volume. With more available space, the molecules strike the walls less often in order to compensate for hitting them harder.

- If the temperature is constant, $PV = k$ (where k is a constant). Therefore, the pressure is inversely proportional to the volume: $P \propto 1/V$

This is known as **Boyle's law**. If the volume decreases, the molecules have less space to move around in. As a result, they'll collide with the walls of the container more often, and the pressure increases. On the other hand, if the volume of the container increases, the gas molecules have more available space and collide with the wall less often, resulting in a lower pressure.

- If the volume is constant, $P/T = k$ (where k is a constant). Therefore, the pressure is proportional to the temperature: $P \propto T$

If the temperature goes up, so does the pressure. This should make sense when you consider the origin of pressure. As the temperature increases, the molecules move faster. As a result, they strike the walls of the container surface more often and with greater speed.

Since each of the two-variable relationships reviewed above are equal to a constant as described, this means that the product or quotient will not change if we meet the specified assumptions (hold the other variables constant). This allows us to generate equations where we compare properties of a gas under two different conditions:

In a system with constant n:

At constant P: $\dfrac{V_1}{T_1} = \dfrac{V_2}{T_2}$

At constant T: $P_1V_1 = P_2V_2$

At constant V: $\dfrac{P_1}{T_1} = \dfrac{P_2}{T_2}$

If only n (which tells us the amount of gas) stays constant, we can combine Boyle's Law and Charles's Law to get the **combined gas law** (which we used to answer Question 2 above):

Combined Gas Law (constant n)

$$\frac{P_1V_1}{T_1} = \frac{P_2V_2}{T_2}$$

Example 8-3: Helium, at a pressure of 3 atm, occupies a 16 L container at a temperature of 30°C. What would be the volume of the gas if the pressure were increased to 5 atm and the temperature lowered to −20°C?

Solution: We use the combined gas law after remembering to convert the given temperatures to kelvin:

$$\frac{P_1V_1}{T_1} = \frac{P_2V_2}{T_2} \implies V_2 = V_1\frac{P_1\,T_2}{P_2\,T_1} = (16\text{ L})\left(\frac{3\text{ atm}}{5\text{ atm}}\right)\left(\frac{253\text{ K}}{303\text{ K}}\right) \approx (16\text{ L})\left(\frac{3}{5}\right)\left(\frac{250\text{ K}}{300\text{ K}}\right) = 8\text{ L}$$

All of these laws follow from the ideal gas law and can be derived easily from it. They tell us what happens when n and P are constant, when n and T are constant, when n and V are constant, and in the case of the combined gas law, when n alone is constant. But what about n when P, V, and T are constant? That law of gases was proposed by Avogadro:

- If two equal-volume containers hold gas at the same pressure and temperature, then they contain the same number of particles (regardless of the identity of the gas).

Avogadro's law can be restated more broadly as **$V/n = k$** (where k is a constant). We can also determine the **standard molar volume** of an ideal gas at STP, which is the volume that one mole of a gas—any *ideal* gas—would occupy at 0°C and 1 atm of pressure:

$$V = \frac{nRT}{P} = \frac{(1 \text{ mol})(0.0821 \frac{\text{L-atm}}{\text{K-mol}})(273 \text{ K})}{1 \text{ atm}} = 22.4 \text{ L}$$

To give you an idea of how much this is, 22.4 L is equal to the total volume of three basketballs.

Avogrado's law and the **standard molar volume** of a gas can be used to simplify some gas law problems. Consider the following questions:

3. Given the Haber process, $3 \text{ H}_2(g) + \text{N}_2(g) \rightarrow 2 \text{ NH}_3(g)$, if you start with 5 L of $\text{H}_2(g)$ and 4 L of $\text{N}_2(g)$ at STP, what will the volume of the three gases be when the reaction is complete?

We can answer this question by using the ideal gas law, or we can recognize that the only thing changing is n (the number of moles of each gas) and use the standard molar volume. If we further recognize that the standard molar volume is the same for all three gases, and it is this value that we'd use to convert each given volume into moles (and then vice versa), we can use the balanced equation to quickly determine the answer.

Since we need 3 L of H_2 for every 1 L of N_2, and we have 4 L of N_2 but only 5 L of H_2, H_2 will be the limiting reagent, and its volume will be zero at the end of the reaction. Since 1 L of N_2 is needed for every 3 L of H_2, we get

$$5 \text{ L of H}_2 \times \frac{1 \text{ L of N}_2}{3 \text{ L of H}_2} = 1.7 \text{ L of N}_2$$

So the amount of N_2 remaining will be $4 - 1.7 = 2.3$ L. The volume of NH_3 produced is

$$5 \text{ L of H}_2 \times \frac{2 \text{ L of NH}_3}{3 \text{ L of H}_2} = 3.3 \text{ L of NH}_3$$

Example 8-4: Three moles of oxygen gas are present in a 10 L chamber at a temperature of 25°C. Which one of the following expressions is equal to the pressure of the gas (in atm)?

A) (3)(0.08)(10) / 25
B) (3)(0.08)(25) / 10
C) (3)(0.08)(10) / 298
D) (3)(0.08)(298) / 10

Solution: Since 25°C = 298 K, the ideal gas law gives

$$P = \frac{nRT}{V} = \frac{(3)(0.08)(298)}{10} \text{ atm}$$

The answer is D.

Example 8-5: An ideal gas at 2 atm occupies a 5-liter tank. It is then transferred to a new tank of volume 12 liters. If temperature is held constant throughout, what is the new pressure?

Solution: Since n and T are constants, we can use Boyle's law to find

$$P_1V_1 = P_2V_2 \quad \Rightarrow \quad P_2 = P_1\frac{V_1}{V_2} = (2 \text{ atm})\frac{5 \text{ L}}{12 \text{ L}} = \frac{5}{6} \text{ atm}$$

Example 8-6: A 6-liter container holds $H_2(g)$ at a temperature of 400 K and a pressure of 3 atm. If the temperature is increased to 600 K, what will be the pressure?

Solution: Since n and V are constants, we can write

$$\frac{P_1}{T_1} = \frac{P_2}{T_2} \quad \Rightarrow \quad P_2 = P_1\frac{T_2}{T_1} = (3 \text{ atm})\frac{600 \text{ K}}{400 \text{ K}} = 4.5 \text{ atm}$$

Example 8-7: How many atoms of helium are present in 11.2 liters of the gas at $P = 1$ atm and $T = 273$ K?

A) 3.01×10^{23}
B) 6.02×10^{23}
C) 1.20×10^{24}
D) Cannot be determined from the information given

Solution: $P = 1$ atm and $T = 273$ K define STP, so 1 mole of an ideal gas would occupy 22.4 L. A volume of 11.2 L is exactly half this so it must correspond to a 0.5 mole sample. Since 1 mole of helium contains 6.02×10^{23} atoms, 0.5 mole contains half this many: 3.01×10^{23} (choice A).

8.3 DEVIATIONS FROM IDEAL-GAS BEHAVIOR

Let's review two of the assumptions that were listed for the kinetic-molecular theory:

1) The particles of an ideal gas experience no intermolecular forces.
2) The volume of the individual particles of an ideal gas is negligible compared to the volume of the gas container.

Under some conditions, namely high pressures and low temperatures, these assumptions don't hold up very well, and the laws for ideal gases don't rigorously apply to real gases.

To determine the effect of non-ideality on gases on a macroscopic level, work though the following thought experiments, which examine each assumption above independently:

1) *No intermolecular forces:*

Imagine blowing up a balloon to a given volume with an ideal gas. Now, fix the volume of the container and allow the gas to behave as a real gas with strongly attractive intermolecular forces (e.g., like water vapor would have). How will the pressure change? Remember that the number of collisions gas particles have with the container walls (and their momentum) determines pressure. While the particles in a real gas have attractive intermolecular forces, they do not have the same attractive forces with the walls. Increased particle interactions therefore lead to fewer collisions with the walls of the container, and the collisions that do occur will involve a smaller transfer of momentum than they would have if the gas were ideal and all collisions perfectly elastic. The resulting pressure of the real gas is therefore smaller than if the gas were ideal, or $P_{real} < P_{ideal}$.

2) *Volumeless particles:*

Imagine blowing up a balloon with an ideal gas somewhere half-way through the atmosphere of Jupiter (with its high pressures), then fix the pressure of the ideal gas system after it equilibrates with external pressure. Now, instead of the ideal volumeless particles, give the individual gas particles finite volumes. How does the volume of the gas change? The tricky part here is that the volume of a gas is defined as the free space the particles have in which to move around. For an ideal gas this volume is simply the volume of the container, since there is no volume taken up by individual particles. However, at high pressures the volume occupied by each gas particle becomes a greater proportion of the gas sample, so it is no longer negligible, and reduces the free space available for particle movement. The overall effect is to decrease the volume, making $V_{real} < V_{ideal}$.

From these two thought experiments we see that the attractive forces between particles cause a decrease in pressure if the volume of the container is fixed, and accounting for particle volume causes a decrease in free space (system volume) if the pressure is fixed. As these two variables interact with many others in a real system, we can sometimes see deviations from the general principles outlined here, especially at exceedingly high pressures.[1] However, complex situations like this are beyond the scope of the MCAT, so we will focus our analysis on the deviations as described above.

---

[1] For example, at pressures > 300 atm, gas particles are pushed so close together that they begin to repel one another, which can result in an increase in the volume of real gases over what would be predicted by the ideal gas law.

8.3

To make accurate predictions about the deviations real gases show from ideal-gas behavior, the ideal gas law must be altered. The **van der Waals equation** includes terms to account for the differences in the observed behavior of real gases and calculated properties of ideal gases, while maintaining the same form as the ideal gas law:

---

van der Waals Equation

$$\left(P + \frac{an^2}{V^2}\right)(V - nb) = nRT$$

The an^2/V^2 term serves as a correction for the intermolecular forces that generally result in lower pressures for real gases, while the nb term corrects for the physical volume that the individual particles occupy in a real gas. Both a and b are known as van der Waals constants and are generally larger for gases that experience greater intermolecular forces (a) and have larger molecular weights, and therefore volumes (b).

To illustrate the impact of intermolecular forces on real gas pressure, let's compare the pressures of two moles of oxygen and two moles of water, each in separate 5 L containers at a moderate temperature (500 K). Using the ideal gas law, we predict the following:

$$P_{\text{ideal}} = \frac{nRT}{V} = \frac{2\,\text{moles} \times 0.0821\dfrac{\text{L}\cdot\text{atm}}{\text{mol}\cdot\text{K}} \times 500\,\text{K}}{5\,\text{L}} = 16.4\,\text{atm}$$

To use the van der Waals equation to predict the actual pressures, we can rearrange and solve for P.

$$P = \left(\frac{nRT}{V - nb}\right) - \left(\frac{an^2}{V^2}\right)$$

Therefore for oxygen (where $a = 1.34\ \text{atm}\cdot\text{L}^2\cdot\text{mol}^{-2}$ and $b = 0.0318\ \text{L}\cdot\text{mol}^{-1}$):

$$P_{O_2} = \left(\frac{2\,\text{mol} \times 0.0821\dfrac{\text{L}\cdot\text{atm}}{\text{mol}\cdot\text{K}} \times 500\,\text{K}}{5\,\text{L} - 2\,\text{mol} \times 0.0318\,\text{L}\cdot\text{mol}^{-1}}\right) - \left(\frac{1.34\ \text{atm}\cdot\text{L}^2\cdot\text{mol}^{-2} \times (2\,\text{mol})^2}{(5\ \text{L})^2}\right)$$

$$= 16.6\ \text{atm} - 0.2\ \text{atm} = 16.4\ \text{atm}$$

Notice that the pressure, due to oxygen's lack of substantial intermolecular forces, is effectively the same as was predicted by the ideal gas law. If we select a gas with significantly stronger intermolecular forces, the deviation from ideal gas behavior becomes more pronounced. For instance, the van der Waals "a" constant for water is significantly higher than that of oxygen due to water's ability to hydrogen bond ($a = 5.47\ \text{atm}\cdot\text{L}^2\cdot\text{mole}^{-2}$ and $b = 0.0305\ \text{L}\cdot\text{mol}^{-1}$).

$$P_{H_2O} = \left(\frac{2\,\text{mol} \times 0.0821\dfrac{\text{L}\cdot\text{atm}}{\text{mol}\cdot\text{K}} \times 500\,\text{K}}{5\,\text{L} - 2\,\text{mol} \times 0.0305\,\text{L}\cdot\text{mol}^{-1}}\right) - \left(\frac{5.47\ \text{atm}\cdot\text{L}^2\cdot\text{mol}^{-2} \times (2\,\text{mol})^2}{(5\ \text{L})^2}\right)$$

$$= 16.6\ \text{atm} - 0.9\ \text{atm} = 15.7\ \text{atm}$$

This represents a 4% decrease in pressure from that predicted by the ideal gas law.

To underscore the concept that gases behave more ideally at higher temperatures, if we increase the temperature of the system for any gas, the first term in the van der Waals equation approaches the pressure of the ideal gas while the second term remains unchanged. For example, if the temperature of our systems above is increased by 100 K (to 600 K), two moles of an ideal gas would exert 19.7 atm of pressure, while the van der Waals equation predicts pressures of 19.7 atm and 19.1 atm for oxygen and water, respectively. Therefore, we can see that at increased temperature the real gas (H_2O) behaves more ideally since it now deviates by only 3% from the pressure predicted by the ideal gas law.

So conceptually, why do higher pressures and lower temperatures cause larger deviations from ideal behavior? As pressure increases, gas particles become closer to one another. This accentuates the effects of attractive intermolecular forces, causing a decrease in observed pressure ($P_{real} < P_{ideal}$). Similarly, at low temperatures intermolecular forces become more important, and when taken to an extreme, cause condensation to occur. Liquids aren't very ideal gases. In addition, when gas particles are packed closer to one another at high pressures, particle volume of the gas itself begins to limit the free space in which the gas particles can move ($V_{real} < V_{ideal}$). However under extremely high pressure, these particles can begin to repel one another leading to an increase in volume.

To summarize, those gases that behave most ideally have the weakest intermolecular forces and the smallest molecular weights (and volumes). Furthermore, by maintaining conditions of high temperature and low pressure, the potential interactions between particles are minimized and particle volume remains insignificant compared to the container size, helping to favor more ideal behavior for all gases.

Example 8-8: Of the following, which gas would likely *deviate* the most from ideal behavior at high pressure and low temperature?

A) $He(g)$
B) $H_2(g)$
C) $O_2(g)$
D) $H_2O(g)$

Solution: Since H_2O molecules will experience hydrogen bonding, they feel significantly stronger intermolecular forces than the other gases do. Therefore, of the choices given, $H_2O(g)$ will deviate the most from ideal behavior at high pressure and low temperature.

Example 8-9: Of the following, which gas would behave most like an ideal gas if all were at the same temperature and pressure?

A) $O_2(g)$
B) $CH_4(g)$
C) $Ar(g)$
D) $Cl_2(g)$

Solution: The molecules of a perfect (ideal) gas take up zero volume, so the gas in this list that will behave most like an ideal gas will be the one that takes up the smallest volume. O_2, CH_4, and Cl_2 are all polyatomic molecules that occupy more space than atomic argon. Therefore, choice C is the answer.

Example 8-10: Of the following, which gas would behave most like an ideal gas if all were at the same temperature and pressure?

A) $H_2O(g)$
B) $CH_4(g)$
C) $HF(g)$
D) $NH_3(g)$

Solution: The molecules of a perfect (ideal) gas experience no intermolecular forces, so the gas in this list that will behave most like an ideal gas will be the one that has the weakest intermolecular forces. H_2O, HF, and NH_3 experience hydrogen-bonding, while CH_4 experiences only weak dispersion forces. Therefore, choice B is the answer.

Example 8-11: Under which of the following conditions does the ideal gas law give the most accurate results for a real gas?

A) Low T and low P
B) Low T and high P
C) High T and low P
D) High T and high P

Solution: Real gases can never behave as true ideal gases because 1) their molecules occupy space, and 2) their molecules experience attractive intermolecular forces. However, when gas molecules are spread out, these violations are minimized. The physical conditions that allow for gases to spread out are high temperature and low pressure, choice C.

8.4 DALTON'S LAW OF PARTIAL PRESSURES

Consider a mixture of, say, three gases in a single container.

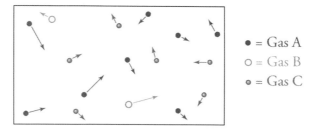

The total pressure is due to the collisions of all three types of molecules with the container walls. The pressure that the molecules of Gas A alone exert is called the **partial pressure** of Gas A, denoted by p_A. Similarly, the pressure exerted by the molecules of Gas B alone and the pressure exerted by the molecules of Gas C alone are p_B and p_C.

Dalton's law of partial pressures says that the total pressure is simply the sum of the partial pressures of all the constituent gases. In this case, then, we'd have

---

Dalton's Law

$$P_{tot} = p_A + p_B + p_C$$

So, if we know the partial pressures, we can determine the total pressure. We can also work backward. Knowing the total pressure, we can figure out the individual partial pressures. All that is required is the mole fraction. For example, in the diagram above, there are a total of 16 molecules: 8 of Gas A, 2 of Gas B, and 6 of Gas C. Therefore, the mole fraction of Gas A is $X_A = 8/16 = 1/2$, the mole fraction of Gas B is $X_B = 2/16 = 1/8$, and the mole fraction of Gas C is $X_C = 6/16 = 3/8$. *The partial pressure of a gas is equal to its mole fraction times the total pressure.* For example, if the total pressure in the container above is 8 atm, then

$$p_A = X_A P_{tot} = \frac{1}{2} P_{tot} = \frac{1}{2}(8 \text{ atm}) = 4 \text{ atm}$$

$$p_B = X_B P_{tot} = \frac{1}{8} P_{tot} = \frac{1}{8}(8 \text{ atm}) = 1 \text{ atm}$$

$$p_C = X_C P_{tot} = \frac{3}{8} P_{tot} = \frac{3}{8}(8 \text{ atm}) = 3 \text{ atm}$$

Example 8-12: A mixture of neon and nitrogen contains 0.5 mol Ne(g) and 2 mol N$_2$(g). If the total pressure is 20 atm, what is the partial pressure of the neon?

Solution: The mole fraction of Ne is

$$X_{Ne} = \frac{n_{Ne}}{n_{Ne} + n_{N_2}} = \frac{0.5}{(0.5+2)} = \frac{0.5}{2.5} = \frac{1}{5}$$

Therefore,

$$p_{Ne} = X_{Ne} P_{tot} = \frac{1}{5} P_{tot} = \frac{1}{5}(20 \text{ atm}) = 4 \text{ atm}$$

Example 8-13: A vessel contains a mixture of three gases: A, B, and C. There is twice as much A as B and half as much C as A. If the total pressure is 300 torr, what is the partial pressure of Gas C?

A)   60 torr
B)   75 torr
C)   100 torr
D)   120 torr

Solution: The question states that there is twice as much A as B, and it also says (backward) there is twice as much A as C. So the amounts of B and C are the same, and each is half the amount of A. Since this is a multiple choice question, instead of doing algebra we'll just plug in the choices and find the one that works. The only one that works is choice B, so that $p_A = 150$ torr, $p_B = 75$ torr, and $p_C = 75$ torr, for a total of 300 torr.

Example 8-14: If the ratio of the partial pressures of a pair of gases mixed together in a sealed vessel is 3:1 at 300 K, what would be the ratio of their partial pressures at 400 K?

- A) 3:1
- B) 4:1
- C) 4:3
- D) 12:1

Solution: Remember that the partial pressure of a gas is the way that we talk about the amount of gas in a mixture. The question states that the ratio of partial pressures of two gases is 3:1. That just means there's three times more of one than the other. Regardless of the temperature, if the vessel is sealed, then there will always be three times more of one than the other. Choice A is the correct answer.

8.5 GRAHAM'S LAW OF EFFUSION

The escape of a gas molecule through a very tiny hole (comparable in size to the molecules themselves) into an evacuated region is called **effusion**:

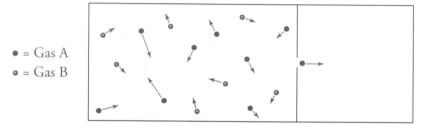

- ● = Gas A
- ○ = Gas B

The gases in the left-hand container are at the same temperature, so their average kinetic energies are the same. If Gas A and Gas B have different molar masses, the heavier molecules will move, on average, slower than the lighter ones will. We can be even more precise. The average kinetic energy of a molecule of Gas A is $\frac{1}{2}m_A(v_A^2)_{avg}$, and the average kinetic energy of a molecule of Gas B is $\frac{1}{2}m_B(v_B^2)_{avg}$. Setting these equal to each other, we get

$$\frac{1}{2}m_A(v_A^2)_{avg} = \frac{1}{2}m_B(v_B^2)_{avg} \quad \Rightarrow \quad \frac{(v_A^2)_{avg}}{(v_B^2)_{avg}} = \frac{m_B}{m_A} \quad \Rightarrow \quad \frac{\text{rms } v_A}{\text{rms } v_B} = \sqrt{\frac{m_B}{m_A}}$$

(The abbreviation **rms** stands for *root-mean-square*; it's the square root of the mean [average] of the square of speed. Therefore, rms v is a convenient measure of the average speed of the molecules.) For example, if Gas A is hydrogen gas (H_2, molecular weight = 2) and Gas B is oxygen gas (O_2, molecular weight = 32), the hydrogen molecules will move, on average,

$$\sqrt{\frac{m_B}{m_A}} = \sqrt{\frac{32}{2}} = \sqrt{16} = 4$$

times faster than the oxygen molecules.

This result—which follows from one of the assumptions of the kinetic-molecular theory (namely that the average kinetic energy of the molecules of a gas is proportional to the temperature)—can be confirmed experimentally by performing an effusion experiment. Which gas should escape faster? The rate at which a gas effuses should depend directly on how fast its molecules move; the faster they travel, the more often they'd "collide" with the hole and escape. So we'd expect that if we compared the effusion rates for Gases A and B, we'd get a ratio equal to the ratio of their average speeds (if the molecules of Gas A travel 4 times faster than those of Gas B, then Gas A should effuse 4 times faster). Since we just figured out that the ratio of their average speeds is equal to the reciprocal of the square root of the ratio of their masses, we'd expect the ratio of their effusion rates to be the same. This result is known as **Graham's law of effusion**:

8.5

Graham's Law of Effusion

$$\frac{\text{rate of effusion of Gas A}}{\text{rate of effusion of Gas B}} = \sqrt{\frac{\text{molar mass of Gas B}}{\text{molar mass of Gas A}}}$$

Let's emphasize the distinction between the relationships of temperature to the kinetic energy and to the speed of the gas. The molecules of two different gases at the same temperature have the same average kinetic energy. But the molecules of two different gases at the same temperature don't have the same average *speed*. Lighter molecules travel faster, because the kinetic energy depends on both the mass and the speed of the molecules.

Also, it's important to remember that not all the molecules of the gas in a container—even if there's only one type of molecule—travel at the same speed. Their speeds cover a wide range. What we *can* say is that as the temperature of the sample is increased, the *average* speed increases. In fact, since $KE \propto T$, the root-mean-square speed is proportional to $\sqrt{T}$. The figure below shows the distribution of molecular speeds for a gas at three different temperatures. Notice that the rms speeds increase as the temperature is increased.

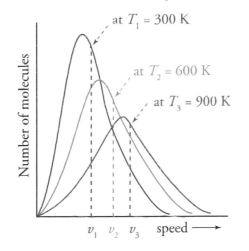

Example 8-15: A container holds methane (CH_4) and sulfur dioxide (SO_2), at a temperature of 227°C. Let v_M denote the rms speed of the methane molecules and v_S the rms speed of the sulfur dioxide molecules. Which of the following best describes the relationship between these speeds?

A) $v_S = 16\, v_M$
B) $v_S = 2\, v_M$
C) $v_M = 2\, v_S$
D) $v_M = 16\, v_S$

Solution: The molecular weight of methane is $12 + 4(1) = 16$, and the molecular weight of sulfur dioxide is $32 + 2(16) = 64$. Therefore

$$\frac{v_M}{v_S} = \sqrt{\frac{m_S}{m_M}} = \sqrt{\frac{64}{16}} = \sqrt{4} = 2 \quad \Rightarrow \quad v_M = 2v_S$$

So, choice C is the answer.

Example 8-16: In a laboratory experiment, Chamber A holds a mixture of four gases: 1 mole each of chlorine, fluorine, nitrogen, and carbon dioxide. A tiny hole is made in the side of the chamber, and the gases are allowed to effuse from Chamber A into an empty container. When 2 moles of gas have escaped, which gas will have the greatest mole fraction in Chamber A?

A) $Cl_2(g)$
B) $F_2(g)$
C) $N_2(g)$
D) $CO_2(g)$

Solution: The gas with the greatest mole fraction remaining in Chamber A will be the gas with the *slowest* rate of effusion. This is the gas with the highest molecular weight. Of the gases in the chamber, Cl_2 has the greatest molecular weight. Therefore, the answer is A.

Example 8-17: A balloon holds a mixture of fluorine, $F_2(g)$, and helium, $He(g)$. If the rms speed of helium atoms is 540 m/s, what is the rms speed of the fluorine molecules?

Solution: The molecular weight of F_2 is $2(19) = 38$, and the molecular weight of He is 4. Therefore,

$$\frac{v_{F_2}}{v_{He}} = \sqrt{\frac{m_{He}}{m_{F_2}}} = \sqrt{\frac{4}{38}} \approx \sqrt{\frac{1}{9}} = \frac{1}{3} \quad \Rightarrow \quad v_{F_2} \approx \frac{1}{3}v_{He} = \frac{1}{3}(540\tfrac{m}{s}) = 180\tfrac{m}{s}$$

Example 8-18: A container holds methane (CH_4) and sulfur dioxide (SO_2) at a temperature of 227°C. Let KE_M denote the average kinetic energy of the methane molecules and KE_S the average kinetic energy of the sulfur dioxide molecules. Which of the following best describes the relationship between these energies?

A) $KE_S = 4\, KE_M$
B) $KE_S = 3\, KE_M$
C) $KE_M = KE_S$
D) $KE_M = 4\, KE_S$

Solution: Since both gases are at the same temperature, the average kinetic energies of their molecules will be the *same* (remember: $KE_{avg} \propto T$). Thus, the answer is C.

Example 8-19: The temperature of neon gas in a glass tube is increased from 10°C to 160°C. As a result, the average kinetic energy of the neon atoms will increase by a factor of:

A) less than 2.
B) 2.
C) 4.
D) 16.

8.5

Solution: We use the fact that $KE_{avg} \propto T$. However, don't fall for the trap of thinking that the temperature has increased by a factor of 16. Calculations involving the gas laws (and that includes the proportionality between KE_{avg} and T from kinetic-molecular theory) must be done with temperatures expressed in *kelvins*. The temperature here increased from 283 K to 433 K, which is less than a factor of 2 increase. Therefore, KE_{avg} will also increase by a factor of less than 2 (choice A).

- The pressure of a gas is due to the collisions gas particles have with the container walls.

- The ideal gas law states that $PV = nRT$.

- Standard temperature and pressure (STP) conditions are at 1 atm and 273 K. Under these conditions, 1 mol of any gas will occupy 22.4 L of space.

- Particles of an ideal gas take up no volume and experience no intermolecular forces. They also have elastic collisions with each other and the walls of their container.

- Real gases approach ideal behavior under most conditions, but deviate most from ideal behavior under conditions of high pressure and low temperature.

- Real gases can be quantified using the van der Waals equation:

$$\left(P + \frac{an^2}{V^2} \right)(V - nb) = nRT$$

- Dalton's law of partial pressures states that the total pressure inside a container is equal to the sum of the partial pressures of each constituent gas. The partial pressure of a gas divided by the total pressure of all gases is equal to its mole fraction within the gaseous mixture.

- Temperature is a measure of the average kinetic energy of molecules within a sample.

- Graham's law of effusion states that the rate of effusion of a gas is inversely proportional to its molecular weight. In other words, lighter gases effuse more quickly than heavier gases.

CHAPTER 8 FREESTANDING PRACTICE QUESTIONS

1. A sample of nitrogen gas is heated in a sealed, rigid container. The pressure inside the container increases because the added energy causes:

A) some of the nitrogen molecules to split, so more particles contribute to increase the pressure.
B) the molecules of gas to move faster, increasing the frequency of intermolecular collisions.
C) the molecules of gas to move faster, increasing the frequency of collisions with the container.
D) the molecules of gas to stick together in clusters that have a greater momentum.

2. Two identical balloons are filled with different gases at STP. Balloon A contains 0.25 moles of neon, and balloon B contains 0.25 moles of oxygen. Which of the following properties would be greater for balloon B?

A) Density
B) Volume
C) Number of particles
D) Average kinetic energy

3. The figure below depicts the relative sizes and mole fractions of two monatomic gases in a closed container.

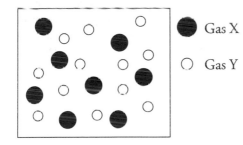

Gas X
Gas Y

Which of the following is true about the gas mixture after a small hole is punched in the container and the gases are allowed to completely effuse?

A) The partial pressure of Gas X will never equal the partial pressure of Gas Y.
B) The partial pressure of Gas Y will decrease faster than the partial pressure of Gas X.
C) The partial pressure of Gas Y will increase because the mole fraction of Gas Y will increase.
D) The partial pressures of each gas will remain unchanged.

4. There are an unknown number of moles of argon in a steel container. A chemist injects two moles of nitrogen into the container. The temperature and volume do not change, but the pressure increases by ten percent. Originally the container held:

A) 16 moles of Ar.
B) 18 moles of Ar.
C) 20 moles of Ar.
D) 22 moles of Ar.

5. Which of the following compounds can best approximate ideal gas behavior?

A) $CH_4(g)$
B) $NH_3(g)$
C) $H_2O(g)$
D) $HF(g)$

6. Which of the following is true for a closed flask containing both 1 mole of ideal Gas X and 1 mole of real Gas Y?

A) The total energy of X is equal to the total energy of Y.
B) The average kinetic energy of X is equal to the average kinetic energy of Y.
C) The total volume available to the gases is the same as the total volume of the flask.
D) Gases X and Y are at different temperatures.

7. Given the following combustion reaction, calculate the mole fraction of hydrocarbon in the reactant solution before combustion. Assume neither starting material is limiting.

$$ZC_xH_y(g) + 8\ O_2(g) \rightarrow 5\ CO_2(g) + 6\ H_2O(l)$$

A) 1/8
B) 1/9
C) 2/9
D) 1/3

CHAPTER 8 PRACTICE PASSAGE

The earth's atmosphere has several layers of gases with different characteristics and temperatures. The atmosphere has a total mass of 5×10^{18} kg, and is composed mainly of nitrogen, oxygen, argon, and carbon dioxide, as well as water vapor to a variable degree. Seventy-five percent of this mass is within 11 km from the earth's surface. Although the limit between outer space and the atmosphere is not definite, the *Kármán Line*, approximately 100 km above sea level, is often taken as the boundary.

Table 1 Composition of atmosphere (dry)

Gas	% of Dry Air
Nitrogen	78.1
Oxygen	20.9
Argon	0.93
Carbon dioxide	0.038

The five main layers of atmosphere are the exosphere, thermosphere, mesosphere, stratosphere, and troposphere. The troposphere is the innermost layer, and extends to approximately 6 km above the earth's surface at the poles and approximately 20 km above sea level at the equator. The next layer is the stratosphere. The ozone layer, which is considered to be a layer of its own because of its unique composition, is within the stratosphere. Approximately 90 percent of the O_3 in the atmosphere is found in the ozone layer, although the actual concentrations are quite low (2–8 ppm). This layer is very important as it absorbs much of the ultraviolet (UV) light emitted from the sun. The mesosphere is the middle layer of the atmosphere with a temperature of approximately 100°C. The thermosphere and exosphere in that order are the outermost layers.

The pressure, density, and temperature of the atmosphere vary with altitude. Both pressure and density decrease with increasing altitude. At sea level, the density of air is 1.2 kg/m^3 and drops by approximately 50 percent every 5.5 km.

The atmosphere contains greenhouse gases, which absorb and emit thermal infrared radiation, leading to the greenhouse effect. Greenhouse gases include water vapor, methane, nitrous oxide, carbon dioxide, and ozone. These gases are needed to maintain the temperature of the earth, which would otherwise be much colder. However, it is thought that an increase in the amount of greenhouse gases in the atmosphere has contributed to the increase in average temperature in the twentieth century. Methane is a very potent greenhouse gas. It can be oxidized in the atmosphere to produce carbon dioxide and water, with a half-life of 7 years.

1. How long would it take for a 1 L sample of methane to decrease to 1 percent of its original amount from atmospheric oxidation?

A) 38 years
B) 42 years
C) 47 years
D) 50 years

2. What is the partial pressure of nitrogen gas in the atmosphere at sea level?

A) 7.91×10^1 Pa
B) 5.96×10^2 Pa
C) 7.91×10^4 Pa
D) 5.96×10^5 Pa

3. The summit of Mount Everest is 8.8 km above sea level. What is the approximate density of air at this point?

A) 0.2 kg/m^3
B) 0.4 kg/m^3
C) 0.8 kg/m^3
D) 1.0 kg/m^3

4. A sample of gas containing oxygen, nitrogen, argon, and carbon dioxide in equal molar proportions is in a closed container. Which of these gases would escape the fastest if a small hole were punctured in the container?

A) Nitrogen
B) Oxygen
C) Argon
D) Carbon dioxide

5. All of the following are true regarding the earth's atmosphere EXCEPT:

A) the boundary between the atmosphere and outer space is indistinct.
B) the ozone layer is primarily composed of ozone gas.
C) more than 3.75×10^{18} kg of atmospheric gases is contained within an 11 km distance from the earth's surface.
D) water vapor contributes to warmer atmospheric temperatures.

6. If a 20 L sample of gas at STP were cooled to mesosphere temperatures at a constant volume, what would the new pressure be?

A) 64 kPa
B) 84 kPa
C) 96 kPa
D) 128 kPa

SOLUTIONS TO CHAPTER 8 FREESTANDING PRACTICE QUESTIONS

1. **C** According to kinetic molecular theory, pressure is defined by the frequency of collisions between gas particles and the walls of their container. While increasing the temperature of the gas will cause more collisions between particles as well, these collisions do not define pressure (eliminate choice B). In addition, collisions between particles are elastic, so unless the particles are highly polar and have a strong attraction for each other (the gas is behaving non-ideally), they will not stick together. Since N_2 is non-polar it should behave ideally, so choice D can be eliminated. Finally, nitrogen is a very stable diatomic element, and heating a sample of nitrogen is not likely to break the strong triple bond between nitrogen atoms, eliminating choice A.

2. **A** Since both balloons contain the same number of moles of gas under identical pressure and temperature conditions (STP), they should have the same volume (in this case 5.6 L since 1 mol = 22.4 L). Eliminate choice B. An identical amount of each gas is added to each balloon, so they should also contain the same number of gas particles (0.25 mol × 6.02 × 10^{23} particles/mol), eliminating choice C. Since the gases are at the same temperature they will have the same average kinetic energy, so by process of elimination, A must be the correct answer. Density is mass/volume. Since the two gases have the same volume, oxygen, with a larger molar mass (O_2 = 32 g/mol vs. Ne = 20 g/mol), will have the greater density.

3. **B** After a hole is punched in the container and the gases begin to escape, the total pressure of the container will decrease, and the individual partial pressures of the gases will therefore also decrease. Eliminate choices C and D. According to Graham's law, the lighter the gas molecule, the faster its rate of effusion through a small hole. Gas Y will effuse faster than Gas X, so its partial pressure will decrease at a faster rate. The gases are allowed to completely effuse and the figure indicates that the mole fraction of Y is slightly larger than X. Therefore there will most likely be a moment in time when the partial pressures of both gases are equal (and this will definitely be the case when the container is finally empty), eliminating choice A.

4. **C** At constant V and T, the pressure of an ideal gas reflects the number of particles (regardless of their identity). It is a simplification of the ideal gas law from $PV = nRT$ to $P \propto n$. So, if the addition of two moles of N_2 into the chamber results in an increase in P of 10 percent, then the moles added must be 10 percent of the initial number of Ar moles. Two moles are 10 percent of 20 moles.

5. **A** Ideal gas behavior requires two assumptions of kinetic molecular theory. The gas is assumed to have infinitesimal molecular size and no intermolecular forces. All of the answer choices have molecules of approximately the same, small size. However, methane experiences only London dispersion forces while the other three molecules experience hydrogen bonding. This H-bonding causes the remaining answer choices to deviate significantly from ideal gas behavior.

6. **B**   Temperature is a measure of average kinetic energy. If gases X and Y are in the same flask they must be at the same temperature, eliminating choice D and making choice B correct. The total energy of a gas is equal to its kinetic energy plus its potential energy. Since Gas Y is a real gas and experiences intermolecular forces, it has potential energy, whereas ideal Gas X does not. Therefore, choice A is eliminated. Real gas molecules occupy some volume in the container, whereas ideal gases have no molecular volume. Since the flask contains a real gas, the total volume available to the gases is slightly less than the total volume of the flask, eliminating choice C.

7. **B**   First, balance the equation:

$$C_5H_{12}(g) + 8\ O_2(g) \rightarrow 5\ CO_2(g) + 6\ H_2O(l)$$

The hydrocarbon must be C_5H_{12} and the coefficient Z is 1. Since the question indicates that neither reactant is limiting, there must be a 1:8 molar ratio of hydrocarbon to oxygen present in the reaction flask, so the mole fraction (X) of hydrocarbon in the reactant solution before combustion is calculated by:

$$X = (\text{moles hydrocarbon})/(\text{total moles})$$

$$X = 1/(1+8) = 1/9$$

SOLUTIONS TO CHAPTER 8 PRACTICE PASSAGE

1. **C**   The passage states that the half-life of methane is 7 years. Starting with 100 percent and dividing by 2 for each half-life, six half-lives would leave 1.5 percent of the methane remaining, and seven half-lives would leave 0.8 percent of the methane remaining. Therefore, it would require 42 to 49 years, making answer choice C the correct answer.

2. **C**   The pressure at sea level is 1 atm ≈ 100 kPa = 1×10^5 Pa. According to Table 1, nitrogen comprises approximately 80 percent of atmospheric air, thus the partial pressure of nitrogen at sea level is approximately $(0.8)(1 \times 10^5\ \text{Pa}) = 8 \times 10^4$ Pa.

3. **B**   The passage states that the density of air is 1.2 kg/m³ and that the density drops by 50 percent every 5.5 km. Therefore, at 8.8 km, the density will be between 25 to 50 percent of the density at sea level, or 0.3–0.6 kg/m³. Choice B is the only answer in this range.

4. **A**   Since rate of effusion is inversely proportional to the square root of mass, the gas with the smallest mass will have the highest rate of effusion. Thus, N_2 (28 g/mol) will escape fastest.

5.   B   The passage states that the limit between outer space and the atmosphere is not definite, so choice A is a true statement. The passage also states that the mass of the atmosphere is 5×10^{18} kg, and 75 percent of this (3.75×10^{18} kg) is 11 km from the surface of the earth. Therefore, choice C is also a true statement. Water vapor was listed as a greenhouse gas in the last paragraph, thus choice D is a true statement. Although the majority of ozone is located in the ozone layer, the passage states that concentrations of ozone are 2–8 ppm. To be the primary component, concentrations would have to exceed 500,000 ppm. Choice B is a false statement and therefore the correct answer.

6.   A   STP is 1 atm $\approx$ 100 kPa and 0°C = 273 K. Solve for the new pressure at the mesosphere temperature given in the passage (–100°C = 173 K) using the combined gas law (since volume is constant, V drops out of the equation):

$$\frac{P_1}{T_1} = \frac{P_2}{T_2}$$

$$P_2 = \frac{T_2 P_1}{T_1} = \frac{(173\,\text{K})(100\,\text{kPa})}{(273\,\text{K})} = (0.6)(100) = 60\,\text{kPa}$$

Note that pressure must decrease at decreased temperature, eliminating choice D.

Chapter 9
Kinetics

9.1 REACTION MECHANISM: AN ANALOGY

Chemical **kinetics** is the study of how reactions take place and how fast they occur. (Kinetics tells us nothing about the *spontaneity* of a reaction, however! We'll study that a little later.)

Consider this scenario: A group of people are washing a pile of dirty dishes and stacking them up as clean, dry dishes. Our "reaction" has dirty dishes as starting material, and clean, dry dishes as the product:

$$\text{dirty dish} \rightarrow \text{clean-and-dry dish}$$

But what about a *soapy* dish? We know it's part of the process, but the equation doesn't include it. When we break down the pathway of a dirty dish to a clean-and-dry dish, we realize that the reaction happens in several steps, a sequence of **elementary** steps that show us the reaction **mechanism**:

1) dirty dish $\rightarrow$ soapy dish
2) soapy dish $\rightarrow$ rinsed dish
3) rinsed dish $\rightarrow$ clean-and-dry dish

The soapy and rinsed dishes are reaction **intermediates**. They are necessary for the conversion of dirty dishes to clean-and-dry dishes, but don't appear either in the starting material or products. If you add up all the reactants and products, the intermediates cancel out, and you'll have the overall equation.

In the same way, we write chemical reactions as if they occur in a single step:

$$2\,NO + O_2 \rightarrow 2\,NO_2$$

But in reality, things are a little more complicated, and reactions often proceed through intermediates that we don't show in the chemical equation. The truth for the reaction above is that it occurs in two steps:

1) $2\,NO \rightarrow N_2O_2$
2) $N_2O_2 + O_2 \rightarrow 2\,NO_2$

The N_2O_2 comes and goes during the reaction, but isn't part of the starting material or products. N_2O_2 is a reaction intermediate.

Just as the soapy dishes and rinsed dishes are produced and then consumed, we can identify an **intermediate** in a series of elementary steps as a substance that is produced in one elementary step and then consumed in a subsequent step. Although the two elementary steps don't need to be sequential, they often are. As above, note that intermediates will not be part of the overall balanced chemical reaction. Depending on the rate of the elementary step that consumes the intermediate, the concentration of the intermediate will vary in solution. As the consuming elementary step becomes faster, the steady-state concentration of the intermediate becomes smaller, and it becomes harder to detect the intermediate.

Rate-Determining Step

What determines the rate of a reaction? Consider our friends doing the dishes.

1) dirty dish → soapy dish   Bingo washes at 5 dishes per minute.

2) soapy dish → rinsed dish   Ringo rinses at 8 dishes per minute.

3) rinsed dish → clean-and-dry dish   Dingo dries at 3 dishes per minute.

What will be the rate of the overall reaction? Thanks to Dingo, the dishes move from dirty to clean-and-dry at only 3 dishes a minute. It doesn't matter how fast Bingo and Ringo wash and rinse; the dishes will pile up behind Dingo. The **rate-determining step** is Dingo's drying step, and true to its name, it determines the overall rate of reaction.

The slowest step in a process determines the overall reaction rate.

This applies to chemical reactions as well. For our chemical reaction given above, we have

$$2\ NO \rightarrow N_2O_2 \quad \text{(fast)}$$

$$N_2O_2 + O_2 \rightarrow 2\ NO_2 \quad \text{(slow)}$$

The second step is the slowest, and it will determine the overall rate of reaction. No matter how fast the first step moves along, the intermediates will pile up in front of the second step as it plods along. The slow step dictates the rate of the overall reaction.

Once again, there's an important difference between our dishes analogy and a chemical reaction: While the dishes pile up behind Dingo, in a chemical reaction the intermediates will not pile up. Rather they will shuttle back and forth between reactants and products until the slow step takes it forward. This would be like taking a rinsed dish and getting it soapy again, until Dingo is ready for it!

Example 9-1: Which of the following is the best example of a rate?

A)   rate = $\Delta[A]/\Delta t$
B)   rate = $\Delta[A]/\Delta[B]$
C)   rate = $\Delta[A]\ \Delta[B]$
D)   rate = $\Delta[A]^2$

Solution: Regardless of the topic, rate is always defined as change in something over change in time. Choice A is the answer.

9.2 REACTION RATE

The **rate** of a reaction indicates how fast reactants are being consumed or how fast products are being formed. The reaction rate depends on several factors. Since the reactant molecules must collide and interact in order for old bonds to be broken and new ones to be formed to generate the product molecules, anything that affects these collisions and interactions will affect the reaction rate. The reaction rate is determined by the following:

1) How frequently the reactant molecules collide
2) The orientation of the colliding molecules
3) Their energy

Activation Energy

Every chemical reaction has an **activation energy** (E_a), or the minimum energy required of reactant molecules during a molecular collision in order for the reaction to proceed to products. If the reactant molecules don't possess this much energy, their collisions won't be able to produce the products and the reaction will not occur. If the reactants possess the necessary activation energy, they can reach a high-energy (and short-lived!) **transition state**, also known as the **activated complex**. For example, if the reaction is $A_2 + B_2 \rightarrow 2\,AB$, say, the activated complex might look something like this:

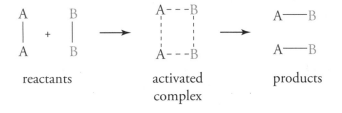

Now that we have introduced all species that might appear throughout the course of a chemical reaction, we can illustrate the energy changes that occur as a reaction occurs in a **reaction coordinate diagram**. Consider the following two-step process and its reaction coordinate graph below:

Step 1: A → X
Step 2: X → B
—————————————————
Overall reaction: A → B

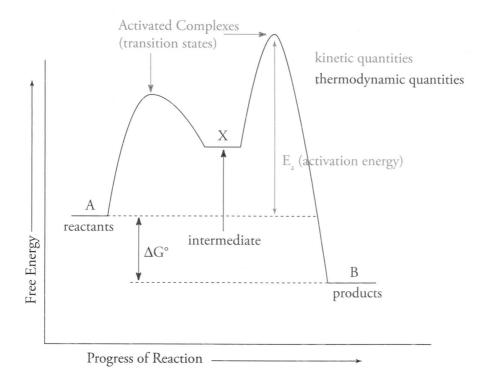

Notice that the transition state is always an energy maximum, and is therefore distinct from an intermediate. Remember that reaction intermediates (shown as X in this case) are produced in an early step of the mechanism, and are later used up so they do not appear as products of the overall reaction. The intermediate is shown here as a local minimum in terms of its energy, but has more energy than either the reactants or products. The high energy intermediate is therefore highly reactive, making it difficult to isolate.

Since the progress of the reaction depends on the reactant molecules colliding with enough energy to generate the activated complex, we can make the following statements concerning the reaction rate:

1) *The lower the activation energy, the faster the reaction rate.* The reaction coordinate above suggests that the second step of the mechanism will therefore be the slow step, or the rate-determining step, since the second "hill" of the diagram is higher.

2) *The greater the concentrations of the reactants, the faster the reaction rate.* Favorable collisions are more likely as the concentrations of reactant molecules increase.

3) *The higher the temperature of the reaction mixture, the faster the reaction rate.* At higher temperatures, more reactant molecules have a sufficient energy to overcome the activation-energy barrier, and molecules collide at a higher frequency, so the reaction can proceed at a faster rate.

Notice in the reaction coordinate diagram above that the $\Delta G°$ of the reaction has no bearing on the rate of the reaction, and vice versa. Thermodynamic factors and kinetic factors *do not affect each other* (a concept the MCAT loves to ask about).

9.3 CATALYSTS

Catalysts provide reactants with a different route, usually a shortcut, to get to products. A **catalyst** will almost always make a reaction go faster by either speeding up the rate-determining step or providing an optimized route to products. A catalyst that accelerates a reaction does so *by lowering the activation energy* of the rate-determining step, and therefore the energy of the highest-energy transition state:

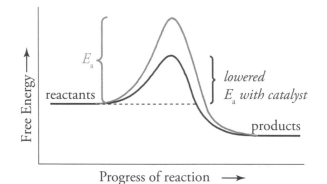

The key difference between a reactant and a catalyst is that the reactants are converted to products, but *a catalyst remains unchanged at the end of a reaction.* A catalyst can undergo a temporary change during a reaction, but it is always converted back to its original state. Like reaction intermediates, catalysts aren't included in the overall reaction equation.

Our dish crew could use a catalyst. Picture Dingo walking to pick up each wet dish, drying it on both sides, and walking back to place it in the clean dish stack. Now imagine a helper, Daisy, who takes the wet dish from Ringo, then walks it over to Dingo, and while he dries and stacks, she returns with another wet dish. This way, Dingo can dry 5 dishes a minute instead of 3, and the overall dish-cleaning rate increases to 5 dishes a minute. Daisy is the catalyst, but the chain of events in the overall reaction remains the same.

In the same way, chemical reactions can be catalyzed. Consider the decomposition of ozone:

$$O_3(g) + O(g) \rightarrow 2\ O_2(g)$$

This reaction actually takes place in two steps and is catalyzed by nitric oxide (NO):

1) $NO(g) + O_3(g) \rightarrow NO_2(g) + O_2(g)$
2) $NO_2(g) + O(g) \rightarrow NO(g) + O_2(g)$

$NO(g)$ is necessary for this reaction to proceed at a noticeable rate, and even undergoes changes itself during the process. But $NO(g)$ remains unchanged at the end of the reaction and makes the reaction occur much faster than it would in its absence. $NO(g)$, a product of automobile exhaust, is a catalyst in ozone destruction.

It is important to note that the addition of a catalyst will affect the rate of a reaction, but not the equilibrium or the thermodynamics of the reaction. A catalyst provides a different pathway for the reactants to get to the products, and lowers the activation energy, E_a. But a catalyst does not change any of the thermodynamic quantities such as ΔG, ΔH, and ΔS of a reaction.

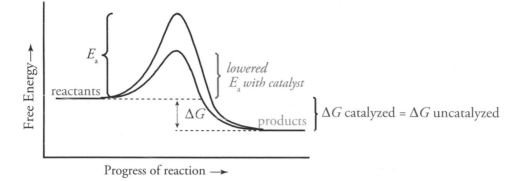

Example 9-2: Which of the following statements is true?

A) Catalysts decrease the activation energy of the forward reaction only.
B) Catalysts decrease the activation energy of the reverse reaction only.
C) Catalysts decrease the activation energy of both the forward and reverse reactions.
D) Catalysts decrease the activation energy of the forward reaction and increase the activation energy of the reverse reaction.

Solution: Catalysts decrease the activation energy of the forward reaction and reverse reaction—that's why they have no net effect on a system that's already at equilibrium. Choice C is the correct choice.

Example 9-3: Which of the following is true about the hypothetical two-step reaction shown below?

1) $A + 2B \rightarrow C + 2D$ (fast)
2) $C \rightarrow A + E$ (slow)

A) A is a catalyst, and C is an intermediate.
B) A is a catalyst, and D is an intermediate.
C) B is a catalyst, and A is an intermediate.
D) B is a catalyst, and C is an intermediate.

Solution: C is an intermediate; it's formed in one step and consumed in the other. This eliminates choices B and C. Now, is A or B the catalyst? Notice that B is consumed but not reformed; therefore, it cannot be the catalyst. The answer is A.

Example 9-4: A reaction is run without a catalyst and is found to have an activation energy of 140 kJ/mol and a heat of reaction, ΔH, of 30 kJ/mol. In the presence of a catalyst, however, the activation energy is reduced to 120 kJ/mol. What will be the heat of reaction in the presence of the catalyst?

A) –10 kJ/mol
B) 10 kJ/mol
C) 30 kJ/mol
D) 50 kJ/mol

Solution: Catalysts affect only the kinetics of a reaction, not the thermodynamics. The heat of the reaction will be the same with or without a catalyst. The answer is C.

9.4 RATE LAWS

On the MCAT, you might be given data about the rate of a particular reaction and be asked to derive the **rate law**. The data for rate laws are determined by the *initial rates* of reaction and typically are given as the **rate at which the reactant disappears**. You'll rarely see products in a rate law expression, usually only reactants. What does a rate law tell us? Although a reaction needs all the reactants to proceed, *only those that are involved in the rate-determining step (the slow step) are part of the rate law expression*. Some reactants may not affect the reaction rate at all, and so they won't be a part of the rate law expression.

Let's look at a generic reaction, $a\,A + b\,B \rightarrow c\,C + d\,D$, and its rate law:

$$\text{rate} = k\,[A]^x[B]^y$$

where

$$x = \text{the } \textbf{order} \text{ of the reaction with respect to A}$$

$$y = \text{the } \textbf{order} \text{ of the reaction with respect to B}$$

$$(x + y) = \text{the } \textbf{overall order} \text{ of the reaction}$$

$$k = \text{the rate constant}$$

The rate law can only be determined *experimentally*. You *can't* get the orders of the reactants, not to mention the rate constant k, just by looking at the balanced equation. The exception to this rule is for an *elementary step* in a reaction mechanism. The rate law is first order for a unimolecular elementary step and second order for a bimolecular elementary step. The individual order of the reactants in a rate law will follow from their stoichiometry in the rate-determining step (similar to the way they're included in an equilibrium constant).

Let's look at a set of reaction rate data and see how to determine the rate law for the reaction

$$A + B + C \rightarrow D + E$$

Experiment	[A]	[B]	[C]	Initial reaction rate [M/s]
1	0.2 *M*	0.1 *M*	0.05 *M*	1×10^{-3}
2	0.4 *M*	0.1 *M*	0.05 *M*	2×10^{-3}
3	0.2 *M*	0.2 *M*	0.05 *M*	4×10^{-3}
4	0.2 *M*	0.1 *M*	0.10 *M*	1×10^{-3}

From the experimental data, we can determine the orders with respect to the reactants—that is, the exponents x, y, and z in the equation

$$\text{rate} = k[A]^x[B]^y[C]^z$$

and the overall order of the reaction, $x + y + z$.

Let's first find the order of the reaction with respect to Reactant A. As we go from Experiment 1 to Experiment 2, only [A] changes, so we can use the data to figure out the order of the reaction with respect to Reactant [A]. We notice that the value of [A] doubled, and the reaction rate doubled. Therefore, the reaction rate is proportional to [A], and $x = 1$.

Next, let's look at [B]. As we go from Experiment 1 to Experiment 3, only [B] changes. When [B] is doubled, the rate is quadrupled. Therefore, the rate is proportional to $[B]^2$, and $y = 2$.

Finally, let's look at [C]. As we go from Experiment 1 to Experiment 4, only [C] changes. When [C] is doubled, the rate is unaffected. This tells us that the reaction rate does not depend on [C], so $z = 0$.

Therefore, the rate law has the form

$$\text{rate} = k[A][B]^2$$

The reaction is first order with respect to [A], second order with respect to [B], zero order with respect to [C], and third order overall. In general, if a reaction rate increases by a factor f when the concentration of a reactant increases by a factor c, and $f = c^x$, then we can say that x is the order with respect to that reactant.

The Rate Constant

From the experimental data, you can also calculate the rate constant, k. For the reaction we looked at above, we found that the rate law is given by: $\text{rate} = k[A][B]^2$. Solving this for k, we get

$$k = \frac{\text{rate}}{[A][B]^2}$$

Now, just pick any experiment in the table, and using the results of Experiment 1, you'd find that

$$k = \frac{\text{rate}}{[A][B]^2} = \frac{1 \times 10^{-3}}{(0.2)(0.1)^2} = 0.5$$

Any of the experiments will give you the same value for k because it's a constant for any given reaction at a given temperature. That is, each reaction has its own rate constant, which takes into account such factors as the frequency of collisions, the fraction of the collisions with the proper orientation to initiate the desired bond changes, and the activation energy. This can be expressed mathematically with the **Arrhenius equation**:

$$k = Ae^{-(E_a/RT)}$$

Here, A is the Arrhenius factor (which takes into account the orientation of the colliding molecules), E_a is the activation energy, R is the gas-law constant, and T is the temperature in kelvins. If we rewrite this equation in the form $\ln k = \ln A - (E_a/RT)$, we can more clearly see that *adding a catalyst* (thus decreasing

E_a) or *increasing the temperature* will increase k. In either case, the expression E_a/RT decreases, and subtracting something smaller gives a greater result, so $\ln k$ (and thus k itself) will increase. (By the way, a rough rule of thumb is that the rate will increase by a factor of about 2 to 4 for every 10-degree (Celsius) increase in temperature.)

The units of the rate constant are not necessarily uniform from one reaction to the next. Reactions of different orders will have rate constants bearing different units. In order to obtain the units of the rate constant one must keep in mind that the rate, on the left side of the equation, must always have units of M/s as it measures the change in concentration of a species in the reaction over time. The units given to the rate constant must, when combined with the units of the concentrations in the rate equation, provide M/sec.

Below is a generic second order rate equation.

$$\text{Rate} = k[A][B]$$

Assuming that the concentrations of both A and B are in molarity (M), then in order to give the left side of the equation units of M/s, the units of the rate constant must be $M^{-1}s^{-1}$. If the rate were third order, the units would be $M^{-2}s^{-1}$, or if first order then simply s^{-1}.

Experiment	[A]	[B]	Initial reaction rate [M/s]
1	0.01 M	0.01 M	4.0×10^{-3}
2	0.01 M	0.02 M	8.0×10^{-3}
3	0.02 M	0.02 M	1.6×10^{-2}
4	0.04 M	0.02 M	3.2×10^{-2}

Example 9-5: Based on the data given above, determine the rate law for the reaction $A + B \rightarrow C$.

A) Rate = $k[B]$
B) Rate = $k[A][B]$
C) Rate = $k[A]^2[B]$
D) Rate = $k[A][B]^2$

Solution: Comparing Experiments 1 and 2, we notice that when [B] doubled (and [A] remained unchanged), the reaction rate doubled. Therefore, the reaction is first order with respect to [B]; this eliminates choice D. Now, comparing Experiments 3 and 4, we notice that when [A] doubled (and [B] remained unchanged), the reaction rate also doubled. This means that the reaction is first order with respect to [A] as well. Therefore, the answer is B.

Example 9-6: Which of the following gives the form of the rate law for the balanced reaction

$$4 A + 2 B \rightarrow C + 3 D?$$

A) Rate = $k[A]^4[B]^2$
B) Rate = $k[A]^2[B]$
C) Rate = $k[C][D]^3/[A]^4[B]^2$
D) Cannot be determined from the information given

Solution: Unless the given reaction is the rate-determining, elementary step, we have no way of knowing what the rate law is. The answer is D.

Experiment	[A]	[B]	Initial reaction rate [M/s]
1	0.1 M	0.2 M	2.0×10^{-5}
2	0.2 M	0.3 M	1.2×10^{-4}
3	0.1 M	0.4 M	4.0×10^{-5}
4	0.2 M	0.4 M	1.6×10^{-4}

Example 9-7: Using the data given above, determine the numerical value of the rate constant for the reaction A + B → C.

Solution: First, let's find the rate law. Comparing Experiments 3 and 4, we notice that when [A] doubled (and [B] remained unchanged), the reaction rate increased by a factor of 4. This means the reaction is second order with respect to [A]. Comparing Experiments 1 and 3, we notice that when [B] doubled (and [A] remained unchanged), the reaction rate increased by a factor of 2. This means the reaction is first order with respect to [B]. Therefore, the rate law is *rate* = $k[A]^2[B]$. Finally, using any of the experiments, we can solve for k; using the data in Experiment 1, say, we find that

$$k = \frac{\text{rate}}{[A]^2[B]} = \frac{2 \times 10^{-5}\, M/s}{2 \times 10^{-3}\, M^3} = 10^{-2}\, M^{-2}\, s^{-1} = 0.01\, M^{-2}\, s^{-1}$$

- Kinetics is the study of how quickly a reaction occurs, but does not determine *whether or not* a reaction will occur.

- All rates are experimentally determined by measuring a change in the concentration of a reactant or product compared to a change in time (often given in *M*/s).

- Molecules must collide in order to react, and the frequency and energy of these collisions determines how fast the reaction occurs.

- Increasing the concentration of reactants *often* increases the reaction rate due to an increased number of collisions.

- Increasing the temperature of a reaction *always* increases the reaction rate since molecules move faster and collide more frequently; the energy of collisions also increases.

- Activation energy (E_a) is the minimum energy required to start a reaction and decreases in the presence of a catalyst, thereby increasing the reaction rate.

- Transition states are at energy maxima, while intermediates are at local energy minima along a reaction coordinate.

- A reaction mechanism must agree with experimental data, and suggests a possible pathway by which reactants and intermediates might collide in order for a chemical reaction to occur.

- The sum of all elementary steps of a mechanism will add to give the overall chemical reaction.

- The slow step of the mechanism is the rate limiting step, and determines the rate of the overall reaction.

- A rate law can only be determined from experimental data or if given a mechanism, and has the general form: Rate = k [reactants]^x, where x is the order of the reaction with respect to the given reactant, and k is the rate constant.

- The overall order of a reaction is the sum of all exponents in the rate law.

- The value of the rate constant, k, depends on temperature and activation energy, and its units will vary depending on the reaction order.

- Coefficients of the reactants in the rate limiting step of a mechanism can be used to determine the order of a reaction in the rate law; coefficients from the overall reaction alone CANNOT be used to find the order of a reaction.

CHAPTER 9 FREESTANDING PRACTICE QUESTIONS

1. In the reaction A + 2 B → C, the rate law is experimentally determined to be rate = $k[B]^2$. What happens to the initial rate of reaction when the concentration of A is doubled?

A) The rate doubles.
B) The rate quadruples.
C) The rate is halved.
D) The rate is unchanged.

2. Which of the following statements is always true about the kinetics of a chemical reaction?

A) The rate law includes all reactants in the balanced overall equation.
B) The overall order equals the sum of the reactant coefficients in the overall reaction.
C) The overall order equals the sum of the reactant coefficients in the slow step of the reaction.
D) The structure of the catalyst remains unchanged throughout the reaction progress.

3. Which of the following is represented by a localized minimum in a reaction coordinate diagram?

A) Transition state
B) Product
C) Activated complex
D) Intermediate

4. Which factor always affects both thermodynamic and kinetic properties?

A) Temperature
B) Transition state energy level
C) Reactant coefficients of the overall reaction
D) No single factor always affects both thermodynamics and kinetics.

5. Which of the following best describes the role of pepsin in the process of proteolysis?

A) It stabilizes the structure of the amino acid end products.
B) It lowers the energy requirement needed for the reaction to proceed.
C) It increases the K_{eq} of proteolysis.
D) It lowers the free energy of the peptide reactant.

6. Based on the reaction mechanism shown below, which of the following statements is correct?

$$2\,NO + O_2 \rightarrow 2\,NO_2$$

1) $2\,NO \rightarrow N_2O_2$ (fast)
2) $N_2O_2 + O_2 \rightarrow 2\,NO_2$ (slow)

A) Step 1 is the rate-determining step and the rate of the overall reaction is $k[N_2O_2]$.
B) Step 1 is the rate-determining step and the rate of the overall reaction is $k[NO]^2$.
C) Step 2 is the rate-determining step and the rate of the overall reaction is $k[NO_2]^2$.
D) Step 2 is the rate-determining step and the rate of the overall reaction is $k[N_2O_2][O_2]$.

7. When table sugar is exposed to air it undergoes the following reaction:

$$C_{12}H_{22}O_{11} + 12\,O_2 \rightarrow 12\,CO_2 + 11\,H_2O$$

$$(\Delta G = -5693 \text{ kJ/mol})$$

When this reaction is observed at the macroscopic level, it appears as though nothing is happening, yet one can detect trace amounts of CO_2 and H_2O being formed. These observations are best explained by the fact that the reaction is:

A) thermodynamically favorable but not kinetically favorable.
B) kinetically favorable but not thermodynamically favorable.
C) neither kinetically nor thermodynamically favorable.
D) both kinetically and thermodynamically favorable.

CHAPTER 9 PRACTICE PASSAGE

One way to determine a rate law is to look at the slowest elementary step in a reaction mechanism. The rate law is equal to the rate constant times the initial concentrations of the reactants in the slowest step raised to the power of their coefficients in the balanced equation. If a chemical appears in the rate law raised to the X power, we say the reaction is X order for that chemical.

In cases where the slow step is not the first step, the rate law will likely depend on the concentration of intermediate species. This is experimentally inconvenient, since the concentration of intermediates is not as straightforward to control as starting materials. As such, rate laws are often rewritten substituting terms consisting solely of starting materials, when possible. For example, consider the decomposition of nitramide:

$$O_2NNH_2(aq) \rightarrow N_2O(g) + H_2O(l)$$

Reaction 1

This reaction consists of three elementary steps (shown below), with step 2 as the slow step.

Step 1 (fast equilibrium):
$$O_2NNH_2(aq) \rightleftharpoons O_2NNH^-(aq) + H^+(aq)$$

Step 2 (slow):
$$O_2NNH^-(aq) \rightarrow N_2O(g) + OH^-(aq)$$

Step 3 (fast):
$$H^+(aq) + OH^-(aq) \rightarrow H_2O(l)$$

One could write a valid rate law for this reaction of the form:

$$\text{rate} = k[O_2NNH^-]$$

However, the inclusion of the intermediate term is not ideal. The fast equilibrium in Step 1 allows the substitution of $[O_2NNH^-]$ according to the equilibrium condition:

$$K_{eq} = \frac{[O_2NNH^-][H^+]}{[O_2NNH_2]}$$

Solving for $[O_2NNH^-]$, and substituting into the rate law gives an equally valid expression, detailing how the rate may be altered by varying the concentration of starting material and the pH of the reaction mixture:

$$\text{rate} = k\left(\frac{K_{eq}[O_2NNH_2]}{[H^+]}\right)$$

The mechanism for this reaction consists of three elementary steps. The first step is an equilibrium reaction with a significant back reaction and the last step is an equilibrium reaction lying so far to the right that we consider it to go to completion:

1. What is the order of the decomposition of nitramide in water with respect to H^+?

    A) Negative first order
    B) One half order
    C) First order
    D) Second order

2. If Step 1 were simply a fast reaction and not a fast equilibrium, what would be the expected rate law for the decomposition of nitramide in water?

    A) Rate $= k[O_2NNH_2]$

    B) Rate $= k[O_2NNH^-]$

    C) Rate $= k[H^+][OH^-]$

    D) Rate $= k\dfrac{\left[O_2NNH_2\right]}{[H^+]}$

3. If separately synthesized $Na^+[O_2NNH^-]$ were added to a reaction in progress (assuming total solubility of the salt), what effect would this have on the rate?

    A) No reaction would be observed.
    B) The rate of the reaction would decrease.
    C) The rate of the reaction would increase.
    D) It is impossible to tell without experimental data.

4. If the $[H^+]$ goes up by a factor of four, the reaction rate will

    A) increase by a factor of four.
    B) increase by a factor of two.
    C) decrease by a factor of two.
    D) decrease by a factor of four.

5. Considering Step 1 in isolation, if a known amount of O_2NNH_2 is dissolved in water, which of the following plays a role in determining how fast the reaction reaches equilibrium?

A) The pH of the solution
B) The reaction temperature
C) The magnitude of the equilibrium constant
D) The stability of O_2NNH_2 compared to O_2NNH^- and H^+

6. What is true regarding the enthalpy and entropy changes for Step 3 of the mechanism?

A) $\Delta H > 0, \Delta S > 0$
B) $\Delta H > 0, \Delta S < 0$
C) $\Delta H < 0, \Delta S > 0$
D) $\Delta H < 0, \Delta S < 0$

7. Which of the following best describes how a catalyst might speed up a reaction?

A) It raises the temperature of the reaction mixture.
B) It raises the activation energy, making it easier to overcome the energy barrier.
C) It increases the rate of the slowest step.
D) It increases the frequency of collisions between molecules.

SOLUTIONS TO CHAPTER 9 FREESTANDING PRACTICE QUESTIONS

1. **D** Since the rate law is independent of [A], (i.e., rate is only dependent on the concentration of B), changing the amount of A will have no effect on the rate.

2. **C** Choice A is incorrect because rate laws are dependent on the slowest step. If a reactant does not participate in the slow step, it will not be included in the overall rate law. Choice B is incorrect because rate laws of overall reactions can only be determined experimentally. Choice D is incorrect because while it is true that a catalyst comes out of a reaction unchanged, it can undergo temporary transformations during the reaction and revert back into its original form at the end. Choice C is the best option because rate laws can be determined from elementary steps of a reaction mechanism by simply raising the reactants to their respective coefficients.

3. **D** It should be noted that choices A and C are the same and should therefore be eliminated. Additionally, transition states are localized maximums, not minimums. Choice B is incorrect because the product for a spontaneous reaction is the absolute minimum and not a localized minimum. Intermediates are formed and then used. They have a certain lifespan represented by a local minimum on the reaction coordinate diagram.

4. **A** Choice B is purely a kinetic factor and can be eliminated. Choice C is eliminated because it dictates the thermodynamic quantity K_{eq} but not necessarily the kinetics of the overall reaction (only of the rate limiting step). Gibbs free energy, a thermodynamic property, is defined as $\Delta G = \Delta H - T\Delta S$, and the Arrhenius equation defines the rate constant k, a kinetic property, as $k = Ae^{(-E_a/RT)}$. Both equations contain the T variable representing temperature. Therefore, choice A is correct and choice D must be incorrect.

5. **B** Pepsin is an enzyme, a biological catalyst. Catalysts lower the activation energy by providing the correct orientation of reactants for a reaction to proceed. Enzymes make a reaction go faster and affect the kinetics of the reaction, making choice B the best answer. Stability of the products, K_{eq}, and free energy of the reactants are all thermodynamic properties, so choices A, C, and D are eliminated.

6. **D** The rate-determining step (RDS) of a reaction mechanism is the slowest step of that mechanism, eliminating choices A and B. The rate law of an elementary step can be determined from the coefficients of the reactants in the elementary step. Because Step 2 is the RDS, the overall rate law will be equivalent to the rate law for the RDS. Therefore, rate = $k[N_2O_2][O_2]$.

7. **A** Given the very negative ΔG value, this is a very thermodynamically favorable, spontaneous chemical reaction (eliminate choices B and C). It is important to make the distinction in this case between kinetics and thermodynamics. The reason only trace amounts of products are formed is that the reaction proceeds at an incredibly slow rate (therefore NOT kinetically favorable) due to a high activation energy.

SOLUTIONS TO CHAPTER 9 PRACTICE PASSAGE

1. **A** The passage states that if a chemical is raised to the X power, the reaction is X order with respect to that chemical. The rate law can be written as Rate $= k[O_2NNH_2][H^+]^{-1}$, so the reaction is negative first order with respect to H^+.

2. **B** If the first step was simply a fast step, then we would be able to make the normal assumptions about elementary steps and rate laws. More specifically, the rate law could be determined by the stoichiometry of the slow Step 2, which would yield the rate law in choice B.

3. **C** Recall that re-writing the rate law in terms of observable starting conditions does not make the rate including $[O_2NNH^-]$ invalid. The two rate laws are equivalent to one another. As such, increasing the concentration of $[O_2NNH^-]$ will increase the reaction rate.

4. **D** Since $[H^+]$ is in the denominator of the rate law expression and raised to the first power, if $[H^+]$ goes up by a factor of four, the rate will go down by a factor of four.

5. **B** The question requires an answer related to the kinetics of the reaction. Choices A, C, and D are not kinetic factors. The temperature of a reaction is factored into the rate constant $(k = Ae^{(-Ea/RT)})$, so it will play a role in determining the speed of progress to equilibrium.

6. **D** Neutralization reactions release large amounts of heat, so ΔH must be less than zero, eliminating choices A and B. From the point of view of entropy, two molecules become one, increasing the order of the system. Moreover, two aqueous species turning into a pure liquid increases order. Therefore, disorder decreases and ΔS must be less than zero.

7. **C** Catalysts don't work by raising the temperature of the reaction mixture, so choice A is eliminated. They lower the activation energy, not raise it, so choice B is wrong. Catalysts sometimes work by speeding up the slowest step (and sometimes by providing an alternate, faster reaction mechanism), so choice C is a viable answer. Catalysts can't change the frequency of collisions between molecules, leaving choice C as the best answer.

Chapter 10
Equilibrium

10.1 EQUILIBRIUM

Many reactions are reversible, and situations can occur in which the forward and reverse reactions come into a balance called **equilibrium**. How does equilibrium come about? Before any bonds are broken or made, the reaction flask contains only reactants and no products. As the reaction proceeds, products begin to form and eventually build up, and some of them begin to revert to reactants. That is, once products are formed, both the forward and reverse reactions will occur. Ultimately, the reaction will come to equilibrium, a state at which both the forward and reverse reactions occur at the same constant rate. At equilibrium, the overall concentration of reactants and products remains the same, but at the molecular level, they are continually interconverting. Because the forward and reverse processes balance one another perfectly, we don't observe any net change in concentrations.

> *When a reaction is at equilibrium (and only at equilibrium), the rate of the forward reaction is equal to the rate of the reverse reaction.*

Equilibria occur for *closed systems* (which means no new reactants, products, or other changes are imposed).

The Equilibrium Constant

Each reaction will tend towards its own equilibrium and, for a given temperature, will have an **equilibrium constant**, K_{eq}. For the generic, balanced reaction

$$a\,A + b\,B \;\rightleftharpoons\; c\,C + d\,D$$

the equilibrium expression is given by:

$$K_{eq} = \frac{[C]^c [D]^d}{[A]^a [B]^b}$$

This is known as the **mass-action ratio**, where the square brackets represent the molar concentrations at equilibrium.

The constant K is often given a subscript to indicate the type of reaction it represents. For example, K_a (for acids), K_b (for bases), and K_{sp} (for solubility product) are all equilibrium constants. The equilibrium expression is derived from the ratio of the concentration of products to reactants at equilibrium, as follows:

1) Products are in the numerator, and reactants are in the denominator. They are in brackets because the equilibrium expression comes from the *concentrations* (at equilibrium) of the species in the reaction. For two or more reactants or products, multiply the concentrations of each species together.

2) The coefficient of each species in the reaction becomes an exponent on its concentration in the equilibrium expression.

3) Solids and pure liquids are *not* included, because their concentrations don't change. (A substance that's a solid or pure liquid in the reaction is often indicated by an "(s)" or "(l)" subscript, respectively. We're also allowed to omit solvents in dilute solutions because the solvents are in vast excess and their concentrations do not change.)

4) Aqueous dissolved particles are included.

5) If the reaction is gaseous, we can use the partial pressure of each gas as its concentration. The value of the equilibrium constant determined with pressures will be different than with concentrations because of their different units. The constant using partial pressures is often termed K_p.

The value of K_{eq} is constant at a given temperature for a particular reaction, no matter what ratio of reactants and products are given at the beginning of the reaction. That is, any closed system will proceed towards its equilibrium ratio of products and reactants even if you start with all products, or a mixture of some reactants and some products. You can even open the flask and add more of any reactant or product, and the system will change until it has reached the K_{eq} ratio. We'll discuss this idea in detail in just a moment, but right now focus on this:

The value of K_{eq} for a given reaction is a constant at a given temperature.

If the temperature changes, then a reaction's K_{eq} value will change.

The value of K_{eq} tells you the direction the reaction favors:

$K_{eq} < 1 \rightarrow$ reaction favors the reactants (i.e., there are more reactants than products at equilibrium)

$K_{eq} = 1 \rightarrow$ reaction has roughly equal amounts of reactants and products

$K_{eq} > 1 \rightarrow$ reaction favors the products (i.e., there are more products than reactants at equilibrium)

Example 10-1: Which of the following expressions gives the equilibrium constant for this reaction:

$$2\ NO \rightleftharpoons N_2 + O_2?$$

A) $[N_2][O_2]/[2\ NO]$
B) $[N_2][O_2]/[NO]^2$
C) $[NO]/[N_2][O_2]$
D) $[NO]^2/[N_2][O_2]$

Solution: The mass-action ratio is products over reactants, so we can immediately eliminate choices C and D. Stoichiometric coefficients become exponents on the concentrations, not coefficients inside the square brackets. Therefore the coefficient of 2 for the reactant NO means the denominator will be $[NO]^2$, so the answer is B.

Example 10-2: A certain reversible reaction comes to equilibrium with high concentration of products and low concentration of reactants. Of the following, which is the most likely value of the equilibrium constant for this reaction?

A) $K_{eq} = -1 \times 10^{-5}$
B) $K_{eq} = 1 \times 10^{-5}$
C) $K_{eq} = 1$
D) $K_{eq} = 1 \times 10^{5}$

Solution: First, eliminate choice A since equilibrium constants are never negative. If the concentration of products is high and the concentration of reactants is low at equilibrium, then the ratio "products over reactants" will have a large value certainly greater than 1. Therefore, choice D is the answer.

Example 10-3: When the reaction $2\,A + B \rightleftharpoons 2\,C$ reaches equilibrium, $[A] = 0.1\,M$ and $[C] = 0.2\,M$. If the value of K_{eq} for this reaction is 8, what is $[B]$ at equilibrium?

A) $0.1\,M$
B) $0.2\,M$
C) $0.4\,M$
D) $0.5\,M$

Solution: The expression for K_{eq} is $\dfrac{[C]^2}{[A]^2[B]}$. We now solve for $[B]$ and substitute in the given values:

$$K_{eq} = \frac{[C]^2}{[A]^2[B]} \rightarrow [B] = \frac{[C]^2}{[A]^2 K_{eq}} = \frac{(0.2)^2}{(0.1)^2(8)} = \frac{2^2}{8} = 0.5$$

The answer is D.

Example 10-4: Which of the following illustrates a chemical system that is at equilibrium?

I.   Bubbles forming in solution
II. A solution saturated with solute
III. The ratio of products to reactants remains constant

A) I only
B) II only
C) I and II only
D) II and III only

Solution: *Equilibrium* means that the system no longer changes with time. Both II and III illustrate this; therefore, choice D is best.

Example 10-5: The term *chemical equilibrium* applies to a system:

A) where the forward and reverse reaction have stopped.
B) whose rate law is of zero order.
C) where individual molecules are still reacting, but there is no net change in the system.
D) in which all components are in the same phase.

Solution: A *chemical equilibrium* is a dynamic equilibrium, which means that molecules are still reacting, but there is no net change in the composition of the system. Choice C is the best choice. Choice A describes a static equilibrium, but all chemical equilibria are dynamic. Choice B refers to rate, but all closed reactions may come to equilibrium, regardless of the order of the reaction. Finally, the term describing choice D is *homogeneous*, not *equilibrium*.

10.2   THE REACTION QUOTIENT

The equilibrium constant expression is a ratio: the concentration of the products divided by those of the reactants, each raised to the power equal to its stoichiometric coefficient in the balanced equation. If the reaction is not at equilibrium, the same expression is known simply as the **reaction quotient, Q**. For the generic, balanced reaction

$$a\,A + b\,B \rightleftharpoons c\,C + d\,D$$

the reaction quotient is given by:

$$Q = \frac{[C]^c\,[D]^d}{[A]^a\,[B]^b}$$

where the square brackets represent the molar concentrations of the species. The point now is that the concentrations in the expression Q do *not* have to be the concentrations at equilibrium. (If the concentrations are the equilibrium concentrations, the Q will equal K_{eq}.)

Comparing the value of Q to K_{eq} tells us in what direction the reaction will proceed. The reaction will strive to reach a state in which $Q = K_{eq}$. So, if Q is less than K_{eq}, then the reaction will proceed in the forward direction (in order to increase the concentration of the products and decrease the concentration of the reactants) to increase Q to the K_{eq} value. On the other hand, if Q is greater than K_{eq}, then the reaction will proceed in the reverse direction (in order to increase the concentrations of the reactants and decrease the concentrations of the products) to reduce Q to K_{eq}.

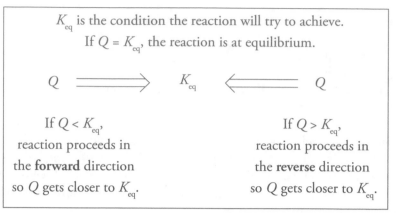

K_{eq} is the condition the reaction will try to achieve.
If $Q = K_{eq}$, the reaction is at equilibrium.

$$Q \implies K_{eq} \impliedby Q$$

If $Q < K_{eq}$,
reaction proceeds in
the **forward** direction
so Q gets closer to K_{eq}.

If $Q > K_{eq}$,
reaction proceeds in
the **reverse** direction
so Q gets closer to K_{eq}.

Example 10-6: The value of the equilibrium constant for the reaction

$$2\ COF_2(g) \rightleftharpoons CO_2(g) + CF_4(g)$$

is $K_{eq} = 2$. If a 1 L reaction container currently holds 1 mole each of CO_2 and CF_4 and 0.5 mole of COF_2, then:

A) the reaction is at equilibrium.
B) the forward reaction will be favored.
C) the reverse reaction will be favored.
D) no prediction can be made without knowing the pressure of the container.

Solution: The expression for Q is $\dfrac{[CO_2][CF_4]}{[COF_2]^2}$. Therefore, the value of Q is:

$$\frac{(1)(1)}{(0.5)^2} = 4$$

Since $Q > K_{eq}$, the reverse reaction will be favored (choice C).

10.3 LE CHÂTELIER'S PRINCIPLE

Le Châtelier's principle states that a system at equilibrium will try to neutralize any imposed change (or stress) in order to reestablish equilibrium. For example, if you add more reactant to a system that is at equilibrium, the system will react by favoring the forward reaction in order to consume that reactant and reestablish equilibrium.

To illustrate, let's look at the Haber process for making ammonia:

$$N_2(g) + 3\ H_2(g) \rightleftharpoons 2\ NH_3(g) + heat$$

Let's assume the reaction is at equilibrium, and see how it reacts to disturbances to the equilibrium by changing the concentration of the species, the pressure, or the temperature.

Adding Ammonia

If we add ammonia, the system is no longer at equilibrium, and there is an excess of product. How can the reaction reestablish equilibrium? By consuming some of the added ammonia, the ratio of products to reactant would decrease towards the equilibrium ratio, so the reverse reaction will be favored (we say the system "shifts to the left"), converting ammonia into nitrogen and hydrogen, until equilibrium is restored.

You can see how this follows from comparing the reaction quotient of the disturbed system to the equilibrium constant. If we add ammonia to the reaction mixture, then $[NH_3]$ increases, and the reaction quotient, Q, becomes greater than K_{eq}. As a result, the reaction will proceed in the reverse direction in order to reduce Q to K_{eq}.

Removing Ammonia

If we remove the product, ammonia, then the forward reaction will be favored—the reaction "shifts to the right"—in order to reach equilibrium again. Again, you can see how this follows from comparing the reaction quotient of the disturbed system to the equilibrium constant. If we remove ammonia from the reaction mixture, then $[NH_3]$ decreases, and the reaction quotient, Q, becomes smaller than K_{eq}. As a result, the reaction will proceed in the forward direction in order to increase Q to K_{eq}.

Adding Hydrogen

If we add some reactant, say $H_2(g)$, then the forward reaction will be favored—the reaction "shifts to the right"—in order to reach equilibrium again. This follows from comparing the reaction quotient of the disturbed system to the equilibrium constant. If we add hydrogen to the reaction mixture, the $[H_2]$ increases, and the reaction quotient, Q, becomes smaller than K_{eq}. As a result, the reaction will proceed in the forward direction in order to increase Q to K_{eq}.

Removing Nitrogen

If we remove some reactant, say $N_2(g)$, then the reverse reaction will be favored—the reaction "shifts to the left"—in order to reach equilibrium again. Again, this follows from comparing the reaction quotient of the disturbed system to the equilibrium constant. If we remove nitrogen from the reaction mixture, then $[N_2]$ decreases, and the reaction quotient, Q, becomes larger than K_{eq}. As a result, the reaction will proceed in the reverse direction in order to decrease Q to K_{eq}.

Changing the Volume of the Reaction Container

The Haber process is a gaseous reaction, so a change in volume will cause the partial pressures of the gases to change. Specifically, a decrease in volume of the reaction container will cause the partial pressures of the gases to increase; an increase in volume reduces the partial pressures of the gases in the mixture. If the number of moles of gas on the left side of the reaction does not equal the number of moles of gas on the right, then a change in pressure due to a change in volume will disrupt the equilibrium ratio, and the system will react to reestablish equilibrium.

How does the system react? Let's first assume the volume is reduced so that the pressure increases. Look back at the equation for the Haber process: There are 4 moles of gas on the reactant side (3 of H_2 plus 1 of N_2) for every 2 moles of NH_3 gas formed. If the reaction shifts to the right, four moles of gas can be condensed into 2 moles, reducing the pressure to reestablish equilibrium. On the other hand, if the volume

10.3

is increased so that the pressure decreases, the reaction will shift to the left, increasing the pressure to reestablish equilibrium.

To summarize: Consider a gaseous reaction (at equilibrium) with unequal numbers of moles of gas of reactants and products. If the volume is reduced, increasing the pressure, a net reaction occurs favoring the side with the smaller total number of moles of gas. If the volume is expanded, decreasing the pressure, a net reaction occurs favoring the side with the greater total number of moles of gas. (This is only true for reactions involving gases.)

Changing the Temperature of the Reaction Mixture

Heat can be treated as a reactant or a product just like all the chemical reactants and products. Adding or removing heat (by increasing or decreasing the temperature) is like adding or removing any other reagent. Exothermic reactions release heat (which we note on the right side of the equation like a product), and the ΔH will be negative. Endothermic reactions consume heat (which we note on the left side of the equation like a reactant), and the ΔH will be positive.

The Haber process is an exothermic reaction. So, if you increase the temperature at which the reaction takes place once it's reached equilibrium, the reaction will shift to the left in order to consume the extra heat, thereby producing more reactants. If you decrease the temperature at which the reaction takes place once it's reached equilibrium, the reaction will shift to the right in order to produce extra heat, thereby producing more product.

Since the reverse of an exothermic reaction is an endothermic one (and vice versa), every equilibrium reaction involves an exothermic reaction and an endothermic reaction. We can then say this: *Lowering the temperature favors the exothermic reaction, while raising the temperature favors the endothermic one.* Keep in mind that, unlike changes in concentration or pressure, changes in temperature *will* affect the reaction's K_{eq} value, depending on the direction the reaction shifts to reestablish equilibrium.

Note that the above changes are specific to the system *once it is at equilibrium*. The kinetics of the reaction are a different matter. Remember, all reactions proceed faster when the temperature is increased, and this is true for the Haber process. Indeed, in industry this reaction is typically run at around 500°C, despite the fact that the reaction is exothermic. The reason is that a fast reaction with a 10 percent yield of ammonia may end up being better overall than a painfully slow reaction with a 90 percent yield of ammonia. Heating a reaction gets it to equilibrium faster. Once it's there, adding or taking away heat will affect the equilibrium as predicted by Le Châtelier's principle.

Adding an Inert (or Non-Reactive) Gas

What if we injected some helium into a constant volume reaction container? This inert gas doesn't participate in the reaction (and for the MCAT, inert gases don't participate in *any* reaction), so it will change neither the partial pressure nor the concentration of the products or reactants. If neither of these values change, then there is no change in equilibrium.

Adding a Catalyst

Adding a catalyst to a reaction that's already at equilibrium has no effect. Because it increases the rate of both the forward and reverse reactions equally, the equilibrium amounts of the species are unchanged. So, the introduction of a catalyst would cause no disturbance. Remember that a catalyst increases the reaction rate but does *not* affect the equilibrium.

Example 10-7: Nitrogen dioxide gas can be formed by the endothermic reaction shown below. Which of the following changes to the equilibrium would *not* increase the formation of NO_2?

$$N_2O_4(g) \rightleftharpoons 2\ NO_2(g) \qquad \Delta H = +58\ kJ$$

A) An increase in the temperature
B) A decrease in the volume of the container
C) Adding additional N_2O_4
D) Removing NO_2 as it is formed

Solution: Since ΔH is positive, this reaction is endothermic, and we can think of heat as a reactant. So if we increase the temperature (thereby "adding a reactant," namely heat), the equilibrium would shift to the right, thus increasing the formation of NO_2. This eliminates choice A. Adding reactant (choice C) or removing product (choice D) would also shift the equilibrium to the right. The answer must be B. A decrease in the volume of the container would increase the pressure of the gases, causing the equilibrium to shift in favor of the side with the fewer number of moles of gases; in this case, that would be to the left.

Example 10-8: If the following endothermic reaction is at equilibrium in a rigid reaction vessel,

$$CH_4(g) + H_2O(g) \rightleftharpoons CO(g) + 3\ H_2(g)$$

which one of the following changes would cause the equilibrium to shift to the right?

A) Adding $Ne(g)$
B) Removing some $H_2O(g)$
C) Increasing the pressure
D) Increasing the temperature

Solution: Choice A would have no effect, since neon is an inert gas and the question states the reaction vessel is rigid, therefore the volume does not change. Removing some reactant (choice B) would shift the equilibrium to the left. An increase in pressure (choice C) would cause the equilibrium to shift in favor of the side with the fewer number of moles of gases; in this case, that would be to the left. The answer must be D. Increasing the temperature of an endothermic reaction will shift the equilibrium toward the products.

Example 10-9: If the reaction

$$2\ NO(g) + O_2(g) \rightleftharpoons 2\ NO_2(g) \qquad \Delta H = -120\ kJ$$

is at equilibrium, which one of the following changes would cause the formation of additional $NO_2(g)$?

A) Increasing the temperature
B) Adding a catalyst
C) Reducing the volume of the reaction container
D) Removing some $NO(g)$

10.4

Solution: First, eliminate choice B; adding a catalyst to a reaction that's already at equilibrium has no effect. Now, because ΔH is negative, the reaction is exothermic (that is, we can consider heat to be a product). Increasing the temperature would therefore shift the equilibrium to the left; this eliminates choice A. Also, choice D can be eliminated since removing a reactant shifts the equilibrium to the left. The answer is C: Reducing the volume of the reaction container will increase the pressure, and the equilibrium responds to this stress by favoring the side with the fewer number of moles of gas. In this case, that would mean a shift to the right.

Example 10-10: The Haber process takes place in a container of fixed volume and is at equilibrium:

$$N_2(g) + 3\,H_2(g) \rightleftharpoons 2NH_3(g) + heat$$

The amounts of the gases present are measured and recorded. Some additional $N_2(g)$ is then injected into the container, and the system is allowed to return to equilibrium. When it does:

A) the amount of H_2 will be smaller than before, and the amounts of N_2 and NH_3 will be greater than before.
B) the amount of N_2 will be smaller than before, and the amounts of H_2 and NH_3 will be greater than before.
C) the amount of NH_3 will be smaller than before, and the amounts of N_2 and H_2 will be greater than before.
D) the amounts of all three gases will be the same as before.

Solution: The system will respond to this change by shifting to the right to reestablish equilibrium. The added N_2 will mean there's more N_2 in the reaction container, even after equilibrium has been reestablished. Also, the shift toward the product side means there'll be more NH_3 than before as well. And in the shifting of the equilibrium in an attempt to reestablish equilibrium, some of the H_2 got used. As a result, we'd expect that the amount of H_2 will be smaller than before, while the amounts of N_2 and NH_3 are greater than before the injection of the extra N_2 (choice A).

10.4 SOLUTIONS AND SOLUBILITY

Solutions

A **solution** forms when one substance **dissolves** into another, forming a *homogeneous* mixture. The process of dissolving is known as **dissolution**. For example, sugar dissolved into iced tea is a solution (though so is unsweetened tea). A substance present in a relatively smaller proportion is called a **solute**, and a substance present in a relatively greater proportion is called a **solvent**. The process that occurs when the solvent molecules surround the solute molecules is known as **solvation**; if the solvent is water, the process is called **hydration**.

Solutions can involve any of the three phases of matter. For example, you can have a solution of two gases, of a gas in a liquid, of a solid in a liquid, or of a solid in a solid (an **alloy**). However, most of the solutions with which you're familiar have a liquid as the solvent. Salt water has solid salt (NaCl) dissolved into water, seltzer water has carbon dioxide gas dissolved in water, and vinegar has liquid acetic acid dissolved in water. In fact, most of the solutions that you commonly see have water as the solvent: lemonade, tea, soda pop, and corn syrup are examples. When a solution has water as the solvent, it is called an **aqueous** solution.

How do we know which solutes are soluble in which solvents? Well, that's easy:

Like dissolves like.

Solutes will dissolve best in solvents where the intermolecular forces being broken in the solute are being replaced by equal (or stronger) intermolecular forces between the solvent and the solute.

Electrolytes

When ionic substances dissolve, they **dissociate** into ions. Free ions in a solution are called **electrolytes** because the solution can conduct electricity. Some salts dissociate completely into individual ions, while others only partially dissociate (that is, a certain percentage of the ions will remain paired, sticking close to each other rather than being independent and fully surrounded by solvent). Solutes that dissociate completely (like ionic substances) are called **strong electrolytes**, and those that remain ion-paired to some extent are called **weak electrolytes**. (Covalent compounds that don't dissociate into ions are **nonelectrolytes**.) Solutions of strong electrolytes are better conductors of electricity than those of weak electrolytes.

Different ionic compounds will dissociate into different numbers of particles. Some won't dissociate at all, and others will break up into several ions. The **van't Hoff** (or **ionizability**) **factor** (i) tells us how many ions one unit of a substance will produce in a solution. For example,

- $C_6H_{12}O_6$ is non-ionic, so it does not dissociate. Therefore, $i = 1$.
  (Note: The van't Hoff factor for almost all biomolecules—hormones, proteins, steroids—is 1.)
- NaCl dissociates into Na^+ and Cl^-. Therefore, $i = 2$.
- HNO_3 dissociates into H^+ and NO_3^-. Therefore, $i = 2$.
- $CaCl_2$ dissociates into Ca^{2+} and 2 Cl^-. Therefore, $i = 3$.

Example 10-11: Of the following, which is the *weakest* electrolyte?

A) NH_4I
B) LiF
C) AgBr
D) H_2O_2

Solution: All ionic compounds, whether soluble or not, are defined as strong electrolytes, so choices A, B, and C are eliminated. Choice D, hydrogen peroxide, is a covalent compound that does not produce an appreciable number of ions upon dissolution and thus is a weak electrolyte. Choice D is the best answer.

The **concentration** of a solution tells you how much solute is dissolved in the solvent (see Section 3.8). A **concentrated** solution has a greater amount of solute per unit volume than a solution that is **dilute**. A **saturated** solution is one in which no more solute will dissolve. At this point, we have reached the **molar solubility** of the solute for that particular solvent, and the reverse process of dissolution, called **precipitation**, occurs at the same rate as dissolving. Both the solid form and the dissolved form of the solute are said to be in **dynamic equilibrium**.

Example 10-12: A researcher adds 0.4 kg of $CaBr_2$ (MW = 200 g/mol) to a large flask and adds enough water to make 10 L of solution.

   A)   What is the molarity of the calcium bromide in the solution?
   B)   What is the concentration of bromide ion in the solution?
   C)   How much water would the researcher need to add to the solution in order to decrease the concentration by a factor of 4?

Solution:

   A)   Since the molecular weight of $CaBr_2$ is 0.2 kg/mol, a 0.4 kg sample represents 2 moles. Then by definition we have

$$\text{Molarity } (M) = \frac{\text{\# moles of solute}}{\text{\# L of solution}} = \frac{2 \text{ mol}}{10 \text{ L}} = 0.2 \ M$$

   B)   Since $CaBr_2$ dissociates into one Ca^{2+} ion and 2 Br^- ions, the concentration of bromide ion in the solution is 2(0.2 M) = 0.4 M.
   C)   Let x be the number of liters of additional water added to the solution. If the concentration is to be decreased by a factor of 4 (that is, to 0.05 M), then

$$\frac{2 \text{ mol}}{10 \text{ L} + x \text{ L}} = 0.05M \quad \Rightarrow \quad \frac{2}{10 + x} = \frac{5}{100} \quad \Rightarrow \quad x = 30$$

Solubility

Solubility refers to the amount of solute that will saturate a particular solvent. Solubility is specific for the type of solute and solvent. For example, 100 mL of water at 25°C becomes saturated with 40 g of dissolved NaCl, but it would take 150 g of KI to saturate the same volume of water at this temperature. And both of these salts behave differently in methanol than in water. Solubility also varies with temperature, increasing or decreasing with temperature depending upon the solute and solvent as outlined in the first set of solubility rules below.

There are two sets of solubility rules that show up time and time again on the MCAT. The first set governs the general solubility of solids and gases in liquids, as a function of the temperature and pressure. These rules below should be taken as just rules of thumb because they are only 95 percent reliable (still not bad). Memorize the following:

> **Phase Solubility Rules**
> 1. The solubility of solids in liquids tends to increase with increasing temperature.
> 2. The solubility of gases in liquids tends to decrease with increasing temperature.
> 3. The solubility of gases in liquids tends to increase with increasing pressure.

Keep in mind, the solubility of a gas in a liquid is also a function of the partial pressure of that gas above the liquid and the Henry's law constant (Solubility = kP). As partial pressure increases, the quantity of dissolved gas necessarily increases as the equilibrium constant remains unchanged.

The second set governs the solubility of salts in water. Memorize the following too:

> **Salt Solubility Rules**
> 1. All Group I (Li^+, Na^+, K^+, Rb^+, Cs^+) and ammonium (NH_4^+) salts are *soluble*.
> 2. All nitrate (NO_3^-), perchlorate (ClO_4^-), and acetate ($C_2H_3O_2^-$) salts are *soluble*.
> 3. All silver (Ag^+), lead (Pb^{2+}/Pb^{4+}), and mercury (Hg_2^{2+}/Hg^{2+}) salts are *insoluble, except* for their nitrates, perchlorates, and acetates.

Example 10-13: Which of the following salts is expected to be *insoluble* in water?

A) $CsOH$
B) NH_4NO_3
C) $CaCO_3$
D) $AgClO_4$

Solution: According to the solubility rules for salts in water, choices A, B, and D are expected to be soluble. Choice C is therefore the best answer.

Example 10-14: Which of the following acids could be added to an unknown salt solution and NOT cause precipitation?

A) HCl
B) HI
C) H_2SO_4
D) HNO_3

Solution: According to the solubility rules for salts, all nitrate (NO_3^-) salts are soluble. Therefore, only the addition of nitric acid guarantees that any new ion combination would be soluble. Choice D is the correct answer.

Example 10-15: Which one of the following observations is *inconsistent* with the solubility rules given above?

A)   More sugar dissolves in a pot of hot water than in a pot of cold water.
B)   Boiler scales are caused by the precipitation of $CaCO_3$ inside plumbing when hot water heaters heat up cold well water.
C)   After breathing compressed air at depth, scuba divers that ascend to the surface too quickly risk having air bubbles in their body.
D)   Boiling the water before making ice cubes out of it results in clear ice cubes that have no trapped air bubbles.

Solution: Choice A is consistent with phase solubility rule 1, so it is eliminated. Choice C is consistent with phase solubility rule 3, so it is eliminated as well. And finally, choice D is consistent with the second solubility rule 2, so it is also eliminated. Although choice B is a true statement, it is one of those few examples that runs counter to our phase solubility rule 1. Choice B is the correct answer.

Solubility Product Constant

All salts have characteristic solubilities in water. Some, like NaCl, are very soluble, while others, like AgCl, barely dissolve at all. The extent to which a salt will dissolve in water can be determined from its **solubility product constant**, K_{sp}. The solubility product is simply another equilibrium constant, one in which the reactants and products are just the undissolved and dissolved salts.

For example, let's look at the dissolution of magnesium hydroxide in water:

$$Mg(OH)_2(s) \; \rightleftharpoons \; Mg^{2+}(aq) + 2\ OH^-(aq)$$

At equilibrium, the solution is *saturated*; the rate at which ions go into solution is equal to the rate at which they precipitate out. The equilibrium expression is

$$K_{sp} = [Mg^{2+}][OH^-]^2$$

Notice that we leave the $Mg(OH)_2$ out of the equilibrium expression because it's a pure solid. (The "concentration of a solid" is meaningless when discussing the equilibrium between a solid and its ions in a saturated aqueous solution.)

Solubility Computations

Let's say you know the K_{sp} for a solid, and you're asked to find out just how much of it can dissolve into water; that is, you're asked to determine the salt's **molar solubility**, the number of moles of that salt that will saturate a liter of water.

To find the solubility of $Mg(OH)_2$, we begin by figuring out how much of each type of ion we'll have once we have x moles of the salt. Since each molecule dissociates into one magnesium ion and two hydroxide ions, if x moles of this salt have dissolved, the solution contains x moles of Mg^{2+} ions and $2x$ moles of OH^- ions:

$$Mg(OH)_2(s) \rightleftharpoons Mg^{2+}(aq) + 2OH^-(aq)$$

$$x \rightleftharpoons x + 2x$$

So, if x stands for the number of moles of $Mg(OH)_2$ that have dissolved per liter of saturated solution (which is what we're trying to find), then $[Mg^{2+}] = x$ and $[OH^-] = 2x$. Substituting these into the solubility product expression gives us

$$K_{sp} = [Mg^{2+}][OH^-]^2$$

$$= x\,(2x)^2 = x\,(4x^2) = 4x^3$$

It is known that K_{sp} for $Mg(OH)_2$ at 25°C is about 1.6×10^{-11}. So, if we set this equal to $4x^3$, we can solve for x. We get $x \approx 1.6 \times 10^{-4}$. This means that a solution of $Mg(OH)_2$ at 25°C will be saturated at a $Mg(OH)_2$ concentration of $1.6 \times 10^{-4}\ M$.

Example 10-16: The value of the solubility product for copper(I) chloride is $K_{sp} = 1.2 \times 10^{-6}$. Under normal conditions, the maximum concentration of an aqueous CuCl solution will be:

A) less than $10^{-6}\ M$.
B) greater than $10^{-6}\ M$ and less than $10^{-4}\ M$.
C) greater than $10^{-4}\ M$ and less than $10^{-2}\ M$.
D) greater than $10^{-2}\ M$ and less than $10^{-1}\ M$.

Solution: The equilibrium is $CuCl(s) \rightleftharpoons Cu^+(aq) + Cl^-(aq)$. If we let x denote $[Cu^+]$, then we also have $x = [Cl^-]$. Therefore, $K_{sp} = x \times x = x^2$; setting this equal to 1.2×10^{-6}, we find that x is $1.1 \times 10^{-3}\ M$. Therefore, the answer is C.

Example 10-17: The solubility product for lithium phosphate, Li_3PO_4, is $K_{sp} = 2.7 \times 10^{-9}$. How many moles of this salt would be required to form a saturated, 1 L aqueous solution?

Solution: The equilibrium is $Li_3PO_4(s) \rightleftharpoons 3Li^+(aq) + PO_4^{3-}(aq)$. If we let x denote $[PO_4^{3-}]$, then we have $[Li^+] = 3x$. Therefore, $K_{sp} = (3x)^3 \times x = 27x^4$; setting this equal to $2.7 \times 10^{-9} = 27 \times 10^{-10}$ we find that

$$27x^4 = 27 \times 10^{-10} \quad \rightarrow \quad x = (10^{-10})^{1/4} = 10^{-2.5} = 10^{0.5} \times 10^{-3} \approx 3.2 \times 10^{-3}$$

Therefore, 3.2×10^{-3} mol will be required.

10.5   ION PRODUCT

The **ion product** is the reaction quotient for a solubility reaction. That is, while K_{sp} is equal to the product of the concentrations of the ions in solution when the solution is saturated (that is, *at equilibrium*), the ion product—which we'll denote by Q_{sp}—has exactly the same form as the K_{sp} expression, but the concentrations don't have to be those at equilibrium. The reaction quotient allows us to make predictions about what the reaction will do:

$$Q_{sp} < K_{sp} \rightarrow \text{more salt can be dissolved}$$
$$Q_{sp} = K_{sp} \rightarrow \text{solution is saturated}$$
$$Q_{sp} > K_{sp} \rightarrow \text{excess salt will precipitate}$$

For example, let's say we had a liter of solution containing 10^{-4} mol of barium chloride and 10^{-3} mol of sodium sulfate, both of which are soluble salts:

$$BaCl_2(s) \rightarrow Ba^{2+}(aq) + 2Cl^-(aq)$$

$$Na_2SO_4(s) \rightarrow 2Na^+(aq) + SO_4^{2-}(aq)$$

When you mix two salts in solution, ions can recombine to form new salts, and you have to consider the new salt's K_{sp}. Barium sulfate, $BaSO_4$, is a slightly soluble salt, and at 25°C, its K_{sp} is 1.1×10^{-10}. Its dissolution equilibrium is

$$BaSO_4(s) \rightleftharpoons Ba^{2+}(aq) + SO_4^{2-}(aq)$$

Its ion product is $Q_{sp} = [Ba^{2+}][SO_4^{2-}]$, so in this solution, we have $Q_{sp} = (10^{-4})(10^{-3}) = 10^{-7}$, which is much greater than its K_{sp}. Since $Q_{sp} > K_{sp}$, the reverse reaction would be favored, and $BaSO_4$ would precipitate out of solution.

10.6   THE COMMON-ION EFFECT

Let's consider again a saturated solution of magnesium hydroxide:

$$Mg(OH)_2(s) \rightleftharpoons Mg^{2+}(aq) + 2OH^-(aq)$$

What would happen if we now added some sodium hydroxide, NaOH, to this solution? Since NaOH is very soluble in water, it will dissociate completely:

$$NaOH(s) \rightarrow Na^+(aq) + OH^-(aq)$$

The addition of NaOH has caused the amount of hydroxide ion—the **common ion**—in the solution to increase. This disturbs the equilibrium of magnesium hydroxide; since the concentration of a product of that equilibrium is increased, Le Châtelier's principle tells us that the system will react by favoring the reverse reaction, producing solid $Mg(OH)_2$, which will precipitate. Therefore, the molar solubility of the slightly soluble salt [in this case, $Mg(OH)_2$] is decreased by the presence of another solute (in this case, NaOH) that supplies a common ion. This is the **common-ion effect**.

Example 10-18: Barium chromate solid ($K_{sp} = 1.2 \times 10^{-10}$) is at equilibrium with its dissociated ions in an aqueous solution. If calcium chromate ($K_{sp} = 7.1 \times 10^{-4}$) is introduced into the solution, it will cause the molar quantity of:

A) solid barium chromate to increase and barium ion to decrease.
B) solid barium chromate to increase and barium ion to increase.
C) solid barium chromate to decrease and barium ion to decrease.
D) solid barium chromate to decrease and barium ion to increase.

Solution: The answer is A. The introduction of additional chromate ion (CrO_4^{2-})—the common ion—will cause the amount of barium ion in solution to decrease (since the solubility equilibrium of $BaCrO_4$ will be shifted to the left, consuming Ba^{2+}). And, as a result, the amount of solid barium chromate will increase, because some will precipitate.

Example 10-19: A researcher wishes to prepare a saturated solution of a lead compound that contains the greatest concentration of lead(II) ions. Of the following, which should she use?

A) $Pb(OH)_2$ ($K_{sp} = 2.8 \times 10^{-16}$)
B) $PbCl_2$ ($K_{sp} = 1.7 \times 10^{-5}$)
C) PbI_2 ($K_{sp} = 8.7 \times 10^{-9}$)
D) $PbBr_2$ ($K_{sp} = 6.3 \times 10^{-6}$)

Solution: Since the equilibrium had the form $PbX_2(s) \rightleftharpoons Pb^{2+}(aq) + 2 X^-(aq)$, we have $K_{sp} = [Pb^{2+}][X^-]^2$. Therefore, to maximize $[Pb^{2+}]$, the researcher would want to maximize K_{sp}. Of the choices given, $PbCl_2$ (choice B) has the largest K_{sp} value.

10.7 COMPLEX ION FORMATION AND SOLUBILITY

Complex ions consist of metallic ions surrounded by generally two, four, or six ligands, also known as Lewis bases. Complexed metal ions may have extremely different solubility properties than the "naked," hydrated metal ions. Therefore, the addition of ligands may substantially alter the solubility of simple metal salts. For example, as described by the solubility rules in Section 10.4 above, silver chloride (AgCl) is largely insoluble in water as is evident by its extremely low K_{sp} (1.7×10^{-10}). However, addition of AgCl to an aqueous solution containing ammonia (NH_3) results in greater solubility, owing to the formation of the complex ion $[Ag(NH_3)_2]^+$. The overall effect is described by the equations below:

$$AgCl(s) \rightleftharpoons Ag^+(aq) + Cl^-(aq) \qquad K_{sp} = 1.6 \times 10^{-10}$$

$$Ag^+(aq) + 2 NH_3(aq) \rightleftharpoons [Ag(NH_3)_2]^+ (aq) \qquad K_{eq} = 1.5 \times 10^7$$

Overall: $$AgCl(s) + 2 NH_3(aq) \rightleftharpoons [Ag(NH_3)_2]^+ (aq) + Cl^-(aq) \qquad K_{overall} \approx 10^{-3}$$

The inclusion of ammonia in the system greatly increases the propensity of the AgCl(s) to exist as ions in solution. While the final value of K (10^{-3}) is still less than 1, it is several orders of magnitude greater than the initial K_{sp} of AgCl. The dissolution of the initial silver salt can be favored even more by taking advantage of Le Châtelier's Principle through the simple addition of excess ammonia.

10.7

One biological application of complex ion formation is metal-chelation therapy; one of the most commonly used metal chelation agents, ethylenediaminetetraacetic acid (EDTA) is approved by the FDA for the treatment of acute lead poisoning. After the administration of EDTA (generally as a mixed calcium/sodium salt), an equilibrium is established, sequestering the toxic Pb^{2+} ions in the patient's system in a very stable EDTA complex. The following reaction demonstrates the association of fully deprotonated EDTA and Pb^{2+} to form the complex ion:

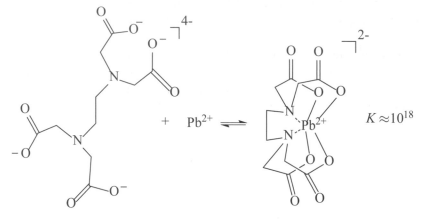

The extremely high equilibrium constant for the formation of the complexed Pb^{2+} ensures that it is prevented from further deleterious interactions with other biological functionalities, and allows its speedy excretion from the body.

10.8 THERMODYNAMICS AND EQUILIBRIUM

In Section 6.5 on Gibbs Free Energy, we saw that if ΔG was negative we could expect a reaction to proceed spontaneously in the forward direction, with the opposite being true for the case in which ΔG is positive. When a system proceeds in one direction or another there is necessarily a change in the relative values of products and reactants that redefine ΔG, and the reaction proceeds until ΔG is equal to 0 and equilibrium is achieved. Therefore, there must be a relationship between ΔG and the reaction quotient Q, as well as the equilibrium constant K_{eq}. This relationship is given in the following equation.

$$\Delta G = \Delta G° + RT \ln Q$$

As the superscript denotes, $\Delta G°$ is the Gibbs free energy for a reaction under standard conditions. You may recall from Section 10.2 that when $Q = K$ the reaction is at equilibrium. Since ΔG is always equal to zero at equilibrium we can change the equation to

$$0 = \Delta G° + RT \ln K_{eq}$$

or

$$\Delta G° = -RT \ln K_{eq}$$

It is important to draw the distinction between ΔG and $\Delta G°$. Whereas ΔG is a statement of spontaneity of a reaction in one direction or another, $\Delta G°$ is, as seen in its relation to K_{eq}, a statement of the relative proportions of products and reactants present at equilibrium. The standard state $\Delta G°$ for a reaction only describes a reaction at one specific temperature, pressure, and set of concentrations, whereas ΔG changes with changing reaction composition until it reaches zero. From the above relationship, we can surmise the following:

$\Delta G° < 0$; $K_{eq} > 1$, products are favored at equilibrium
$\Delta G° = 0$; $K_{eq} = 1$, products and reactants are present in roughly equal amounts at equilibrium
$\Delta G° > 0$; $K_{eq} < 1$, reactants are favored at equilibrium

The difference between the heights of the reactants and products on any reaction coordinate diagram is $\Delta G°$. As we know from analyzing these plots if the reactants are higher than the products, we expect the products to be favored. This would give us the expected negative value of $\Delta G°$, and likewise a value of K_{eq} greater than 1.

10.8

- The equilibrium constant dictates the relative ratios of products to reactant when a system is at equilibrium.

- For $aA + bB \rightarrow cC + dD$: $K_{eq} = [[C]^c[D]^d]/[[A]^a[B]^b]$

- Pure solids and liquids are not included in the equilbrium expression.

- If $K > 1$, products are favored. If $K < 1$ reactants are favored.

- The reaction quotient, Q, is a ratio of products and reactants with the same form as K, but can be used when the reaction isn't at equilibrium. If $Q < K$, the reaction will proceed in the forward reaction; if $Q > K$, the reaction will proceed in the reverse direction until equilibrium is achieved.

- The only factor that changes the equilibrium constant is temperature.

- Changing the concentrations of the products or reactants of a reaction at equilibrium will force the system to shift according to Le Châtelier's principle.

- Increasing the temperature of a system at equilibrium favors the products in an endothermic reaction and the reactants in an exothermic reaction. Decreasing the temperature will have the opposite effect on both types of reactions.

- In a gaseous reaction, increasing the pressure by decreasing the volume favors the side of the reaction with fewer moles of gas. Decreasing the pressure has the opposite effect.

- An electrolyte is a solute that produces free ions in solution. Strong electrolytes produce more ions in solution than weak electrolytes.

- The van't Hoff (or ionizability) factor, i, tells us how many ions one unit of a substance will produce in solution.

- All Group I, ammonium, nitrate, perchlorate, and acetate salts are completely soluble. All silver, lead, and mercury salts are insoluble, except when they are paired with nitrate, perchlorate, or acetate.

- The solubility of solids in liquids increases with increasing temperature.

- The solubility of gases in liquids decreases with increasing temperature and increases with increasing pressure.

- The amount of a salt that can be dissolved in a solute is given by its solubility product constant (K_{sp}).

- For a reaction at equilibrium under standard conditions, $\Delta G° = -RT\ln K_{eq}$.

- For a reaction under non-standard conditions, ΔG can be calculated using $\Delta G = \Delta G° + RT\ln Q$.

CHAPTER 10 FREESTANDING PRACTICE QUESTIONS

1. Which of the following manipulations is capable of changing the K_{eq} of the reaction shown below?

$$N_2(g) + 3\,H_2(g) \rightleftharpoons 2\,NH_3(g)$$

A) Doubling the concentrations of $N_2(g)$, $H_2(g)$, and $NH_3(g)$
B) Tripling the volume of the reaction container
C) Increasing the pressure from 1 to 2 atm
D) Decreasing the temperature to from 298 K to 273 K

2. A group of scientists is studying the dynamics of the acetic acid dissociation below and bring the process to equilibrium under standard conditions. If the scientists then add 35 g of sodium acetate to the reaction container, which of the following will be true?

$$CH_3COOH(aq) \rightleftharpoons CH_3COO^-(aq) + H^+\,(aq)$$

A) $Q > K_{eq}$ and the reaction will move in reverse.
B) $Q < K_{eq}$ and the reaction will move forward.
C) $Q > K_{eq}$ and the reaction will move forward.
D) $Q < K_{eq}$ and the reaction will move in reverse.

3. Given the following equilibrium:

$$N_2(g) + 3\,H_2(g) \rightleftharpoons 2\,NH_3(g) \quad \Delta H = -91.8\,kJ$$

How would an increase in temperature affect the concentration of N_2 at equilibrium?

A) The concentration of N_2 will increase because of an increase in K_{eq}.
B) The concentration of N_2 will decrease because of an increase in K_{eq}.
C) The concentration of N_2 will increase because of a decrease in K_{eq}.
D) The concentration of N_2 will remain unchanged.

4. Na_2SO_4 is soluble in water. If $NaCl(s)$ is added to a solution of $Na_2SO_4(aq)$ so that the concentration of Na^+ doubles, then the:

A) solubility constant of Na_2SO_4 increases while that of NaCl decreases.
B) solubility constants of Na_2SO_4 and NaCl both decrease.
C) solubility of Na_2SO_4 and NaCl both decrease.
D) solubility of Na_2SO_4 decreases while that of NaCl increases.

5. The equilibrium expression below corresponds to which of the following reactions?

$$K_{eq} = \frac{(P_{SO_2})^2 \cdot P_{O_2}}{(P_{SO_3})^2}$$

A) $2\,SO_2(aq) + O_2(g) \rightleftharpoons 2\,SO_3(aq)$
B) $2\,SO_3(aq) \rightleftharpoons 2\,SO_2(aq) + O_2(g)$
C) $2\,SO_2(g) + O_2(g) \rightleftharpoons 2\,SO_3(g)$
D) $2\,SO_3(g) \rightleftharpoons 2\,SO_2(g) + O_2(g)$

6. Which of the following salts is least soluble in water?

A) PbI_2 ($K_{sp} = 7.9 \times 10^{-9}$)
B) $Mg(OH)_2$ ($K_{sp} = 6.3 \times 10^{-10}$)
C) $Zn(IO_3)_2$ ($K_{sp} = 3.9 \times 10^{-6}$)
D) SrF_2 ($K_{sp} = 2.6 \times 10^{-9}$)

7. The water solubility of $MgSO_4$ is approximately 25 g/100 mL at 20°C. Compared to a 0.25 g/mL solution of $MgSO_4$ prepared at 20°C, a 0.25 g/mL solution prepared at 37°C will:

A) dissolve faster and have the same concentration of ions in solution.
B) dissolve faster and have a higher concentration of ions in solution.
C) dissolve slower and have a lower concentration of ions in solution.
D) dissolve slower and have the same concentration of ions in solution.

8. If the K_{sp} of KI is 1.45×10^{-6} in propanol at 25°C, what would the K_{sp} of KI be in propane at the same temperature?

A) 1.84
B) 2.90×10^{-3}
C) 1.81×10^{-6}
D) 7.56×10^{-23}

9. The K_{sp} of NaCl in water is 35.9 at 25°C. If 500 mL of 12 M NaOH(aq) and 500 mL of 12 M HCl(aq) solution both at 25°C are combined, what would best describe the resulting solution?

A) A small amount of NaCl(s) would precipitate.
B) There will be a 6 M aqueous solution of NaCl.
C) Enthalpy and entropy would increase.
D) The resulting solution would be slightly basic.

CHAPTER 10 PRACTICE PASSAGE

Many caves trace their roots back to chemical principles. Some caves, called solutional caves, are formed as a result of acidic water flowing through rock such as limestone ($CaCO_3$, $K_{sp} = 3.4 \times 10^{-9}$ at 25°C). In this process limestone is dissolved, resulting in cave formation.

Solutional caves often contain spectacular rock formations. They are the products of equilibria involving water, carbon dioxide and limestone. The process begins when surface water flowing into the caves encounters soil with a higher P_{CO_2} than found in the atmosphere. This high CO_2 content is a result of CO_2 release from the earth's mantle, in a process called *outgassing*. Equation 1 describes the dissolution of CO_2 in water:

$$CO_2(g) + H_2O(l) \rightleftharpoons CO_2(aq) + H_2O(l)$$

Equation 1

Once solubilized, $CO_2(aq)$ causes the acidification of water via Equation 2:

$$CO_2(aq) + H_2O(l) \rightleftharpoons H_2CO_3(aq) \rightleftharpoons H_3O^+(aq) + HCO_3^-(aq)$$

Equation 2

The acidic water causes dissolution of limestone according to the following equilibrium:

$$CaCO_3(s) + H_3O^+(aq) \rightleftharpoons Ca^{2+}(aq) + HCO_3^-(aq) + H_2O(l)$$

Equation 3

When acidic solution finally flows through the roof and into the cave, it encounters ambient air with a lower P_{CO_2} than that in the soil. As such, dissolved $CO_2(aq)$ is released as a gas, eventually causing the precipitation of $CaCO_3(s)$. This precipitate forms *stalagmites*, an upward spike formed from water striking the ground in the cave, and *stalactites*, which are downward spikes created from water flowing down from the roofs toward the ground. Eventually, in a process that can take thousands of years, the two can meet to form a column in the cave.

1. A local factory accidentally pollutes groundwater supplies near a cave with $(NH_4)_2CO_3$. How would the cave most likely be affected?

   A) Stalagmite and stalactite formation would likely not be affected.
   B) Increased groundwater acidity would increase stalagmite and stalactite formation.
   C) Increased groundwater acidity would decrease stalagmite and stalactite formation.
   D) Cannot be determined from the information given.

2. As the ground temperature surrounding a cave increases, stalactite and stalagmite growth is found to decrease. What is the best explanation for this?

   A) Increased heat causes $CaCO_3$ to melt.
   B) Formation of stalactites and stalagmites is endothermic.
   C) Increasing temperature decreases the aqueous solubility of $CaCO_3$.
   D) The concentration of $CO_2(g)$ in water increases as temperature increases.

3. What is the approximate concentration of CO_3^{-2} when enough $CaCO_3(s)$ is dissolved in water to form a saturated solution?

   A) 2.5×10^{-9} M
   B) 5.0×10^{-9} M
   C) 6.0×10^{-5} M
   D) 1.0×10^{-4} M

4. Which of the following will form a buffer when combined with $CaCO_3(aq)$?

   A) $C_2H_4O_2$
   B) K_2CO_3
   C) $NaHCO_3$
   D) CO_2

5. The shape of the carbonate ion is:

A) trigonal planar and the carbon atom is sp^3 hybridized.
B) trigonal planar and the carbon atom is sp^2 hybridized.
C) tetrahedral and the carbon atom is sp^2 hybridized.
D) tetrahedral and the carbon atom is sp^3 hybridized.

6. A stalagmite in a cave suffers damage and researchers want it repaired naturally as quickly as possible. Which of the following will help this process?

A) Adding $CaCl_2$ to groundwater.
B) Adding chemical compounds in the cave that absorb CO_2 from the air.
C) Increasing the pH of the groundwater supply.
D) Spraying the stalagmite with compressed CO_2.

SOLUTIONS TO CHAPTER 10 FREESTANDING PRACTICE QUESTIONS

1. **D** Equilibrium constants are specific to a single temperature and standard state free energy change according to: $\Delta G° = -RT\ln K$. Altering temperature is the only answer choice that can change the reaction's K_{eq}.

2. **A** K_{eq} = [products]/[reactants] when both reactant and product concentrations are those at equilibrium. Q = [products]/[reactants] regardless of whether reactant and product concentrations are those at equilibrium. The addition of sodium acetate essentially translates into the addition of acetate ion, a product in this equilibrium. As a result of such an addition, $Q > K_{eq}$ and products are present in excess of equilibrium values. Le Châtelier's principle states that net reverse movement is created when the concentration of products is increased in an equilibrium system.

3. **C** Since the reaction is exothermic, an increase in temperature will shift the equilibrium to the left, and the concentration of N_2 will increase, eliminating choices B and D. For exothermic reactions, an increase in temperature will decrease the K_{eq}, eliminating choice A and making choice C the correct answer.

4. **C** Solubility constants, like all equilibrium constants, are functions of temperature only. This eliminates choices A and B. Given the equilibria:

$$Na_2SO_4(s) \rightleftharpoons 2\,Na^+\,(aq) + SO_4^{2-}\,(aq)$$
$$NaCl(s) \rightleftharpoons Na^+\,(aq) + Cl^-\,(aq)$$

    Na^+ is a common ion to both systems. Increasing Na^+ concentration will decrease the solubility of both salts, eliminating choice D and making choice C the best answer.

5. **D** The expression is in terms of partial pressure, so all components must be gaseous, eliminating choices A and B. An equilibrium expression has products in the numerator and reactants in the denominator, eliminating choice C. The exponents correspond to the stoichiometric coefficients of the balanced equation, so choice D is correct.

6. **B** All of the compounds are composed of one cation and two anions, so comparing K_{sp} values will give relative solubility. Since the question asks for an extreme, the middle values of the variable cannot be correct, eliminating choices A and D. The compound with the lowest K_{sp} value will have the lowest solubility because for all the compounds, K_{sp} = [cation][anion]^2. Therefore, choice B is correct.

7. **A** This is a two-by-two problem. First, consider rate. Any time temperature is increased, the reaction kinetics increase. In this case, the salt will dissolve faster, eliminating choices C and D. An increase in temperature generally causes an increase in the solubility of solids in liquids. However, both solutions contain the same amount of $MgSO_4$ that does not exceed the maximum solubility at either temperature. Therefore, the concentrations of ions will be the same, eliminating choice B.

8. **D** The golden rule of solubility is "like dissolves like." Potassium iodide is a salt held together by ionic forces and therefore comprised of charged ions. A salt will dissolve in a polar solvent better than a non-polar solvent. Propanol has a polar –OH group whereas propane is completely non-polar. Therefore, KI must have a smaller K_{sp} in propane than in propanol. The only answer that has a smaller K_{sp} value is choice D.

9. **B** Neutralizations are exothermic and form salt and water. The starting 500 mL solutions contain 6 moles each of NaOH and HCl. The final solution will be 1 L of 6 M NaCl(aq):

$$6\ HCl(aq) + 6\ NaOH(aq) \rightarrow 6\ NaCl(aq) + 6\ H_2O(l)$$

Although the reaction quotient of NaCl in this resulting solution will slightly exceed K_{sp}:

$$Q = [Na^+][Cl^-] = [6][6] = 36$$

the temperature will be significantly increased, allowing more NaCl to dissolve (K_{sp} will increase with temperature), eliminating choice A. Choice C is eliminated because enthalpy significantly decreases as heat is given off in this exothermic reaction. Choice D is eliminated because NaCl is a neutral salt.

SOLUTIONS TO CHAPTER 10 PRACTICE PASSAGE

1. **D** NH_4^+ is an acidic ion and CO_3^{2-} is a basic ion. Both could potentially affect the equilibrium described in Equation 3, so choice A seems unlikely. Although ammonium carbonate is a basic salt, eliminating choices B and C, this could not be determined without knowing the relative pK_b and pK_a values of NH_3 and HCO_3^- respectively. Given the rise in pH of groundwater and that CO_3^{2-} would likely have a common ion effect on the $CaCO_3$ solubility, less limestone would be expected to dissolve, leading to decreased formations in the cave.

2. **C** This question is best answered by Process of Elimination, because the answer is unexpected. $CaCO_3$ is an ionic compound with a melting point greater than 800°C, making choice A unlikely. If formation of stalactites and stalagmites were endothermic, increased temperature would favor their formation, eliminating choice B. Increased temperature decreases the concentration of dissolved gases in liquids, eliminating choice D. $CaCO_3$ is one of the exceptions to general solubility rules because its solubility in water actually decreases with increasing temperature. If less $CaCO_3$ gets dissolved, less will be available to precipitate in the cave as a stalactite or stalagmite.

3. **C** Calcium carbonate dissolves in water as follows:

$$CaCO_3(s) \rightleftharpoons Ca^{2+} + CO_3^{2-}$$

The K_{sp} defines the maximum solubility of a saturated solution. Solve the solubility expression for the maximum theoretical concentration of CO_3^{2-}:

$$K_{sp} = [Ca^{2+}][CO_3^{2-}]$$
$$3.4 \times 10^{-9} = [x][x]$$
$$x^2 = 34 \times 10^{-10}$$
$$x \approx 6 \times 10^{-5}M$$

4. **C** A buffer must contain a conjugate acid-base pair. CO_3^{2-} is a basic ion so adding the conjugate acid, HCO_3^-, would be required to form a buffer solution. $NaHCO_3^-$ will most readily supply this.

5. **B** The carbonate ion is trigonal planar and the carbon atom is sp^2 hybridized:

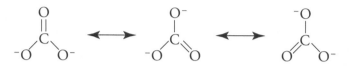

With three total substituents, the carbon atom cannot be sp^3 hybridized, eliminating choices A and D. Tetrahedral shapes require four substituents, eliminating choice C.

6. **B** According to the passage, increasing the amount of dissolved $CaCO_3$ that makes it to the ground/cave interface or maximizing the difference in ground and cave CO_2 levels will increase stalagmite formation. Choice A would decrease $CaCO_3$ solubility in groundwater by the common ion effect. Choice C would decrease $CaCO_3$ solubility in groundwater because the passage states acidic solutions dissolve $CaCO_3$. Choices B and D are opposite answers, which often means one is correct. The passage states that lower CO_2 levels in the cave compared to the leaking water lead to precipitation of $CaCO_3$. Therefore, choice D is eliminated and choice B is the best answer.

Chapter 11
Acids and Bases

11.1 DEFINITIONS

There are three different definitions of acids and bases.

Arrhenius Acids and Bases

Arrhenius gave us the most straightforward definitions of acids and bases, though they are the oldest and narrowest definitions so they are the least commonly used:

Acids ionize in water to produce hydrogen (H^+) ions.
Bases ionize in water to produce hydroxide (OH^-) ions.

For example, HCl is an acid,

$$HCl \rightarrow H^+ + Cl^-$$

and NaOH is a base:

$$NaOH \rightarrow Na^+ + OH^-$$

It's important to remember that H^+ does not exist by itself. Rather, it will combine with a molecule of water to give H_3O^+. However, for purposes of the MCAT, it doesn't matter which of the two you use: H^+ or H_3O^+.

Brønsted-Lowry Acids and Bases

Brønsted and Lowry offered the following definitions:

Acids are proton (H^+) donors.
Bases are proton (H^+) acceptors.

This definition of an acid is essentially the same idea as put forth by Arrhenius. The subtlety is apparent in their definition of a base. A Brønsted-Lowry base is a substance that is capable of accepting a proton. While hydroxide ions qualify as Brønsted-Lowry bases, many other compounds fit this definition as well.

If we consider the reversible reaction below:

$$H_2CO_3 + H_2O \rightleftharpoons H_3O^+ + HCO_3^-$$

then according to the Brønsted-Lowry definition, H_2CO_3 and H_3O^+ are acids; HCO_3^- and H_2O are bases. The Arrhenius and Brønsted-Lowry definitions of acid and bases are the most important ones for MCAT General Chemistry.

Lewis Acids and Bases

Lewis's definitions of acids and bases are the broadest of all:

> *Lewis acids are electron-pair acceptors.*
> *Lewis bases are electron-pair donors.*

If we consider the reversible reaction below:

$$AlCl_3 + H_2O \rightleftharpoons (AlCl_3OH)^- + H^+$$

then according to the Lewis definition, $AlCl_3$ and H^+ are acids because they accept electron pairs; H_2O and $(AlCl_3OH)^-$ are bases because they donate electron pairs. Lewis acid/base reactions frequently result in the formation of coordinate covalent bonds, as discussed in Chapter 5. For example, in the reaction above, water acts as a Lewis base since it donates both of the electrons involved in the coordinate covalent bond between OH^- and $AlCl_3$. $AlCl_3$ acts as a Lewis acid, since it accepts the electrons involved in this bond.

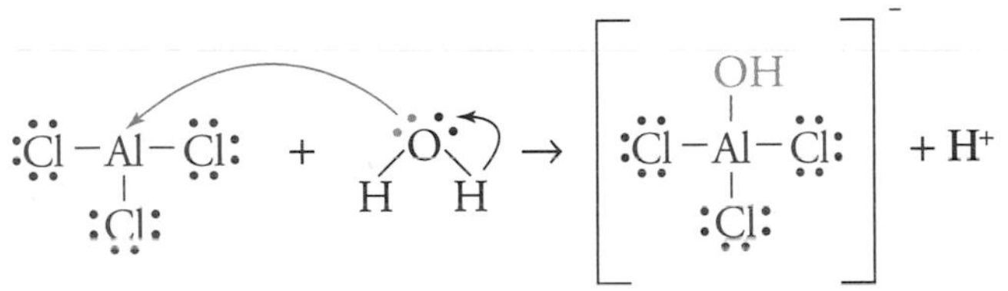

11.2 CONJUGATE ACIDS AND BASES

When a Brønsted-Lowry acid donates an H^+, the remaining structure is called the conjugate base of the acid. Likewise, when a Brønsted-Lowry base bonds with an H^+ in solution, this new species is called the **conjugate acid** of the base. To illustrate these definitions, consider this reaction:

acid–base conjugates

$$NH_3 + H_2O \rightleftharpoons NH_4^+ + OH^-$$

acid–base conjugates

Considering only the forward direction, NH_3 is the base and H_2O is the acid. The products are the conjugate acid and conjugate base of the reactants: NH_4^+ is the conjugate acid of NH_3, and OH^- is the conjugate base of H_2O:

acid ------------> conjugate base

$$NH_3 + H_2O \rightleftharpoons NH_4^+ + OH^-$$

base ------------> conjugate acid

Now consider the reverse reaction in which NH_4^+ is the acid and OH^- is the base. The conjugates are the same as for the forward reaction: NH_3 is the conjugate base of NH_4^+, and H_2O is the conjugate acid of OH^-:

$$\begin{array}{c} \text{conjugate} \\ \text{base} \longleftarrow \cdots \cdots \text{acid} \\ NH_3 + H_2O \rightleftharpoons NH_4^+ + OH^- \\ \text{conjugate} \\ \text{acid} \longleftarrow \cdots \cdots \text{base} \end{array}$$

The difference between a Brønsted-Lowry acid and its conjugate base is that the base is missing an H^+. The difference between a Brønsted-Lowry base and its conjugate acid is that the acid has an extra H^+.

forming conjugates:

$$\text{acid} \underset{+ H^+}{\overset{- H^+}{\rightleftharpoons}} \text{base}$$

Example 11-1: Which one of the following can behave as a Brønsted-Lowry acid but not a Lewis acid?

A) CF_4
B) $NaAlCl_4$
C) HF
D) Br_2

Solution: A Brønsted-Lowry acid donates an H^+, while a Lewis acid accepts a pair of electrons. Since a Brønsted-Lowry acid must have an H in the first place, only choice C can be the answer.

Example 11-2: What is the conjugate base of HBrO (hypobromous acid)?

A) H^+
B) H_2BrO_2
C) H_2BrO^+
D) BrO^-

Solution: To form the conjugate base of an acid, simply remove an H^+. Therefore, the conjugate base of HBrO is BrO^-, choice D.

11.3 THE STRENGTHS OF ACIDS AND BASES

Brønsted-Lowry acids can be placed into two big categories: *strong* and *weak*. Whether an acid is strong or weak depends on how completely it ionizes in water. A **strong** acid is one that dissociates completely (or very nearly so) in water; hydrochloric acid, HCl, is an example:

$$HCl(aq) + H_2O(l) \rightarrow H_3O^+(aq) + Cl^-(aq)$$

This reaction goes essentially to completion.

On the other hand, hydrofluoric acid, HF, is an example of a **weak** acid, since its dissociation in water,

$$HF(aq) + H_2O(l) \rightleftharpoons H_3O^+(aq) + F^-(aq)$$

does not go to completion; most of the HF remains undissociated.

If we use HA to denote a generic acid, its dissociation in water has the form

$$HA(aq) + H_2O(l) \rightleftharpoons H_3O^+(aq) + A^-(aq)$$

The strength of the acid is directly related to how much the products are favored over the reactants. The equilibrium expression for this reaction is

$$K_a = \frac{[H_3O^+][A^-]}{[HA]}$$

This is written as K_a, rather than K_{eq}, to emphasize that this is the equilibrium expression for an acid-dissociation reaction. In fact, K_a is known as the **acid-ionization** (or **acid-dissociation**) **constant** of the acid (HA). If $K_a > 1$, then the products are favored, and we say the acid is strong; if $K_a < 1$ then the reactants are favored and the acid is weak. We can also rank the relative strengths of acids by comparing their K_a values: The larger the K_a value, the stronger the acid; the smaller the K_a value, the weaker the acid.

The acids for which $K_a > 1$—the strong acids—are so few that you should memorize them:

Common Strong Acids	
Hydroiodic acid	HI
Hydrobromic acid	HBr
Hydrochloric acid	HCl
Perchloric acid	$HClO_4$
Sulfuric acid	H_2SO_4
Nitric acid	HNO_3

The values of K_a for these acids are so large that most tables of acid ionization constants don't even list them. On the MCAT, you may assume that any acid that's not in this list is a weak acid. (Other acids that fit the definition of *strong* are so uncommon that it's very unlikely they'd appear on the test. For example, $HClO_3$ has a pK_a of –1, and could be considered strong, but it is definitely one of the weaker strong acids and is not likely to appear on the MCAT.)

Example 11-3: In a 1 M aqueous solution of boric acid (H_3BO_3, $K_a = 5.8 \times 10^{-10}$), which of the following species will be present in solution in the greatest quantity?

A) H_3BO_3
B) $H_2BO_3^-$
C) HBO_3^{2-}
D) H_3O^+

Solution: The equilibrium here is $H_3BO_3(aq) + H_2O(l) \rightleftharpoons H_3O^+(aq) + H_2BO_3^-(aq)$. Boric acid is a weak acid (it's not on the list of strong acids), so the equilibrium lies to the left (also, notice how small its K_a value is). So, there'll be very few H_3O^+ or $H_2BO_3^-$ ions in solution but plenty of undissociated H_3BO_3. The answer is A.

Example 11-4: Of the following, which statement best explains why HF is a weak acid, but HCl, HBr, and HI are strong acids?

A) F has a greater ionization energy than Cl, Br, or I.
B) F has a larger radius than Cl, Br, or I.
C) F^- has a larger radius than Cl^-, Br^-, I^-.
D) F^- has a smaller radius than Cl^-, Br^-, I^-.

Solution: F is smaller than Cl, Br, or I (eliminating choices B and C). Ionization energy is associated with forming a cation from a neutral atom, and has no bearing here. Choice D is therefore correct. The more stable an acid's conjugate base is, the stronger the acid. Larger anions are better able to spread out their negative charge, making them more stable. HF is the weakest of the H-X acids because it has the least stable conjugate base due to its size.

Example 11-5: Of the following acids, which one would dissociate to the greatest extent (in water)?

A) HCN (hydrocyanic acid), $K_a = 6.2 \times 10^{-10}$
B) HNCO (cyanic acid), $K_a = 3.3 \times 10^{-4}$
C) HClO (hypochlorous acid), $K_a = 2.9 \times 10^{-8}$
D) HBrO (hypobromous acid), $K_a = 2.2 \times 10^{-9}$

Solution: The acid that would dissociate to the greatest extent would have the greatest K_a value. Of the choices given, HNCO (choice B) has the greatest K_a value.

We can apply the same ideas as above to identify strong and weak *bases*. If we use B to denote a generic base, its dissolution in water has the form

$$B(aq) + H_2O(l) \rightleftharpoons HB^+(aq) + OH^-(aq)$$

The strength of the base is directly related to how much the products are favored over the reactants. If we write the equilibrium constant for this reaction, we get

$$K_b = \frac{[HB^+][OH^-]}{[B]}$$

This is written as K_b, rather than K_{eq}, to emphasize that this is the equilibrium expression for a base-dissociation reaction. In fact, K_b is known as the **base-ionization** (or **base-dissociation**) **constant**. We can rank the relative strengths of bases by comparing their K_b values: The larger the K_b value, the stronger the base; the smaller the K_b value, the weaker the base.

For the MCAT and general chemistry, you should know about the following strong bases that may be used in aqueous solutions:

Common Strong Bases
Group 1 hydroxides (For example, NaOH)
Group 1 oxides (For example, Li_2O)
Some group 2 hydroxides ($Ba(OH)_2$, $Sr(OH)_2$, $Ca(OH)_2$)
Metal amides (For example, $NaNH_2$)

Weak bases include ammonia (NH_3) and amines, as well as the conjugate bases of many weak acids, as we'll discuss on the following page.

The Relative Strengths of Conjugate Acid-Base Pairs

Let's once again look at the dissociation of HCl in water:

$$HCl(aq) + H_2O(l) \rightarrow H_3O^+(aq) + Cl^-(aq)$$

no basic properties

The chloride ion (Cl^-) is the conjugate base of HCl. Since this reaction goes to completion, there must be no reverse reaction. Therefore, Cl^- has no tendency to accept a proton and thus does not act as a base. The conjugate base of a strong acid has no basic properties in water.

On the other hand, hydrofluoric acid, HF, is a weak acid since its dissociation is not complete:

$$HF(aq) + H_2O(l) \rightleftharpoons H_3O^+(aq) + F^-(aq)$$

Since the reverse reaction does take place to a significant extent, the conjugate base of HF, the fluoride ion, F^-, *does* have some tendency to accept a proton, and so behaves as a weak base. The conjugate base of a weak acid is a weak base.

In fact, the weaker the acid, the more the reverse reaction is favored, and the stronger its conjugate base. For example, hydrocyanic acid (HCN) has a K_a value of about 5×10^{-10}, which is much smaller than that of hydrofluoric acid ($K_a \approx 7 \times 10^{-4}$). Therefore, the conjugate base of HCN, the cyanide ion, CN^-, is a stronger base than F^-.

The same ideas can be applied to bases:

1) The conjugate acid of a strong base has no acidic properties in water. For example, the conjugate acid of LiOH is Li^+, which does not act as an acid in water.
2) The conjugate acid of a weak base is a weak acid (and the weaker the base, the stronger the conjugate acid). For example, the conjugate acid of NH_3 is NH_4^+, which is a weak acid.

Example 11-6: Of the following anions, which is the strongest base?

A) I^-
B) CN^-
C) NO_3^-
D) Br^-

Solution: Here's another way to ask the same question: Which of the following anions has the weakest conjugate acid? Since HI, HNO_3, and HBr are all strong acids, while HCN is a weak acid, CN^- (choice B) has the weakest conjugate acid, and is thus the strongest base.

Example 11-7: Of the following, which acid has the weakest conjugate base?

A) $HClO_4$
B) HCOOH
C) H_3PO_4
D) H_2CO_3

Solution: Here's another way to ask the same question: Which of the following acids is the strongest? Thought about this way, the answer's easy. Perchloric acid, choice A, is the only strong acid in the list.

Amphoteric Substances

Take a look at the dissociation of carbonic acid (H_2CO_3), a weak acid:

$$H_2CO_3(aq) + H_2O(l) \rightleftharpoons H_3O^+(aq) + HCO_3^-(aq) \quad (K_a = 4.5 \times 10^{-7})$$

The conjugate base of carbonic acid is HCO_3^-, which also has an ionizable proton. Carbonic acid is said to be **polyprotic**, because it has more than one proton to donate.

Let's look at how the conjugate base of carbonic acid dissociates:

$$HCO_3^-(aq) + H_2O(l) \rightleftharpoons H_3O^+(aq) + CO_3^{2-}(aq) \quad (K_a = 4.8 \times 10^{-11})$$

In the first reaction, HCO_3^- acts as a base, but in the second reaction it acts as an acid. Whenever a substance can act as either an acid or a base, we say that it is **amphoteric**. The conjugate base of a weak polyprotic acid is always amphoteric, because it can either donate or accept another proton. Also notice that HCO_3^- is a weaker acid than H_2CO_3; in general, every time a polyprotic acid donates a proton, the resulting species will be a weaker acid than its predecessor.

11.4   THE ION-PRODUCT CONSTANT OF WATER

Water is amphoteric. It reacts with itself in a Brønsted-Lowry acid-base reaction, one molecule acting as the acid, the other as the base:

$$H_2O(l) + H_2O(l) \rightleftharpoons H_3O^+(aq) + OH^-(aq)$$

This is called the autoionization (or self-ionization) of water. The equilibrium expression is

$$K_w = [H_3O^+][OH^-]$$

This is written as K_w, rather than K_{eq}, to emphasize that this is the equilibrium expression for the autoionization of _water_; K_w is known as the ion-product constant of water. Only a very small fraction of the water molecules will undergo this reaction, and it's known that at 25°C,

$$K_w = 1.0 \times 10^{-14}$$

(Like all other equilibrium constants, K_w varies with temperature; it increases as the temperature increases. However, because 25°C is so common, this is the value you should memorize.) Since the number of H_3O^+ ions in pure water will be equal to the number of OH^- ions, if we call each of their concentrations x, then $x^2 = K_w$, which gives $x = 1 \times 10^{-7}$. That is, the concentration of both types of ions in pure water is 1×10^{-7} M. (In addition, K_w is constant at a given temperature, regardless of the H_3O^+ concentration.)

If the introduction of an acid increases the concentration of H_3O^+ ions, then the equilibrium is disturbed, and the reverse reaction is favored, decreasing the concentration of OH^- ions. Similarly, if the introduction of a base increases the concentration of OH^- ions, then the equilibrium is again disturbed; the reverse reaction is favored, decreasing the concentration of H_3O^+ ions. However, in either case, the product of $[H_3O^+]$ and $[OH^-]$ will remain equal to K_w.

For example, suppose we add 0.002 moles of HCl to water to create a 1-liter solution. Since the dissociation of HCl goes to completion (it's a strong acid), it will create 0.002 moles of H_3O^+ ions, so $[H_3O^+] = 0.002$ M. Since H_3O^+ concentration has been increased, we expect the OH^- concentration to decrease, which it does:

$$[OH^-] = \frac{K_w}{[H_3O^+]} = \frac{1 \times 10^{-14}}{2 \times 10^{-3}} = 5 \times 10^{-12} \, M$$

11.5 pH

The pH scale measures the concentration of H^+ (or H_3O^+) ions in a solution. Because the molarity of H^+ tends to be quite small and can vary over many orders of magnitude, the pH scale is logarithmic:

$$pH = -\log[H^+]$$

This formula implies that $[H^+] = 10^{-pH}$. Since $[H^+] = 10^{-7}$ M in pure water, the pH of water is 7. At 25°C, this defines a pH neutral solution. If $[H^+]$ is greater than 10^{-7} M, then the pH will be less than 7, and the solution is said to be acidic. If $[H^+]$ is less than 10^{-7} M, the pH will be greater than 7, and the solution is basic (or alkaline). Notice that a *low* pH means a *high* $[H^+]$ and the solution is *acidic*; a *high* pH means a *low* $[H^+]$ and the solution is basic.

pH > 7	basic solution
pH = 7	neutral solution
pH < 7	acidic solution

The range of the pH scale for most solutions falls between 0 and 14, but some strong acids and bases extend the scale past this range. For example, a 10 M solution of HCl will fully dissociate into H^+ and Cl^-. Therefore, the $[H^+] = 10$ M, and the pH = –1.

An alternate measurement expresses the acidity or basicity in terms of the hydroxide ion concentration, $[OH^-]$, by using pOH. The same formula applies for hydroxide ions as for hydrogen ions.

$$pOH = -\log[OH^-]$$

This formula implies that $[OH^-] = 10^{-pOH}$.

Acids and bases are inversely related: the greater the concentration of H^+ ions, the lower the concentration of OH^- ions, and vice versa. Since $[H^+][OH^-] = 10^{-14}$ at 25°C, the values of pH and pOH satisfy a special relationship at 25°C:

$$pH + pOH = 14$$

So, if you know the pOH of a solution, you can find the pH, and vice versa. For example, if the pH of a solution is 5, then the pOH must be 9. If the pOH of a solution is 2, then the pH must be 12.

On the MCAT, it will be helpful to be able to figure out the pH even in cases where the H^+ concentration isn't exactly equal to the whole-number power of 10. In general, if y is a number between 1 and 10, and you're told that $[H^+] = y \times 10^{-n}$ (where n is a whole number) then the pH will be between $(n-1)$ and n. For example, if $[H^+] = 6.2 \times 10^{-5}$, then the pH is between 4 and 5.

Relationships Between Conjugates

pK_a and pK_b

The definitions of pH and pOH both involved the opposite of a logarithm. In general, "p" of something is equal to the –log of that something. Therefore, the following definitions won't be surprising:

$$pK_a = -\log K_a$$

$$pK_b = -\log K_b$$

Because H$^+$ concentrations are generally very small and can vary over such a wide range, the pH scale gives us more convenient numbers to work with. The same is true for pK_a and pK_b. Remember that the larger the K_a value, the stronger the acid. Since "p" means "take the negative log of…," the *lower* the pK_a value, the stronger the acid. For example, acetic acid (CH$_3$COOH) has a K_a of 1.75×10^{-5}, and hypochlorous acid (HClO) has a K_a of 2.9×10^{-8}. Since the K_a of acetic acid is larger than that of hypochlorous acid, we know this means that more molecules of acetic acid than hypochlorous acid will dissociate into ions in aqueous solution. In other words, acetic acid is stronger than hypochlorous acid. The pK_a of acetic acid is 4.8, and the pK_a of hypochlorous acid is 7.5. The acid with the lower pK_a value is the stronger acid. The same logic applies to pK_b: the lower the pK_b value, the stronger the base.

K_a and K_b

Let's now look at the relationship between the K_a and the K_b for an acid-base conjugate pair by working through an example question. Let K_a be the acid-dissociation constant for formic acid (HCOOH) and let K_b stand for the base-dissociation constant of its conjugate base (the formate ion, HCOO$^-$). If K_a is equal to 5.6×10^{-11}, what is $K_a \times K_b$?

The equilibrium for the dissociation of HCOOH is

$$HCOOH(aq) + H_2O(l) \rightleftharpoons H_3O^+(aq) + HCOO^-(aq)$$

so

$$K_a = \frac{[H_3O^+][HCOO^-]}{[HCOOH]}$$

The equilibrium for the dissociation of HCOO$^-$ is

$$HCOO^-(aq) + H_2O(l) \rightleftharpoons HCOOH(aq) + OH^-(aq)$$

so

$$K_b = \frac{[HCOOH][OH^-]}{[HCOO^-]}$$

Therefore,

$$K_a K_b = \frac{[H_3O^+][HCOO^-]}{[HCOOH]} \times \frac{[HCOOH][OH^-]}{[HCOO^-]} = [H_3O^+][OH^-]$$

We now immediately recognize this product as K_w, the ion-product constant of water, whose value (at 25°C) is 1×10^{-14}.

This calculation wasn't special for HCOOH; we can see that the same thing will happen for any acid and its conjugate base. So, for any acid-base conjugate pair, we'll have

$$K_a K_b = K_w = 1 \times 10^{-14}$$

This gives us a way to quantitatively relate the strength of an acid and its conjugate base. For example, the value of K_a for HF is about 7×10^{-4}; therefore, the value of K_b for its conjugate base, F^-, is about 1.4×10^{-11}. For HCN, $K_a \approx 5 \times 10^{-10}$, so K_b for CN^- is 2×10^{-5}.

It also follows from our definitions and logarithm algebra that for an acid-base conjugate pair at 25°C, we'll have

$$pK_a + pK_b = 14$$

Example 11-8: Of the following liquids, which one contains the lowest concentration of H_3O^+ ions?

A) Lemon juice (pH = 2.3)
B) Blood (pH = 7.4)
C) Seawater (pH = 8.5)
D) Coffee (pH = 5.1)

Solution: Since $pH = -\log [H_3O^+]$, we know that $[H_3O^+] = 1/10^{pH}$. This fraction is smallest when the pH is greatest. Of the choices given, seawater (choice C) has the highest pH.

Example 11-9: What is the pH of a solution at 25°C whose hydroxide ion concentration is 1×10^{-4} M?

Solution: Since $pOH = -\log[OH^-]$, we know that $pOH = 4$. Therefore, the pH is 10.

Example 11-10: Orange juice has a pH of 3.5. What is its $[H^+]$?

Solution: Because $pH = -\log[H^+]$, we know that $[H^+] = 10^{-pH}$. For orange juice, then, we have $[H^+] = 10^{-3.5} = 10^{0.5-4} = 10^{0.5} \times 10^{-4} = \sqrt{10} \times 10^{-4} \approx 3.2 \times 10^{-4}$ M.

Example 11-11: If 99% of the H_3O^+ ions are removed from a solution whose pH was originally 3, what will be its new pH?

Solution: If 99% of the H_3O^+ ions are removed, then only 1% remain. This means that the number of H_3O^+ ions is now only 1/100 of the original. If $[H_3O^+]$ is decreased by a factor of 100, then the pH is *increased* by 2—to pH 5 in this case—since $\log 100 = 2$.

Example 11-12: Given that the self-ionization of water is endothermic, what is the value of the sum pH + pOH at 50°C?

$$H_2O(l) + H_2O(l) \rightleftharpoons H_3O^+(aq) + OH^-(aq)$$

A)   Less than 14
B)   Equal to 14
C)   Greater than 14
D)   Cannot determine from the information given

Solution: This is a Le Châtelier's principle question in disguise. Imagine we start at equilibrium at 25°C; which way would the self-ionization reaction shift if we increase the temperature to 50°C? Since the question tells us this reaction is endothermic, we can consider heat as one of the reactants, and therefore an increase in temperature would cause the system to shift to the right. Shifting to the right means that at equilibrium, [H⁺] and [OH⁻] will increase. So pH and pOH will both be *lower* than 7 at 50°C, and the sum of pH and pOH will be less than 14 at 50°C. Choice A is the correct answer.

pH Calculations

For Strong Acids

Strong acids dissociate completely, so the hydrogen ion concentration will be the same as the concentration of the acid. That means that you can calculate the pH directly from the molarity of the solution. For example, a 0.01 M solution of HCl will have [H⁺] = 0.01 M and pH = 2.

For Weak Acids

Weak acids come to equilibrium with their dissociated ions. In fact, for a weak acid at equilibrium, the concentration of undissociated acid will be much greater than the concentration of hydrogen ion. To get the pH of a weak acid solution, you need to use the equilibrium expression.

Let's say you add 0.2 mol of HCN (hydrocyanic acid, a weak acid) to water to create a 1-liter solution, and you want to find the pH. Initially, [HCN] = 0.2 M, and none of it has dissociated. If x moles of HCN are dissociated at equilibrium, then the equilibrium concentration of HCN is 0.2 − x. Now, since each molecule of HCN dissociates into one H⁺ ion and one CN⁻ ion, if x moles of HCN have dissociated, there'll be x moles of H⁺ and x moles of CN⁻:

	HCN	$\rightleftharpoons$	H⁺	+	CN
initial:	0.2 M		0 M		0 M
at equilibrium:	(0.2 − x) M		x M		x M

(Actually, the initial concentration of H^+ is 10^{-7} M, but it's so small that it can be neglected for this calculation.) Our goal is to find x, because once we know $[H^+]$, we'll know the pH. So, we set up the equilibrium expression:

$$K_a = \frac{[H^+][CN^-]}{[HCN]} = \frac{x^2}{0.2 - x}$$

11.5

It's known that the value of K_a for HCN is 4.9×10^{-10}. Because the K_a is so small, not that much of the HCN is going to dissociate. (This assumption, that x added to or subtracted from a number is negligible, is always a good one when $K < 10^{-4}$ [the usual case found on the MCAT].) That is, we can assume that x is going to be a very small number, insignificant compared to 0.2; therefore, the value $(0.2 - x)$ is almost exactly the same as 0.2. By substituting 0.2 for $(0.2 - x)$, we can solve the equation above for x:

$$\frac{x^2}{0.2} \approx 4.9 \times 10^{-10}$$
$$x^2 \approx 1 \times 10^{-10}$$
$$\therefore x \approx 1 \times 10^{-5}$$

Since $[H^+]$ is approximately 1×10^{-5} M, the pH is about 5.

We simplified the computation by assuming that the concentration of hydrogen ion $[H^+]$ was insignificant compared to the concentration of undissociated acid $[HCN]$. Since it turned out that $[H^+] \approx 10^{-5}$ M, which is much less than $[HCN] = 0.2$ M, our assumption was valid. On the MCAT, you should always simplify the math wherever possible.

Example 11-13: If 0.7 mol of benzoic acid (C_6H_5COOH, $K_a = 6.6 \times 10^{-5}$) is added to water to create a 1-liter solution, what will be the pH?

Solution: Initially $[C_6H_5COOH] = 0.7$ M, and none of it has dissociated. If x moles of C_6H_5COOH are dissociated at equilibrium, then the equilibrium concentration of C_6H_5COOH is $0.7 - x$. Now, since each molecule of C_6H_5COOH dissociates into one H^+ ion and one $C_6H_5COO^-$ ion, if x moles of C_6H_5COOH have dissociated, there'll be x moles of H^+ and x moles of $C_6H_5COO^-$:

	C_6H_5COOH	$\rightleftharpoons$	H^+	+	$C_6H_5COO^-$
initial:	0.7 M		0 M		0 M
at equilibrium:	$(0.7 - x)$ M		x M		x M

(Again, the initial concentration of H^+ is 10^{-7} M, but it's so small that it can be neglected.) Our goal is to find x, because once we know $[H^+]$, we'll know the pH. So, we set up the equilibrium expression:

$$K_a = \frac{[H^+][C_6H_5COO^-]}{[C_6H_5COOH]} = \frac{x^2}{0.7 - x} \approx \frac{x^2}{0.7}$$

and then solve the equation for x:

$$\frac{x^2}{0.7} \approx 6.6 \times 10^{-5}$$
$$x^2 \approx 4.6 \times 10^{-5} = 46 \times 10^{-6}$$
$$\therefore x \approx 7 \times 10^{-3}$$

Since $[H^+]$ is approximately $7 \times 10^{-3}\ M \approx 10^{-2}\ M$, the pH is a little more than 2, say 2.2.

11.6 NEUTRALIZATION REACTIONS

When an acid and a base are combined, they will react in what is called a **neutralization reaction**. Often-times this reaction will produce a salt and water. Here's an example:

$$HCl\ +\ NaOH\ \rightarrow\ NaCl\ +\ H_2O$$

acid   base   salt   water

This type of reaction takes place when, for example, you take an antacid to relieve excess stomach acid. The antacid is a weak base, usually carbonate, that reacts in the stomach to neutralize acid.

If a strong acid and strong base react (as in the example above), the resulting solution will be pH neutral (which is why we call it a neutralization reaction). However, if the reaction involves a weak acid or weak base, the resulting solution will generally not be pH neutral.

No matter how weak an acid or base is, when mixed with an equimolar amount of a strong base or acid, we can expect complete neutralization. It has been found experimentally that all neutralizations have the same exothermic "heat of neutralization," the energy released from the reaction that is the same for all neutralizations: $H^+ + OH^- \rightarrow H_2O$.

As you can see from the reaction above, equal molar amounts of HCl and NaOH are needed to complete the neutralization. To determine just how much base (B) to add to an acidic solution (or how much acid (A) to add to a basic solution) in order to cause complete neutralization, we just use the following formula:

$$a \times [A] \times V_A = b \times [B] \times V_B$$

where a is the number of acidic hydrogens per formula unit and b is a constant that tells us how many H_3O^+ ions the base can accept.

For example, let's calculate how much 0.1 M NaOH solution is needed to neutralize 40 mL of a 0.3 M HCl solution:

$$V_B = \frac{a \times [A] \times V_A}{b \times [B]} = \frac{1 \times (0.3M) \times (40mL)}{1 \times (0.1M)} = 120\ mL$$

Example 11-14: Binary mixtures of equal moles of which of the following acid-base combinations will lead to a complete (99+%) neutralization reaction?

    I.   HCl and NaOH
    II.   HF and NH_3
   III. HNO_3 and $NaHCO_3$

    A)   I only
    B)   I and II only
    C)   II and III only
    D)   I, II, and III

Solution: Remember, regardless of the strengths of the acids and bases, all neutralization reactions go to completion. Choice D is the correct answer.

11.7

11.7   HYDROLYSIS OF SALTS

A **salt** is an ionic compound, consisting of a cation and an anion. In water, the salt dissociates into ions, and depending on how these ions react with water, the resulting solution will be either acidic, basic, or pH neutral. To make the prediction, we notice that there are essentially two possibilities for both the cation and the anion in a salt:

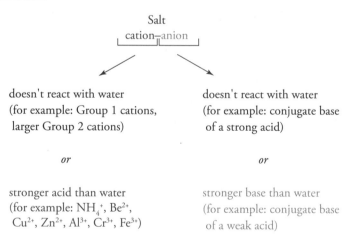

Whether the salt solution will be acidic, basic, or pH neutral depends on which combination of possibilities (four total) from the diagram above applies. The reaction of a substance—such as a salt or an ion—with water is called a hydrolysis reaction, a more general use of the term since the water molecule may not be split. Let's look at some examples.

If we dissolve NaCl in water, Na^+ and Cl^- ions go into solution. Na^+ ions are Group 1 ions and do not react with water. Since Cl^- is the conjugate base of a strong acid (HCl), it also doesn't react with water. These ions just become hydrated (surrounded by water molecules). Therefore, the solution will be pH neutral.

How about NH_4Cl? In solution it will break into NH_4^+ and Cl^-. The ammonium ion is a stronger acid than water (it's the conjugate acid of NH_3, a weak base), and Cl^- will not react with water. As a result, a solution of this salt will be acidic and have a pH less than 7, and NH_4Cl is called an acidic salt.

Now let's consider sodium acetate, $Na(CH_3COO)$. In solution it will break into Na^+ and CH_3COO^-. Na^+ is a Group 1 cation and does not react with water. However, CH_3COO^- is a stronger base than water since it's the conjugate base of acetic acid (CH_3COOH), a weak acid. Therefore, a solution of the salt will be basic and have a pH greater than 7, and $NaCH_3COO$ is a basic salt.

Finally, let's consider NH_4CN. In solution it will break into NH_4^+ and CN^-. NH_4^+ is a stronger acid than water, and CN^- is a stronger base than water (it's the conjugate base of HCN, a weak acid). So, which one wins? In a case like this, we need to know the K_a value for the reaction of the cation with water with the K_b value for the reaction of the anion with water and compare these values. Since

$$NH_4^+(aq) + H_2O(l) \rightleftharpoons NH_3(aq) + H_3O^+(aq) \quad (K_a = 6.3 \times 10^{-10})$$

$$CN^-(aq) + H_2O(l) \rightleftharpoons HCN(aq) + OH^-(aq) \quad (K_b = 1.6 \times 10^{-5})$$

we see that in this case K_b of $CN^- > K_a$ of NH_4^+, so the forward reaction of the second reaction will dominate the forward reaction of the first reaction, and the solution will be basic.

Example 11-15: Which of the following salts will produce a basic solution when added to pure water?

A)   KCl
B)   NaClO
C) NH_4Cl
D) $MgBr_2$

Solution: NaClO (choice B) will dissociate into Na^+ and ClO^-. Na^+ is a Group 1 cation, so it has no effect on the pH. However, ClO^-, the hypochlorite ion, is the conjugate base of a weak acid, HClO (hypochlorous acid). Therefore, the solution will be basic. The salt in choices A will have no effect on the pH, and the salts in choice C and D will leave the solution acidic (since NH_4^+ is the conjugate acid of a weak base, NH_3, and Mg^{2+} will react with water to form the weak base $Mg(OH)_2$).

Example 11-16: Which of the following is an acidic salt?

A) KNO_3
B) $SrCl_2$
C) $CuCl_2$
D) $Ba(CH_3COO)_2$

Solution: Cu^{2+} is a stronger acid than water, so $CuCl_2$ (choice C) is an acidic salt. The salts in choices A and B are neither acidic nor basic, and choice D is a basic salt.

11.8 BUFFER SOLUTIONS

A **buffer** is a solution that resists changing pH when a small amount of acid or base is added. The buffering capacity comes from the presence of a weak acid and its conjugate base (or a weak base and its conjugate acid) in roughly equal concentrations.

One type of buffer is made from a weak acid and a salt of its conjugate base. To illustrate how a buffer works, let's look at a specific example and add 0.1 mol of acetic acid (CH_3COOH) and 0.1 mol of sodium acetate ($NaCH_3COO$) to water to obtain a 1-liter solution. Since acetic acid is a weak acid ($K_a = 1.75 \times 10^{-5}$), it will partially dissociate to give some acetate (CH_3COO^-) ions. However, the salt is soluble and will dissociate completely to give plenty of acetate ions. The addition of this common ion will shift the acid dissociation to the left, so the equilibrium concentrations of undissociated acetic acid molecules and acetate ions will be essentially equal to their initial concentrations, 0.1 M.

$$CH_3COOH + H_2O \rightleftharpoons H_3O^+ + CH_3COO^-$$

Since buffer solutions are designed to resist changes in pH, let's first figure out the pH of this solution. Writing the expression for the equilibrium constant gives

$$K_a = \frac{[H_3O^+][CH_3COO^-]}{[CH_3COOH]}$$

which we can solve for $[H_3O^+]$:

$$[H_3O^+] = \frac{K_a[CH_3COOH]}{[CH_3COO^-]} \qquad \text{(Equation 1)}$$

Since the equilibrium concentrations of both CH_3COOH and CH_3COO^- are 0.1 M, this equation tells us that

$$[H_3O^+] = \frac{K_a[CH_3COOH]}{[CH_3COO^-]} = \frac{K_a(0.1M)}{0.1M} = 1.75 \times 10^{-5}$$

and pH = $-\log[H_3O^+]$, so

$$pH = -\log(1.75 \times 10^{-5})$$
$$pH = 4.76$$

Okay, now let's see what happens if we add a little bit of strong acid—HCl, for example. If we add, say, 0.005 mol of HCl, it will dissociate completely in solution into 0.005 mol of H^+ ions and 0.005 mol of Cl^- ions. The Cl^- ions will have no effect on the equilibrium, but the added H^+ (or H_3O^+) ions will. Adding a product shifts the equilibrium to the left, and the acetate ions react with the additional H_3O^+ ions to produce additional acetic acid molecules. As a result, the concentration of acetate ions will drop by 0.005, from 0.1 M to 0.095 M; the concentration of acetic acid will increase by 0.005, from 0.1 M to 0.105 M. Let's now use Equation (1) above to find the new pH:

$$[H_3O^+] = \frac{K_a[CH_3COOH]}{[CH_3COO^-]} = \frac{K_a(0.105\ M)}{0.095\ M} = 1.75 \times 10^{-5}(1.105) = 1.93 \times 10^{-5}$$

11.8

and

$$pH = -\log(1.93 \times 10^{-5})$$
$$pH = 4.71$$

Notice that the pH dropped from 4.76 to 4.71, a decrease of just 0.05. If we had added this HCl to a liter of pure water, the pH would have dropped from 7 to 2.3, a *much* larger decrease! The buffer solution we created was effective at resisting a large drop in pH because it had enough base (in the form of acetate ions in this case) to neutralize the added acid.

Now let's see what happens if we add a little bit of strong base—KOH, for example. If we add, say, 0.005 mol of KOH, it will dissociate completely in solution into 0.005 mol of K^+ ions and 0.005 mol of OH^- ions. The K^+ ions will have no effect, but the added OH^- ions will shift the equilibrium to the right, since they'll react with acetic acid molecules to produce more acetate ions ($CH_3COOH + OH^- \rightarrow CH_3COO^- + H_2O$). As a result, the concentration of acetic acid will drop by 0.005, from 0.1 M to 0.095 M; the concentration of acetate ions will increase by 0.005, from 0.1 M to 0.105 M. Let's again use Equation (1) above to find the new pH:

$$[H_3O^+] = \frac{K_a[CH_3COOH]}{[CH_3COO^-]} = \frac{K_a(0.095\ M)}{0.105\ M} = 1.75 \times 10^{-5}(0.905) = 1.58 \times 10^{-5}$$

11.8

and

$$pH = -\log(1.58 \times 10^{-5})$$
$$pH = 4.80$$

Notice that the pH increased from 4.76 to 4.80, an increase of just 0.04. If we had added this KOH to a liter of pure water, the pH would have increased from 7 to 11.7, a much larger increase! The buffer solution we created was effective at resisting a large rise in pH because it had enough acid to neutralize the added base.

If we generalize Equation (1) to any buffer solution containing a weak acid and a salt of its conjugate base, we get $[H_3O^+] = K_a([\text{weak acid}]/[\text{conjugate base}])$. Taking the $-\log$ of both sides give us the

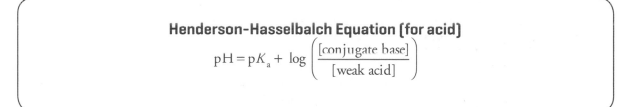

Henderson-Hasselbalch Equation (for acid)

$$pH = pK_a + \log\left(\frac{[\text{conjugate base}]}{[\text{weak acid}]}\right)$$

To design a buffer solution, we choose a weak acid whose pK_a is as close to the desired pH as possible. An ideal buffer would have [weak acid] = [conjugate base], so pH = pK_a. If no weak acid has the exact pK_a needed, just adjust the initial concentrations of the weak acid and conjugate base accordingly.

We can also design a buffer solution by choosing a weak base (and a salt of its conjugate acid) such that the pK_b value of the base is as close to the desired pOH as possible. The version of the Henderson-Hasselbalch equation in this situation looks like this:

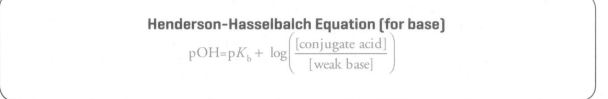

Henderson-Hasselbalch Equation (for base)

$$pOH = pK_b + \log\left(\frac{[\text{conjugate acid}]}{[\text{weak base}]}\right)$$

Example 11-17: Which of the following compounds could be added to a solution of HCN to create a buffer?

A) HNO_3
B) $CaCl_2$
C) $NaCN$
D) KOH

Solution: HCN is a weak acid, so we'd look for a salt of its conjugate base, CN^-. Choice C, NaCN, is such a salt.

Example 11-18: As hydrogen ions are added to an acidic buffer solution, what happens to the concentrations of undissociated acid and conjugate base?

Solution: The conjugate base, A^-, reacts with the added H^+ to form HA, so the conjugate base decreases and the undissociated acid increases.

Example 11-19: As hydrogen ions are added to an alkaline buffer solution, what happens to the concentrations of base and conjugate acid?

Solution: The base, B, reacts with the added H^+ to form HB^+, so the base decreases and the conjugate acid increases.

11.9 INDICATORS

An **indicator** is a weak acid that undergoes a color change when it's converted to its conjugate base. Let HA denote a generic indicator. In its non-ionized form, it has a particular color, which we'll call color #1. When it has donated a proton to become its conjugate base, A^-, it has a different color, which we'll call color #2.

Indicator

$$HA + H_2O \rightleftharpoons H_3O^+ + A^-$$

color #1   color #2

11.9

Under what conditions would an indicator change its color? What if an indicator were added to an acidic solution—that is, one whose pH were quite low due to a high concentration of H_3O^+ ions? Then according to Le Châtelier, the indicator's equilibrium would shift to the left, and the indicator would display color #1. Conversely, if the indicator were added to a basic solution (that is, one with plenty of OH^- ions), the amount of H_3O^+ would decrease, and the indicator's equilibrium would be shifted to the right, causing it to display color #2. We can make this discussion a little more precise.

Take the expression for the indicator's equilibrium constant, $K_a = [H_3O^+][A^-]/[HA]$ and easily rearrange it into

$$\frac{[H_3O^+]}{K_a} = \frac{[HA]}{[A^-]}$$

Written this way, we can see that

- If $[H_3O^+] \gg K_a$, then $[HA] \gg [A^-]$, so we'd see color #1.
- If $[H_3O^+] \approx K_a$, then $[HA] \approx [A^-]$, so we'd see a mix of colors #1 & #2.
- If $[H_3O^+] \ll K_a$, then $[HA] \ll [A^-]$, so we'd see color #2.

Note that the indicator changes color within a fairly short pH range, about 2 units:

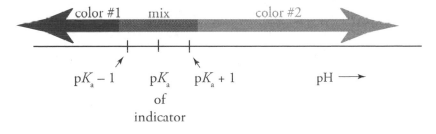

Therefore, if we want our indicator to be useful, we need to select one whose pK_a value is convenient for our purposes. For example, phenolphthalein is an indicator with a pK_a value of about 9.0. When added to a solution whose pH is less than 8, it remains colorless. However, if the solution's pH is above 10, it will turn red. (For $8 < pH < 10$, the solution will be pink.) Thus, phenolphthalein can be used to differentiate between a solution whose pH is, say, 7 from one whose pH is 11. However, the indicator methyl orange could not distinguish between two such solutions: It would be yellow at pH 7 and yellow at pH 11. Methyl orange has a pK_a of about 3.8, so it changes color around pH 4.

Note: The $pK_a \pm 1$ range for an indicator's color change is convenient and typical, but it's not a hard-and-fast rule. Some indicators (like methyl orange) have a color-change range of only 1.2 (rather than 2) pH units. Also, some indicators have more than just two colors. Polyprotic indicators, like thymol blue and bromocesol green, can change color more than once, and can therefore exhibit more than two distinct colors.

11.10 ACID-BASE TITRATIONS

An **acid-base titration** is an experimental technique used to determine the identity of an unknown weak acid (or weak base) by determining its pK_a (or pK_b). Titrations can also be used to determine the concentration of *any* acid or base solution (whether it be known or unknown). The procedure consists of adding a strong acid (or a strong base) of *known* identity and concentration—the **titrant**—to a solution containing the unknown base (or acid). (One never titrates an acid with an acid or a base with a base.) While the titrant is added in small, discrete amounts, the pH of the solution is recorded (with a pH meter).

If we plot the data points (the pH value vs. the volume of titrant added), we obtain a graph called a titration curve. Let's consider a specific example: the titration of HF (a weak acid) with NaOH (a strong base).

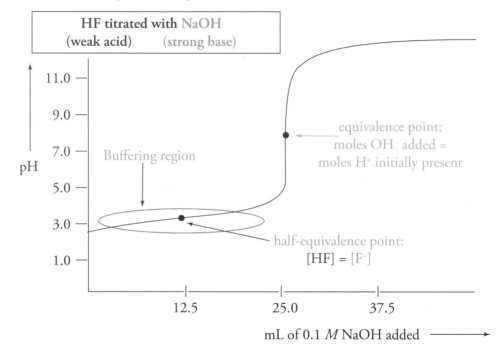

When the amount of titrant added is 0, the pH is of course just the pH of the original, pure solution of HF. Then, as NaOH is added, an equivalent amount of HF will be neutralized according to the reaction

$$NaOH + HF \rightarrow Na^+ + F^- + H_2O$$

As HF is neutralized, the pH will increase. But from the titration curve, we can see that the pH is certainly not increasing very rapidly as we add the first 20 or so mL of NaOH. This should tell you that at the beginning of this titration the solution is behaving as a buffer. As HF is being converted into F⁻, we are forming a solution that contains a weak acid and its conjugate base. This section of the titration curve, where the pH changes very gradually, is called the buffering domain (or buffering region).

Now, as the experiment continues, the solution suddenly loses its buffering capability and the pH increases dramatically. At some point during this drastic increase, all HF is neutralized and no acid remains in solution. Every new molecule of OH⁻ that is added remains in solution. Therefore, the pH continues to increase rapidly until the OH⁻ concentration in solution is not that much different from the NaOH concentration in the titrant. From here on, the pH doesn't change very much and the curve levels off.

There is a point during the drastic pH increase at which just enough NaOH has been added to completely neutralize all the HF. This is called the acid-base equivalence point. At this point, we simply have Na^+ ions and F^- ions in solution. Note that the solution should be *basic* here. In fact, from what we know about the behavior of conjugates, we can state the following facts about the equivalence point of different titrations:

- For a weak acid (titrated with a strong base), the equivalence point will occur at a pH > 7.
- For a weak base (titrated with a strong acid), the equivalence point will occur at a pH < 7.
- For a strong acid (titrated with a strong base) or for a strong base (titrated with a strong acid), the equivalence point will occur at pH = 7.

Therefore, by just looking at the pH at the equivalence point of our titration, we can tell whether the acid (or base) we were titrating was weak or strong.

Recall the purpose of this titration experiment: to determine the pK_a (or pK_b) of the unknown weak acid (or weak base). From the titration curve, determine the volume of titrant added at the equivalence point; call it $V_{at\ equiv}$. A key question is this: What's in solution when the volume of added titrant is $1/2\ V_{at\ equiv}$? Let's return to our titration of HF by NaOH. We can read from its titration curve that $V_{at\ equiv} = 25$ mL. When the amount of NaOH added was $1/2\ V_{at\ equiv} = 12.5$ mL, the solution consisted of equal concentrations of HF and F^-, i.e., enough NaOH was added to convert 1/2 of the HF to F^-. (After all, when the amount of titrant added was twice as much, $V_{at\ equiv} = 25$ mL, *all* of the HF had been converted to F^-. So naturally, when 1/2 as much was added, only 1/2 was converted.) Therefore, at this point—called the half-equivalence point—we have

$$[HF]_{at\ half-equiv} = [F^-]_{at\ half-equiv}$$

The Henderson-Hasselbalch equation then tells us that

$$pH_{at\ half-equiv} = pK_a' + \log\left(\frac{[F^-]_{at\ half-equiv}}{[HF]_{at\ half-equiv}}\right) = pK_a' + \log 1 = pK_a'$$

The pK_a of HF equals the pH at the half-equivalence point. For our curve, we see that this occurs around pH 3.2, so we conclude that the pK_a of HF is about 3.2.

11.10

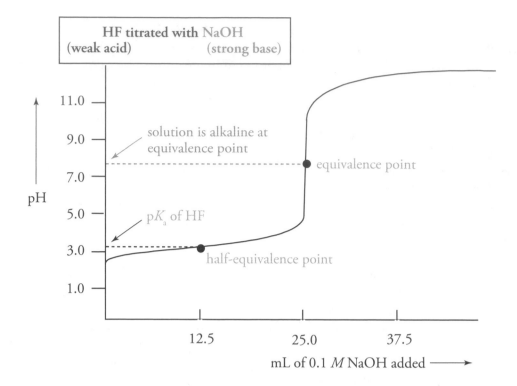

11.10

Compare the sample titration curves for a weak base titrated with a strong acid to the one for a weak acid titrated with a strong base (like the one we just looked at). Note the pH at the equivalence point (relative to pH 7) for each curve.

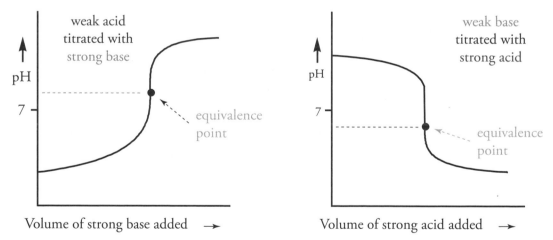

As mentioned above, the titration curve for a strong acid-strong base titration would have the equivalence point at a neutral pH of 7, as shown below.

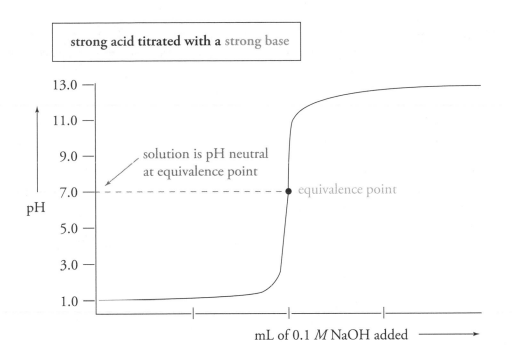

strong acid titrated with a strong base

The titration curve for the titration of a polyprotic acid (like H_2SO_4 or H_3PO_4) will have more than one equivalence point. The number of equivalence points is equal to the number of ionizable hydrogens the acid can donate.

11.10

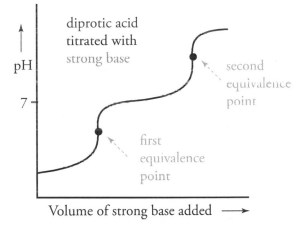

Example 11-20: A fifty mL solution of HCOOH (formic acid) is titrated with 0.2 M NaOH. The equivalence point is reached when 40 mL of the NaOH solution has been added. What was the original concentration of the formic acid solution?

Solution: Using our formula $a \times [A] \times V_A = b \times [B] \times V_B$, we find that

$$[A] = \frac{b \times [B] \times V_B}{a \times V_A} = \frac{1 \times (0.2 \ M) \times (40 \ mL)}{1 \times (50 \ mL)} = 0.16 \ M$$

Example 11-21: Methyl red is an indicator that changes from red to yellow in the pH range 4.4–6.2. For which of the following titrations would methyl red be useful for indicating the equivalence point?

A) HCN titrated with KOH
B) NaOH titrated with HI
C) C_6H_5COOH (benzoic acid) titrated with LiOH
D) $C_6H_5NH_2$ (aniline) titrated with HNO_3

Solution: Since methyl red changes color in a range of *acidic* pH values, it would be an appropriate indicator for a titration whose equivalence point occurs at a pH less than 7. For a weak base titrated with a strong acid, the equivalence point occurs at a pH less than 7. Only choice D describes such a titration.

11.10

- Acids are proton donors and electron acceptors; bases are proton acceptors and electron donors.

- Strong acids completely dissociate in water ($K_a > 1$). You should memorize the list of strong acids and bases.

- The higher the K_a (lower the pK_a), the stronger the acid. The higher the K_b (lower the pK_b), the stronger the base.

- For any conjugate acid and base pair, $K_a K_b = K_w$. Therefore, it follows that the stronger the acid, the weaker its conjugate base. Conjugates of strong acids and bases have no acid/base properties in water.

- Amphoteric substances may act as either acids or bases.

- Water is amphoteric, and autoionizes into OH^- and H_3O^+. The equilibrium constant for the autoionization of water is $K_w = [OH^-][H_3O^+]$. At 25°C, $K_w = 1 \times 10^{-14}$.

- $pH = -\log[H_3O^+]$. For a concentration of H_3O^+ given in a 10^{-x} M notation, simply take the negative exponent to find the pH. The same is true for the relationship between $[OH^-]$ and pOH, K_a and pK_a, and K_b and pK_b.

- At 25°C, $pK_a + pK_b = 14$.

- If a salt is dissolved in water and the cation is a stronger acid than water, the resulting solution will have a pH < 7. If the anion is a base stronger than water, the resulting solution will have a pH > 7.

- Buffers resist pH change upon the addition of a small amount of strong acid or base. A higher concentration of buffer resists pH change better than a lower concentration of buffer (that is, the solution has a higher buffering capacity).

- A buffer consists of approximately equal molar amounts of a weak acid and its conjugate base, and maintains a pH close to its pK_a.

- The Henderson-Hasselbalch equation can be used to determine the pH of a buffer solution.

- Indicators are weak acids that change color upon conversion to their conjugate base. An indicator changes color in the range +/− 1 pH unit from its pK_a.

· In a titration, the equivalence point is the point at which all of the original acid or base has been neutralized.

· When a strong acid is titrated against a weak base, the pH at the equivalence point is < 7. When a strong base is titrated against a weak acid, the pH at the equivalence point is > 7. When a strong base is titrated against a strong acid, the pH at the equivalence point is = 7.

· At the half equivalence point of a titration of a weak plus a strong acid or base, the solution has equal concentrations of acid and conjugate base, and pH = pK_a.

CHAPTER 11 FREESTANDING PRACTICE QUESTIONS

1. The pH of a CH_3COOH solution is < 7 because when this compound is added to water:

   A) CH_3COOH donates H^+, making $[H^+] > [OH^-]$.
   B) CH_3COOH loses OH^-, making $[H^+] < [OH^-]$.
   C) CH_3COO^- deprotonates H_2O, increasing $[OH^-]$.
   D) CH_3COOH dissociation increases $[H^+]$, thereby increasing K_w.

2. All of the following are amphoteric EXCEPT:

   A) HCO_3^-
   B) $H_2PO_4^-$
   C) SO_4^{2-}
   D) $HOOCCOO^-$

3. A graph depicting a titration of a weak acid with a strong base will start at a:

   A) high pH and slope downwards with an equivalence pH equal to 7.
   B) high pH and slope downwards with an equivalence pH below 7.
   C) low pH and slope upwards with an equivalence pH equal to 7.
   D) low pH and slope upwards with an equivalence pH above 7.

4. List the following compounds by increasing pK_a:

   I. H_2SO_4
   II. NH_3
   III. CH_3CH_2COOH
   IV. HF

   A) $I < III < II < IV$
   B) $I < IV < III < II$
   C) $III < I < IV < II$
   D) $II < III < IV < I$

5. The amino and carboxyl terminals of alanine lose protons according to the following equilibrium:

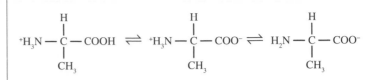

   Which of the following indicators would be best used to determine the second equivalence point when alanine is titrated with sodium hydroxide?

   A) Methyl violet ($pK_b = 13.0$)
   B) Methyl yellow ($pK_b = 10.5$)
   C) Thymol blue ($pK_b = 12.0$)
   D) Phenolphthalein ($pK_b = 4.9$)

6. The K_a of HSCN is equal to 1×10^{-4}. The pH of a HSCN solution:

   A) will be approximately 4.
   B) will be approximately 10.
   C) will increase as [HSCN] increases.
   D) cannot be determined from the information given.

7. A 25.0 mL solution of 0.2 M acetic acid ($pK_a - 4.76$) is mixed with 50 mL of 1.0 M sodium acetate ($pK_b = 9.24$). What is the final pH?

   A) 4.8
   B) 5.8
   C) 9.2
   D) 10.2

CHAPTER 11 PRACTICE PASSAGE

Blood pH homeostasis is the result of several systems operating within the bloodstream. They collectively maintain blood plasma pH at 7.4, since a drop in pH below 6.8 or rise above 7.8 may result in death.

One component of this system is the enzyme *carbonic anhydrase*, which catalyzes the conversion of CO_2 in the blood to carbonic acid. Carbonic acid, in turn, ionizes to form the carbonic acid-bicarbonate buffer. The interdependence of these reactions is shown below in Equation 1.

$$CO_2(g) + H_2O(l) \rightleftharpoons H_2CO_3(aq) \rightleftharpoons H^+(aq) + HCO_3^-(aq)$$

Equation 1

Uncatalyzed blood CO_2 and H^+ can be found binding to hemoglobin after oxygen liberation in peripheral tissues. As the blood reaches the lungs these actions reverse themselves; hemoglobin binds with oxygen, releasing the CO_2 and H^+ ions. The exchange of gases between the lungs and the blood and other tissues in the body is a physiologic process known as respiration.

A second system, the phosphoric acid buffer, plays a minor role compared to the carbonic acid-bicarbonate buffer. Phosphoric acid (H_3PO_4), the primary reactant of this system, is a triprotic acid, which can ionize three protons. This three-step process is illustrated below:

Reaction	K_a
1 $H_3PO_4(aq) \rightleftharpoons H^+(aq) + H_2PO_4^-(aq)$	$K_{a1} = 7.5 \times 10^{-3}$
2 $H_2PO_4^-(aq) \rightleftharpoons H^+(aq) + HPO_4^{2-}(aq)$	$K_{a2} = 6.2 \times 10^{-8}$
3 $HPO_4^{2-}(aq) \rightleftharpoons H^+(aq) + PO_4^{3-}(aq)$	$K_{a3} = 1.7 \times 10^{-12}$

1. Carbonic acid is best described as:

A) amphoteric.
B) polyprotic.
C) a strong acid.
D) the conjugate acid for CO_2.

2. If CO_2 gas is bubbled continuously in a beaker of water to form carbonic acid, which of the following would be true?

   I.   Addition of carbonic anhydrase will increase the K_{eq} of the reaction.
   II. Carbonic acid will increase in concentration until K_{eq} is reached.
   III. Addition of bicarbonate will increase the pH of the system.

A) I only
B) II only
C) III only
D) II and III

3. All of the following statements are true regarding human respiration EXCEPT:

A) when a person's breathing is hampered by conditions such as asthma or emphysema, the blood $[H^+]$ increases.
B) exercise stimulates deeper and more rapid breathing, which increases blood plasma pH.
C) slow, shallow breathing allows CO_2 to accumulate in the blood.
D) hyperventilation can result in the loss of too much CO_2, causing the accumulation of bicarbonate ions.

4. In the dissociation of phosphoric acid, the trend $K_{a1} > K_{a2} > K_{a3}$ is predominantly due to:

A) an equilibrium shift towards the reactants side in Reactions 2 and 3 due to the release of H^+ in Reaction 1.
B) a smaller radius in the H^+ liberated in Reaction 1 compared to that in Reactions 2 and 3.
C) a slower rate of reaction after subsequent ionizations.
D) an increasing influence of the anion after subsequent ionizations.

5. What is the relationship between the K_{a1} value for phosphoric acid and the K_{b1} value for dihydrogen phosphate?

A) K_{a1} and K_{b1} are inversely related through the dissociation constant for water, K_w.
B) K_{a1} and K_{b1} are directly related through the dissociation constant for water, K_w.
C) The K_{a1} is less than the K_{b1}.
D) There is no relationship between K_{a1} and K_{b1}.

6. What would be the pH of a solution made from combining 50 mL of 0.030 M acetic acid $(K_a = 1.8 \times 10^{-5})$ and 10 mL of 0.15 M sodium acetate?

A) pH = 1.6
B) pH = 2.5
C) pH = 3.3
D) pH = 4.7

SOLUTIONS TO CHAPTER 11 FREESTANDING PRACTICE QUESTIONS

1. **A** CH_3COOH is acetic acid, a common organic, carboxylic acid. It will dissociate in water to produce H^+ and CH_3COO^-, eliminating choice B. An acidic solution (pH < 7) has more H^+ ions in solution than OH^- ions, making choice A the best answer. Choice C can be eliminated because if $[OH^-]$ were to increase, the pH of the solution would be greater than 7, rather than less than 7. Choice D can be eliminated because the only thing that changes the value of K_w, or any equilibrium constant, is temperature.

2. **C** An amphoteric substance is one that can act as both an acid and a base. This definition fits choices A, B, and D because they can all donate or accept a proton. Choice C has no protons for donation and cannot be acidic.

3. **D** A graph showing the titration of a weak acid will start at a low pH and slope upwards as the titrant (in this case a strong base) is added. Therefore, choices A and B cannot be true. As the weak acid and titrant (strong base) react, water and salt are formed as products. The salt will determine the pH at the equivalence point. The conjugate acid of a strong base has no acidic properties and will be neutral in solution. However, the conjugate base of the weak acid will be weakly basic. Because of this, the pH at the equivalence point will be above 7.

4. **B** A higher pK_a means a weaker acid, while a lower pK_a means a stronger acid. Since this is a ranking question, start with the extremes. Compound I is a strong acid and will have the lowest pK_a, eliminating choices C and D. Compound II is the only base so it will have the largest pK_a and choice A can be eliminated.

5. **D** Alanine is a neutral amino acid with an isoelectric point close to 7. Therefore, the second equivalence point represents when all the ammonium residue of the zwitterion (the middle structure shown in the question) is deprotonated. This must occur at a basic pH. An appropriate indicator will change color if its pK_a is ±1 of the pH at this equivalence point. Therefore, the desired indicator should have a $pK_a > 7$, or $pK_b < 7$, making choice D the best answer. Another approach to this question is to recognize that no numerical data are provided and choice D is the only indicator for a basic region. There would be no other reasonable way to choose between choices A, B, and C.

6. **D** The K_a of an acid is a measure of its ability to dissociate in water, not the pH of a solution (the smaller the K_a the weaker the acid). If we know the $[H^+]$ of a solution we can find the pH by finding $-\log [H^+]$, but we cannot find the pH of a weak acid solution from only the K_a. We must also know the concentration of the acid. Choice A is a trap answer if you confuse pK_a with pH. The greater the concentration of an acid, the more H^+ ions will be in solution. However, this will *decrease* the pH of the solution, not increase it (choices B and C can be eliminated). By process of elimination, choice D is the best answer.

7. **B** The sodium acetate solution will be completely ionized:

$$NaC_2H_3O_2 \rightarrow Na^+ + C_2H_3O_2^-$$

However, acetic acid will have negligible dissociation in solution:

$$HC_2H_3O_2 \rightleftharpoons H^+ + C_2H_3O_2^- \; (K_a \approx 1 \times 10^{-5})$$

Therefore, for the combined solution, it is reasonable to assume that all of the $HC_2H_3O_2$ is contributed from the acid solution, and all of the $C_2H_3O_2^-$ is contributed from the salt solution:

$$(0.2 \; M \; HC_2H_3O_2)(0.025 \; L) = 5 \times 10^{-3} \; mol \; HC_2H_3O_2$$

$$(1 \; M \; NaC_2H_3O_2)(0.05 \; L) - 5 \times 10^{-2} \; mol \; C_2H_3O_2^-$$

The new volume of 0.075 L cancels out when solving for the pH using the Henderson-Hasselbalch equation:

$$pH = pK_a + \log \frac{[C_2H_3O_2^-]}{[HC_2H_3O_2]}$$

$$pH = 4.76 + \log \frac{\left(\dfrac{5 \times 10^{-2} \; mol}{0.075 \; L} \right)}{\left(\dfrac{5 \times 10^{-3} \; mol}{0.075 \; L} \right)}$$

$$pH = 4.76 + \log(10) = 5.76$$

SOLUTIONS TO CHAPTER 11 PRACTICE PASSAGE

1. **B** Even though the bicarbonate ion is amphoteric and can donate and accept a proton, carbonic acid cannot (eliminate choice A). Choice C is eliminated because carbonic acid is not one of the six strong acids you should know for the MCAT (HI, HBr, HCl, $HClO_4$, H_2SO_4, HNO_3). Choice D is false because carbon dioxide and carbonic acid cannot be a conjugate acid-base pair since they differ by more than one H^+. Choice B is correct because carbonic acid has the ability to donate two protons, making it polyprotic.

2. **D** Addition of a catalyst (such as the enzyme carbonic anhydrase) will simply increase the rate of a reaction. It plays no role in shifting the equilibrium, or changing the equilibrium constant making Item I false (eliminate choice A). As carbon dioxide is bubbled through, carbonic acid will form until its equilibrium concentration is attained, making Item II valid (eliminate choice C). Finally, addition of bicarbonate will shift the carbonic acid equilibrium to the reactant side, consuming H^+ in the process. Since the concentration of H^+ will decrease, pH will increase, making Item III valid (eliminate choice B).

3. **D** Choices A and C can be eliminated because they create the same effect. A decrease in breathing rate causes less CO_2 to exchange, leading to an increase in CO_2 remaining in the blood (i.e., increased CO_2 concentration). Consequently, this shifts the equilibria shown in Figure 1 to the right, which results in increased H^+ concentration, and decreased pH. Choice B is the opposite effect. Deeper, more rapid breathing expels more CO_2, decreasing the CO_2 in the blood and increasing pH. Hyperventilation may involve the loss of too much CO_2. This loss will shift the equilibria shown in Equation 1 to the left. Loss of bicarbonate ions will result, making choice D the only statement that is NOT true.

4. **D** Generation of H^+ in Reaction 1 is coupled with a release of $H_2PO_4^-$. Both the product and reactant sides of Reaction 2 are increased proportionally, causing no shift in equilibrium (eliminate choice A). Atomic radius is a function of an atom's position in the periodic table. Thus, the radius of H^+ is the same in all three reactions, eliminating choice B. Equilibrium constants have no relationship to reaction rates, so choice C can be eliminated. The K_a values progressively decrease when removing a proton from a polyprotic acid because it is more difficult to remove a proton from an anion compared to a neutral molecule. In subsequent ionizations, the anion becomes more negative, resulting in greater difficulty liberating a positively charged H^+ ion.

5. **A** The relationship between the K_a value of an acid and the K_b value of its conjugate base is through the dissociation constant of water, where $K_w = (K_a)(K_b)$. Therefore, the relationship between K_{a1} and K_{b1} is $K_{a1} = K_w/K_{b1}$; an inverse relationship.

6. **D** The final solution is composed of $(50 \text{ mL})(0.03 \ M) = 1.5$ mmol of $HC_2H_3O_2$ and (10 mL) $(0.15 \ M) = 1.5$ mmol of $NaC_2H_3O_2$ (or 1.5 mmol of $C_2H_3O_2^-$). The total volume will be 60 mL and the starting concentration of acetic acid will be the same as the starting concentration of its conjugate base. Since acetic acid is a weak acid, any subsequent dissociation will be relatively insignificant and the equilibrium concentrations of acid and base will remain approximately the same. When the concentration of the two species in a conjugate pair are equal, the $pK_a =$ pH from the Henderson-Hasselbalch equation: pH = pK_a + log [conjugate base]/[acid]. The pK_a of acetic acid ($K_a = 1.8 \times 10^{-5}$) is approximately 4.7.

Chapter 12
Electrochemistry

12.1 OXIDATION-REDUCTION REACTIONS

Recall that the **oxidation number** (or **oxidation state**) of each atom in a molecule describes how many electrons it is donating or accepting in the overall bonding of the molecule. Many elements can assume different oxidation states depending on the bonds they make. A reaction in which the oxidation numbers of any of the reactants change is called an **oxidation-reduction** (or **redox**) reaction.

In a redox reaction, atoms gain or lose electrons as new bonds are formed. The total number of electrons does not change, of course; they're just redistributed among the atoms. When an atom loses electrons, its oxidation number increases; this is **oxidation**. When an atom gains electrons, the oxidation number decreases; this is **reduction**. A mnemonic device is helpful:

LEO the lion says GER

LEO: Lose Electrons = Oxidation

GER: Gain Electrons = Reduction

Another popular mnemonic is

OIL RIG

OIL: Oxidation Is electron Loss

RIG: Reduction Is electron Gain

An atom that is oxidized in a reaction loses electrons to another atom. We call the oxidized atom a **reducing agent** or **reductant**, because by giving up electrons, it reduces another atom that gains the electrons. On the other hand, the atom that gains the electrons has been **reduced**. We call the reduced atom an **oxidizing agent** or **oxidant**, because it oxidizes another atom that loses the electrons. (You may want to review Section 3.13 on Oxidation States.)

Example 12-1: In an oxidation-reduction, the oxidation number of an aluminum atom changes from 0 to +3. The aluminum atom has been:

A) reduced, and is a reducing agent.
B) reduced, and is an oxidizing agent.
C) oxidized, and is a reducing agent.
D) oxidized, and is an oxidizing agent.

Solution: Since the oxidation number has increased, the atom's been oxidized. And since it's been oxidized, it reduced something else and thus acted as a reducing agent. Therefore, the answer is C.

Take a look at this redox reaction:

$$Fe + 2 \, HCl \rightarrow FeCl_2 + H_2$$

The oxidation state of iron changes from 0 to +2. The oxidation state of hydrogen changes from +1 to 0. (The oxidation state of chlorine remains at –1.) So, iron has lost two electrons, and two protons (H^+) have gained one electron each. Therefore, the iron has been oxidized, and the hydrogens have been reduced. In order to better see the exchange of electrons, a redox reaction can be broken down into a pair of **half-reactions** that show the oxidation and reduction separately. These **ion-electron** equations show only the actual oxidized or reduced species—and the electrons involved—in an electron-balanced reaction. For the redox reaction shown above, the ion-electron half-reactions are:

$$\text{oxidation:} \quad Fe \rightarrow Fe^{2+} + 2e^-$$

$$\text{reduction:} \quad 2\,H^+ + 2e^- \rightarrow H_2$$

Example 12-2: For the redox reaction

$$3\,MnO_2 + 2\,Al \rightarrow 2\,Al_2O_3 + 3\,Mn$$

which of the following shows the oxidation half-reaction?

A) $Mn^{4+} + 4e^- \rightarrow Mn$
B) $Mn^{2+} + 2e^- \rightarrow Mn$
C) $Al \rightarrow Al^{3+} + 3e^-$
D) $Al^{4+} \rightarrow Al^{6+} + 6e^-$

Solution: First, eliminate choices A and B since they're *reduction* half-reactions. We can then eliminate choice D for two reasons: First, Al^{4+} is not the species of aluminum on the reactant side; second, it's not balanced electrically. The answer must be C.

12.2 GALVANIC CELLS

Because a redox reaction involves the transfer of electrons, and the flow of electrons constitutes an electric current that can do work, we can use a spontaneous redox reaction to generate an electric current. A device for doing this is called a **galvanic** (or **voltaic**) **cell**, the main features of which are shown in the figure below.

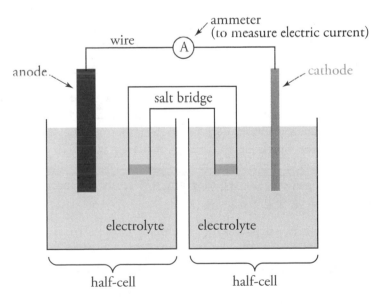

One **electrode**, generally composed of a metal (labeled the **anode**) gets oxidized, and the electrons its atoms lose travel along the wire to a second metal electrode (labeled the **cathode**). It is at the cathode that reduction takes place. In this way, the anode acts as an electron source, while the cathode acts as an electron sink. Electrons always flow through the conducting wire from the anode to the cathode. This electron flow is the electric current that is produced by the spontaneous redox reaction between the electrodes.

Let's look at a specific galvanic cell, with the anode made of zinc, and the cathode made of copper. The anode is immersed in a $ZnSO_4$ solution, the cathode is immersed in a $CuSO_4$ solution, and the half cells are connected by a **salt bridge** containing an aqueous solution of KNO_3. When the electrodes are connected by a wire, zinc atoms in the anode are oxidized ($Zn \rightarrow Zn^{2+} + 2e^-$), and the electrons travel through the wire to the cathode. There, the Cu^{2+} ions in solution pick up these electrons and get reduced to copper metal ($Cu^{2+} + 2e^- \rightarrow Cu$), which accumulates on the copper cathode. The sulfate anions balance the charge on the Zn^{2+}, but do not participate in any redox reaction, and are therefore known as spectator ions.

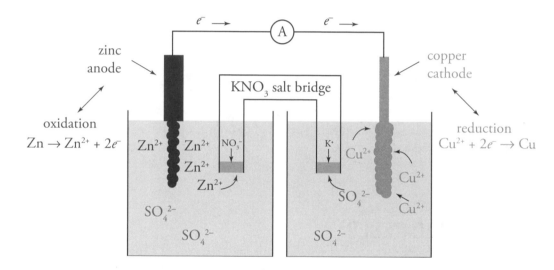

The Zn^{2+} ions that remain in the solution in the zinc half-cell attract NO_3^- ions from the salt bridge, and K^+ ions in the salt bridge are attracted into the copper half-cell. Notice that anions in solution travel from the right cell to the left cell—and cations travel in the opposite direction—using the salt bridge as a conduit. This movement of ions completes the circuit and allows the current in the wire to continue, until the zinc strip is consumed. Remember that anions from the salt bridge go to the anode and cations from the salt bridge go to the cathode.

Notice that the anode is always the site of oxidation, and the cathode is always the site of reduction. One way to help remember this is just to notice that "a" and "o" (anode and oxidation) are both vowels, while "c" and "r" (cathode and reduction) are both consonants. Another popular mnemonic is "an ox, red cat" for "anode = oxidation, reduction = cathode."

We often use a shorthand notation, called a **cell diagram**, to identify the species present in a galvanic cell. Cell diagrams are read as follows:

Anode | Anodic solution (concentration) || Cathodic solution (concentration) | Cathode

If the concentrations are not specified in the cell diagram, you should assume they are 1 M.

Example 12-3: In the electrochemical cell described by the following cell diagram, what reaction occurs at the anode?

$$Zn(s) \mid Zn^{2+}(aq) \mid\mid Cl^-(aq) \mid Cl_2(g)$$

A) $Zn \rightarrow Zn^{2+} + 2e^-$
B) $Zn^{2+} + 2e^- \rightarrow Zn$
C) $2\,Cl^- \rightarrow Cl_2 + 2e^-$
D) $Cl_2 + 2e^- \rightarrow 2\,Cl^-$

Solution: For any electrochemical cell, oxidation occurs at the anode, and reduction occurs at the cathode. Therefore, we're looking for an oxidation, and choices B and D are eliminated. Since Zn is present at the anode, the answer is A.

Example 12-4: In the absence of a salt bridge, charge separation develops. The anode develops a positive charge and the cathode develops a negative charge, quickly halting the flow of electrons. In this state, the battery resembles:

A) a resistor.
B) a capacitor.
C) a transformer.
D) an inductor.

Solution: The question tells us that the result of removing a salt bridge is charge separation. In physics, we learned that a capacitor is a device that stores electrical energy due to the separation of charge on adjacent surfaces. Thus, choice B is the correct choice.

12.3 STANDARD REDUCTION POTENTIALS

To determine whether the redox reaction of a cell is spontaneous and can produce an electric current, we need to figure out the cell voltage. Each half-reaction has a potential (E), which is the cell voltage it would have if the other electrode were the standard reference electrode. (*Note*: We usually consider cells at standard conditions: 25°C, 1 atm pressure, aqueous solutions at $1\,M$ concentrations, and with substances in their standard states. To indicate standard conditions, we use a ° superscript on quantities such as E and ΔG.) By definition, the standard reference electrode is the site of the redox reaction $2\,H^+ + 2e^- \rightarrow H_2$, which is assigned a potential of 0.00 volts. By adding the half-reaction potential for a given pair of electrodes, we get the cell's overall voltage. Tables of half-reaction potentials are usually given for reductions only. Since each cell has a reduction half-reaction and an oxidation half-reaction, we get the potential of the oxidation by simply reversing the sign of the corresponding reduction potential.

For example, the standard reduction potential for the half-reaction $Cu^{2+} + 2e^- \rightarrow Cu$ is +0.34 V. The standard reduction potential for the half-reaction $Zn^{2+} + 2e^- \rightarrow Zn$ is –0.76 V. Reversing the zinc reduction to an oxidation, we get $Zn \rightarrow Zn^{2+} + 2e^-$, with a potential of +0.76 V. Therefore, the overall cell voltage for the zinc-copper cell is (+0.76 V) + (+0.34 V) = +1.10 V:

oxidation:	$Zn \rightarrow Zn^{2+} + 2e^-$		$E° = +0.76$ V
reduction:	$Cu^{2+} + 2e^- \rightarrow Cu$		$E° = +0.34$ V
	$Zn + Cu^{2+} \rightarrow Zn^{2+} + Cu$		$E° = +1.10$ V

The free-energy change, $\Delta G°$, for a redox reaction in which cell voltage is $E°$ is given by the equation

$$\Delta G° = -nFE°$$

where n is the number of moles of electrons transferred and F stands for a **faraday** (the magnitude of the charge of one mole of electrons, approximately 96,500 coulombs). Since a reaction is spontaneous if $\Delta G°$ is negative, this equation tells us that the redox reaction in a cell will be spontaneous if the cell voltage is positive. Since the cell voltage for our zinc-copper cell was +1.10 V, we know the reaction will be spontaneous and produce an electric current that can do work.

> If the cell voltage is positive, then the reaction is spontaneous.
>
> If the cell voltage is negative, then the reaction is nonspontaneous.

Let's do another example and consider what would happen if the zinc electrode in our cell above were replaced by a gold electrode, given that the **standard reduction potential** for the reaction $Au^{3+} + 3e^- \rightarrow Au$ is $E° = +1.50$ V. The redox reaction that we're investigating is

$$Au + Cu^{2+} \rightarrow Au^{3+} + Cu$$

Let's first break this down into half-reactions:

$Au \rightarrow Au^{3+} + 3e^-$	$E° = -1.50$ V
$Cu^{2+} + 2e^- \rightarrow Cu$	$E° = +0.34$ V

The overall reaction is not electron balanced; but by multiplying the first half-reaction by 2 and the second half-reaction by 3, we get

$2\,Au \rightarrow 2\,Au^{3+} + 6e^-$	$E° = -1.50$ V
$3\,Cu^{2+} + 6e^- \rightarrow 3\,Cu$	$E° = +0.34$ V
$2\,Au + 3\,Cu^{2+} \rightarrow 2\,Au^{3+} + 3\,Cu$	$E° = -1.16$ V

The final equation is now electron balanced. Notice that although we multiplied the half-reactions by stoichiometric coefficients, we did *not* multiply the potentials by those coefficients. You never multiply the potential by a coefficient, even if you multiply a half-reaction by a coefficient to get the balanced equation for the reaction. This is because the potentials are *intrinsic* to the identities of the species involved and do not depend on the number of moles of the species.

Because the cell voltage is negative, this reaction would not be spontaneous. However, it would be spontaneous in the other direction; that is, if copper were the *anode* and gold the *cathode*, then the potential of the cell would be +1.16 V, which implies a spontaneous reaction.

Oxidizing and Reducing Agents

We can also use reduction potentials to determine whether reactants are good or poor oxidizing or reducing agents. For example, let's look again at the half-reactions in our original zinc-copper cell. The half-reaction $Zn^{2+} + 2e^- \rightarrow Zn$ has a standard potential of −0.76 V, and the half-reaction $Cu^{2+} + 2e^- \rightarrow Cu$ has a standard potential of +0.34 V. The fact that the reduction of Zn^{2+} is nonspontaneous means that the oxidation of Zn is spontaneous, so Zn would rather give up electrons. If it does, this means that Zn acts as a reducing agent because in giving up electrons it reduces something else. The fact that the reduction of Cu^{2+} has a positive potential tells us that this reaction would be spontaneous at standard conditions. In other words, Cu^{2+} is a good oxidizing agent because it's looking to accept electrons, thereby oxidizing something else. So, in general, if a reduction half-reaction has a large negative potential, then the product is a good reducing agent. On the other hand, if a reduction half-reaction has a large positive potential, then the reactant is a good oxidizing agent. Now, whether something is a "good" oxidizing or reducing agent depends on what it's being compared to. So, to be more precise, we should say this:

> The more negative the reduction potential, the weaker the reactant is as an oxidizing agent, and the stronger the product is as a reducing agent.
>
> The more positive the reduction potential, the stronger the reactant is as an oxidizing agent, and the weaker the product is as a reducing agent.

For example, given that $Pb^{2+} + 2e^- \rightarrow Pb$ has a standard potential of −0.13 V, and $Al^{3+} + 3e^- \rightarrow Al$ has a standard potential of −1.67 V, what could we conclude? Well, since Al^{3+} has a large negative reduction potential, the product, aluminum metal, is a good reducing agent. In fact, because the reduction potential of Al^{3+} is more negative than that of Pb^{2+}, we'd say that aluminum is a stronger reducing agent than lead.

Example 12-5: A galvanic cell is set to operate at standard conditions. If one electrode is made of magnesium and the other is made of copper, then the magnesium electrode will serve as the:

A) anode and be the site of oxidation.
B) anode and be the site of reduction.
C) cathode and be the site of oxidation.
D) cathode and be the site of reduction.

Solution: First, eliminate choices B and C since the anode is always the site of oxidation and the cathode is always the site of reduction. From the table, we see that the reduction of Mg^{2+} is nonspontaneous, whereas the reduction of Cu^{2+} is spontaneous.

Reaction	$E°$ (volts)
$Li^+ + e^- \rightarrow Li$	−3.05
$Mg^{2+} + 2e^- \rightarrow Mg$	−2.36
$Al^{3+} + 3e^- \rightarrow Al$	−1.67
$Zn^{2+} + 2e^- \rightarrow Zn$	−0.76
$Fe^{2+} + 2e^- \rightarrow Fe$	−0.44
$Pb^{2+} + 2e^- \rightarrow Pb$	−0.13
$2 H^+ + 2e^- \rightarrow H_2$	0.00
$Cu^{2+} + 2e^- \rightarrow Cu$	0.34
$Ag^+ + e^- \rightarrow Ag$	0.80
$Pd^{2+} + 2e^- \rightarrow Pd$	0.99
$Pt^{2+} + 2e^- \rightarrow Pt$	1.20
$Au^{3+} + 3e^- \rightarrow Au$	1.50
$F_2 + 2e^- \rightarrow 2 F^-$	2.87

Therefore, the copper electrode will serve as the cathode and be the site of reduction, and the magnesium electrode will serve as the anode and be the site of oxidation (choice A).

Example 12-6: What is the standard cell voltage for the reduction of Ag^+ by Al?

Solution: The half-reactions are

$$Ag^+ + e^- \rightarrow Ag \qquad E° = 0.80 \text{ V}$$
$$Al \rightarrow Al^{3+} + 3e^- \qquad E° = +1.67 \text{ V}$$

Although we'd multiply both sides of the first half-reaction by the stoichiometric coefficient 3 before adding it to the second one to give the overall, electron-balanced redox reaction, we don't bother to do that here. The question is asking only for $E°$, and the potentials of the half-reactions are not affected by stoichiometric coefficients. Adding the potentials of these half-reactions gives us the overall cell voltage: $E° = 2.47$ V.

Example 12-7: For the reaction below, which of the following statements is true?

$$2 \text{ Au} + 3 \text{ Fe}^{2+} \rightarrow 2 \text{ Au}^{3+} + 3 \text{ Fe}$$

A) The reaction is spontaneous, because its cell voltage is positive.
B) The reaction is spontaneous, because its cell voltage is negative.
C) The reaction is not spontaneous, because its cell voltage is positive.
D) The reaction is not spontaneous, because its cell voltage is negative.

Solution: First, eliminate choices B and C. Even without looking at the table of reduction potentials, these choices can't be correct. If the cell voltage $E°$ is negative, then the reaction is nonspontaneous, and if $E°$ is positive, then the reaction is spontaneous. The half-reactions are

$$2 \text{ (Au} \rightarrow \text{Au}^{3+} + 3e^-) \qquad E° = -1.50 \text{ V}$$
$$3 \text{ (Fe}^{2+} + 2e^- \rightarrow \text{Fe)} \qquad E° = -0.44 \text{ V}$$

Notice again that the question is really asking only about $E°$, and the potentials of the half-reactions are *not* affected by stoichiometric coefficients (2 and 3, in this case). Since each of these half-reactions has a negative value for $E°$, the cell voltage (obtained by adding them) will also be negative, so the answer is D.

Example 12-8: Of the following, which is the strongest reducing agent?

A) Zn
B) Fe
C) Pd
D) Pd^{2+}

Solution: Remember the rule: The more negative the reduction potential, the stronger the product is as a reducing agent. Zn (choice A) is the product of a redox half-reaction whose potential is -0.76 V. Fe (choice B) is the product of a redox half-reaction whose potential is -0.44 V. So, we know we can eliminate choice B. Pd (choice C) is the product of a redox half-reaction whose potential is $+0.99$ V, so C is eliminated. Finally, in order for Pd^{2+} to be a reducing agent, it would have to be oxidized—that is, lose more electrons. A cation getting further oxidized? Not likely, especially when there's a neutral metal (choice A) that is happier to do so.

Example 12-9: Of the following, which is the strongest oxidizing agent?

A) Al^{3+}
B) Ag^+
C) Au^{3+}
D) Cu^{2+}

Solution: Remember the rule: The more positive the reduction potential, the stronger the reactant is as an oxidizing agent. Al^{3+} (choice A) is the reactant of a redox half-reaction whose potential is negative, so we can probably eliminate choice A right away. Ag^+ (choice B) is the reactant of a redox half-reaction whose potential is +0.80 V. (Now we know that A can be eliminated). Au^{3+} (choice C) is the reactant of a redox half-reaction whose potential is +1.50 V, so now B is eliminated. Finally, Cu^{2+} (choice D) is the reactant of a redox half-reaction whose potential is only +0.34 V, so choice C is better.

Example 12-10: Which of the following best approximates the value of $\Delta G°$ for this reaction:

$$2\ Al + 3\ Cu^{2+} \rightarrow 2\ Al^{3+} + 3\ Cu?$$

A) $-(12)(96{,}500)$ J
B) $-(6)(96{,}500)$ J
C) $+(6)(96{,}500)$ J
D) $+(12)(96{,}500)$ J

Solution: The half-reactions are

$$2\ (Al \rightarrow Al^{3+} + 3e^-) \qquad E° = +1.67\ V$$
$$3\ (Cu^{2+} + 2e^- \rightarrow Cu) \qquad E° = 0.34\ V$$

so the overall cell voltage is $E° - 2.01\ V \approx 2\ V$. Because the number of electrons transferred is $n = 2 \times 3 = 6$, the equation $\Delta G° = -nFE°$ tells us that choice A is the answer:

$$\Delta G° = -(6)(96{,}500)(2)\ J = -(12)(96{,}500)\ J$$

12.4 NONSTANDARD CONDITIONS

All the previous discussion of potentials assumed the conditions to be standard state, meaning that all aqueous reactants in the mixture were 1 M in concentration. So long as this is true, the tabulated values for reduction potentials apply to each half reaction.

However, since conditions are not always standard we must have a way to alternatively, and more generally, describe the voltage of an electrochemical reaction. To do this we use the Nernst equation.

Recall the following relationship:

$$\Delta G = \Delta G° + RT \ln Q$$

12.4

If we substitute ΔG and $\Delta G°$ with their respective relation to E and $E°$, we arrive at

$$-nFE = -nFE° + RT \ln Q$$

or

$$E = E° - \left(\frac{RT}{nF}\right) \ln Q$$

This is the **Nernst equation**. It describes how deviations in temperature and concentration of reactants can alter the voltage of a reaction under nonstandard conditions. As in the standard chemical systems previously discussed, the concentrations of product and reactants will change until $Q = K_{eq}$, and $E = 0$.

Concentration Cells

A **concentration cell** is a galvanic cell that has identical electrodes but which has half-cells with different ion concentrations. Since the electrodes and relevant ions in the two beakers have the same identities, the *standard* cell voltage, $E°$, would be zero. But, such a cell is *not* standard because both electrolytic solutions in the half-cells are not 1 M. So even though the electrodes are the same, in a concentration cell there *will* be a potential difference between them, and an electric current will be produced. For example, let's say both electrodes are made of zinc, and the $[Zn^{2+}]$ concentrations in the electrolytes were 0.1 M and 0.3 M, respectively. We'd expect electrons to be induced to flow through the conducting wire to the half-cell with the higher concentration of these positive ions. So, the zinc electrode in the 0.1 M solution would serve as the anode, with the liberated electrons flowing across the wire to the zinc electrode in the 0.3 M solution, which serves as the cathode. When the concentrations of the solutions become equal, the reaction will stop.

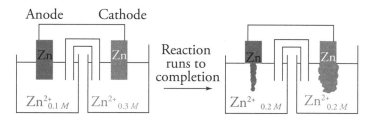

12.5 REDOX TITRATIONS

Just as the titration of an acid with a strong base of known concentration can provide information about the initial acid solution (most notably the concentration and pK_a), titration of a redox active species with a strong oxidant or reductant can be used to determine similar unknowns.

Most redox titrations involve the use of a redox indicator. Much like an indicator in acid/base chemistry, a redox indicator uses a change in color to determine the endpoint. However, in a redox reaction, this change in color is due to a change in oxidation state rather than loss or gain of a proton. One commonly used redox indicator is the Ce^{4+} ion, a strong oxidant according to the equation below:

$$Ce^{4+} + 1\,e^- \rightarrow Ce^{3+} \qquad E^0 \approx 1.5 \text{ V } (1\text{ }M\text{ HCl solution})$$

The Ce^{4+} ion is bright yellow in solution, whereas the reduced Ce^{3+} is colorless. This color change, along with the comparatively high redox potential, make Ce^{4+} an ideal indicator for the determination of the concentration of solutions of oxidizable species.

For example, cerium is known to oxidize secondary alcohols to ketones in aqueous solution. As such, titration with Ce^{4+} is an appropriate method for the determination of alcohol concentration in solution, or for the determination of the number of secondary hydroxyl groups present in a chemical species. As long as the Ce^{4+} added to the solution is consumed, the solution will remain colorless. However, the solution will turn yellow immediately after all oxidizable hydroxyls have been consumed. Knowledge of the concentration of the Ce^{4+} titrant allows for the determination of initial $^-$OH concentration.

A redox titration curve, similar to an acid-base titration curve, can be plotted for any such redox titration. An example is given below where a generic reductant is titrated with Ce^{4+}.

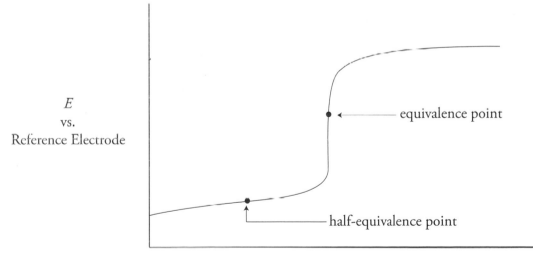

Volume Ce^{4+}

The equivalence point on the plot above will coincide with the solution turning yellow, indicating the completion of the redox reaction and the total consumption of the reductant as described by the system's balanced redox equation. The significance of the half-equivalence point can be seen in the Nernst equation:

$$E = E° - (RT/nF) \ln Q$$

In this case, Q refers to the ratio of oxidized and non-oxidized reactant. At the half-equivalence point these two quantities are equal and $Q = 1$. Since $\ln(1) = 0$, at the half equivalence point the value of E (measured against whichever reference electrode one chooses) is equal to the value of $E°$ for the redox couple being titrated.

12.6 ELECTROLYTIC CELLS

Unlike a galvanic cell, an **electrolytic cell** *uses* an external voltage source (such as a battery) to *create an electric current* that forces a nonspontaneous redox reaction to occur. This is known as **electrolysis**. A typical example of an electrolytic cell is one used to form sodium metal and chlorine gas from molten NaCl.

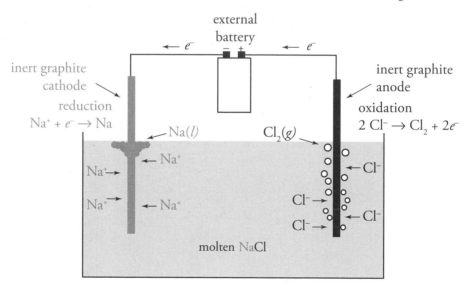

The half-reactions for converting molten Na^+Cl^- into sodium and chlorine are:

$$Na^+ + e^- \rightarrow Na(l) \qquad E° = -2.71 \text{ V}$$
$$2\,Cl^- \rightarrow Cl_2(g) + 2e^- \qquad E° = -1.36 \text{ V}$$

The standard voltage for the overall reaction is −4.07 V, which means the reaction is *not* spontaneous. The electrolytic cell shown above uses an external battery to remove electrons from chloride ions and forces sodium ions to accept them. In so doing, the sodium ions are reduced to sodium metal, and the chloride ions are oxidized to produce chlorine gas, which bubbles out of the electrolyte.

Electrolytic cells are also used for plating a thin layer of metal on top of another material, a process known as **electroplating**. If a fork is used as the cathode in an electrolytic cell whose electrolyte contains silver ions, silver will precipitate onto the fork, producing a silver-plated fork. Other examples of metal plating include gold-plated jewelry, and plating tin or chromium onto steel (for tin cans and car bumpers).

Galvanic vs. Electrolytic Cells

Notice that in both galvanic cells and electrolytic cells, the anode is the site of oxidation and the cathode is the site of reduction. Furthermore, electrons in the external circuit always move from the anode to the cathode. The difference, of course, is that a galvanic cell uses a spontaneous redox reaction to create an electric current, whereas an electrolytic cell uses an electric current to force a nonspontaneous redox reaction to occur.

It follows that in a galvanic cell, the anode is negative and the cathode is positive since electrons are spontaneously moving from a negative to a positive charge. However, in an electrolytic cell the anode is positive and the cathode is negative since electrons are being forced to move where they don't want to go.

Galvanic	Electrolytic
Reduction at cathode	
Oxidation at anode	
Electrons flow from anode to cathode	
Anions migrate to anode	
Cations migrate to cathode	
Spontaneously generates electrical power ($\Delta G° < 0$)	Nonspontaneous, requires an external electric power source ($\Delta G° > 0$)
Total $E°$ of reaction is positive	Total $E°$ of reaction is negative
Anode is negative	Anode is positive
Cathode is positive	Cathode is negative

Example 12-11: The final products of the electrolysis of aqueous NaCl are most likely:

A) Na(s) and Cl_2(g)
B) HOCl(aq) and Na(s)
C) Na(s) and O_2(g)
D) NaOH(aq) and HOCl(aq)

Solution: This is a little tricky, but it provides a good example of using the process of elimination. We're not expected to be able to answer this question outright, since there is virtually no information provided. Instead, realize that choices A, B and C list metallic sodium as a final product. That's a problem because we're in an aqueous medium, and we know that sodium metal reacts violently in water to form NaOH and hydrogen gas and fire. So after eliminating these choices, we're left with choice D.

Common Rechargeable Batteries

One particularly useful galvanic cell uses two different oxidations states of Pb for its constitutive electrodes and sulfuric acid as an electrolyte. Often referred to as lead-acid batteries, these cells constitute the oldest type of rechargeable batteries, and are perhaps most commonly employed as automobile batteries.

12.6

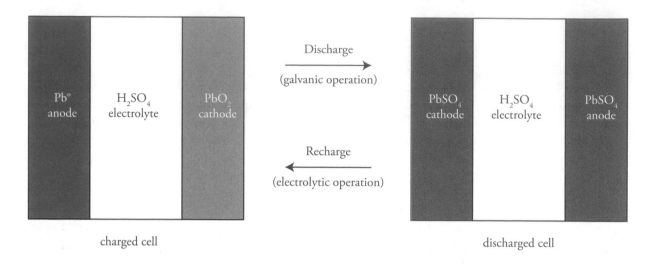

As depicted in the simplified figure above, fully charged lead acid batteries utilize $Pb°$ as an anodic electrode and a cathode consisting of PbO_2. As the battery discharges, $Pb°$ undergoes a two-electron oxidation to $PbSO_4$, while PbO_2 is reduced to the same species, as described by the following equations.

$$Pb° + HSO_4^- \rightarrow PbSO_4 + H^+ + 2\ e^-$$

$$PbO_2 + HSO_4^- + 3\ H^+ + 2e^- \rightarrow PbSO_4 + 2\ H_2O$$

Recharging the battery involves reversing the electron flow of discharge with applied voltage, as an electrolytic cell. The oxidation of $PbSO_4$ back to PbO_2, along with the regeneration of $Pb°$ by the reduction of $PbSO_4$ restores the initial potential of the cell.

Nickel-cadmium batteries, or NiCad batteries, are another common type of rechargeable battery. These cells utilize a metallic $Cd°$ anode and a nickel oxide hydroxide (NiO(OH)) cathode. The redox reactions involved in the discharge of the battery are given below. To facilitate these reactions, NiCad cells contain an alkaline KOH electrolyte.

$$Cd° + 2\ OH^- \rightarrow Cd(OH)_2 + 2\ e^-$$

$$2\ NiO(OH) + 2\ H_2O + 2\ e^- \rightarrow 2\ Ni(OH)_2 + 2\ OH^-$$

Recharging spent NiCad batteries, as one might expect, involves applying a voltage to run these two reactions in reverse (typical electrolytic-cell behavior).

12.7 FARADAY'S LAW OF ELECTROLYSIS

We can determine the amounts of sodium metal and chlorine gas produced at the electrodes in the electrolytic cell shown in Section 12.6 using Faraday's law of electrolysis:

Faraday's Law of Electrolysis

The amount of chemical change is proportional to the amount of electricity that flows through the cell.

For example, let's answer this question: If 5 amps of current flowed in the NaCl electrolytic cell for 1930 seconds, how much sodium metal and chlorine gas would be produced?

Step 1: First determine the amount of electricity (in coulombs, C) that flowed through the cell.
We use the equation $Q = It$ (that is, charge = current × time) to find that

$$Q = (5 \text{ amps})(1930 \text{ sec}) = 9650 \text{ coulombs}$$

Step 2: Use the faraday, F, to convert Q from Step 1 to moles of electrons.
The faraday is the magnitude of the charge on 1 mole of electrons; it's a constant equal to $(1.6 \times 10^{-19} \text{ C}/e^-)(6.02 \times 10^{23} \ e^-/\text{mol}) \approx 96{,}500 \text{ C/mol}$. So, if 9650 C of charge flowed through the cell, this represents

$$9650 \text{ C} \times \frac{1 \text{ mol } e^-}{96{,}500 \text{ C}} = 0.1 \text{ mol } e^-$$

Step 3: Use the stoichiometry of the half-reactions to finish the calculation.
  a) From the stoichiometry of the reaction $Na^+ + e^- \rightarrow Na$, we see that 1 mole of electrons would give 1 mole of Na. Therefore, 0.1 mol of electrons gives 0.1 mol of Na. Since the molar mass of sodium is 23 g/mol, we'd get $(0.1)(23 \text{ g}) = 2.3$ g of sodium metal deposited onto the cathode.
  b) From the stoichiometry of the reaction $2 Cl^- \rightarrow Cl_2(g) + 2e^-$, we see that for every 1 mole of electrons lost, we get $\frac{1}{2}$ mole of $Cl_2(g)$. Since Step 2 told us that 0.1 mol of electrons were liberated at the anode, 0.05 mol of $Cl_2(g)$ was produced. Because the molar mass of Cl_2 is $2(35.5 \text{ g/mol}) = 71$ g/mol, we'd get $(0.05 \text{ mol})(71 \text{ g/mol}) = 3.55$ g of chlorine gas.

Example 12-12: A piece of steel is the cathode in a hot solution of chromic acid (H_2CrO_4) to electroplate it with chromium metal. How much chromium would be deposited onto the steel after 48,250 C of electricity was forced through the cell?

A) $\frac{1}{12}$ mol

B) $\frac{1}{6}$ mol

C) $\frac{1}{4}$ mol

D) 3 mol

Solution: First, we notice that 48,250 C of electricity is equal to $\frac{1}{2}$ faraday (F = 96,500 C/mol). This is equivalent to $\frac{1}{2}$ mole of electrons. In the molecule H_2CrO_4, chromium is in a +6 oxidation state. So, from the stoichiometry of the reaction $Cr^{6+} + 6e^- \rightarrow Cr$, we see that for every 6 moles of electrons gained, we get 1 mole of Cr metal. Another way of looking at this is to say that for every 1 mole of electrons gained, we get just $\frac{1}{6}$ mole of Cr metal. Therefore, if we have a supply of $\frac{1}{2}$ mol of electrons, we'll produce $(\frac{1}{6})(\frac{1}{2}) = \frac{1}{12}$ mol of Cr, choice A.

12.7

- Oxidation is electron loss; reduction is electron gain (remember "OIL RIG").

- A species that is oxidized is a reducing agent, and a species that is reduced is an oxidizing agent.

- In all electrochemical cells, oxidation occurs at the anode and reduction occurs at the cathode.

- Electrons always flow from the anode to the cathode.

- Salt bridge anions always migrate toward the anode, and cations always migrate toward the cathode.

- The free energy of an electrochemical cell can be calculated from its potential based on $\Delta G° = -nFE°$.

- A galvanic cell spontaneously generates electrical power ($-\Delta G$, $+E$).

- An electrolytic cell consists of nonspontaneous reactions and requires an external electrical power source ($+\Delta G$, $-E$).

- In a galvanic cell, electrons spontaneously flow from the negative ($-$) terminal to the positive ($+$) terminal. Therefore, it follows that in a galvanic cell the anode is negatively charged ($-$) and the cathode is positively charged ($+$).

- In an electrolytic cell, electrons are forced from the positive ($+$) terminal to the negative ($-$) terminal, and therefore the anode is positively charged ($+$) and the cathode is negatively charged ($-$).

- Standard reduction and oxidation potentials are intrinsic values and therefore should not be multiplied by molar coefficients in balanced half reactions.

- For a given reduction potential, the reverse reaction, or oxidation potential, has the same magnitude of E but the opposite sign.

- Faraday's law of electrolysis states that the amount of chemical change is proportional to the amount of electricity that flows through the cell.

- Under nonstandard conditions, the potential of an electrochemical cell can be calculated using the Nernst equation: $E = E° - (\frac{RT}{nF})\ln Q$.

CHAPTER 12 FREESTANDING PRACTICE QUESTIONS

1. Typical dry cell batteries contain a zinc anode and a carbon cathode and produce a potential difference of 1.5 V. Given that many electronic devices require additional voltage, which of the following would result in an overall increase in voltage?

    I.   Doubling the quantity of Zn(s)
    II. Placing two batteries in parallel
    III. Replacing Zn(s) with Na(s)

A) I only
B) III only
C) I and II only
D) II and III only

2. Given the following reactions:

$$Pb^{2+} + 2e^- \rightarrow Pb(s) \quad E^\circ = -0.13 \text{ V}$$
$$Fe(s) \rightarrow Fe^{2+} + 2e^- \quad E^\circ = 0.45 \text{ V}$$

Which one of the following is true?

A) Pb(s) is a better reductant than Fe(s)
B) Fe(s) is a worse reductant than Pb(s)
C) Fe^{2+} is a better oxidant than Pb^{2+}
D) Pb^{2+} is a better oxidant than Fe^{2+}

3. Which of the following best characterizes the spontaneous half-reaction below under standard conditions?

$$Pd^{2+} + 2e^- \rightarrow Pd$$

A) $\Delta G^\circ > 0$ and $E^\circ < 0$
B) $\Delta G^\circ < 0$ and $E^\circ < 0$
C) $\Delta G^\circ > 0$ and $E^\circ > 0$
D) $\Delta G^\circ < 0$ and $E^\circ > 0$

4. High valent metals (those with large, positive oxidation states) are often used as strong oxidizing agents. Which of the following compounds would have the most positive reduction potential vs. a standard hydrogen electrode?

A) $FeCl_3$
B) OsO_4
C) $Zn(NO_3)Cl$
D) $W(CO)_6$

5. Which of the following best describes the difference between a galvanic cell and an electrolytic cell?

A) In a galvanic cell, the anode is the site of oxidation, whereas in an electrolytic cell the anode is the site of reduction.
B) In a galvanic cell, the cathode is the negative electrode, whereas in an electrolytic cell the cathode is the positive electrode.
C) In a galvanic cell, spontaneous reactions generate a current, whereas in an electrolytic cell a current forces nonspontaneous reactions to occur.
D) In a galvanic cell, the electrons flow from anode to cathode, whereas in an electrolytic cell the electrons flow from cathode to anode.

6. To give "white gold" a white appearance, it is plated with rhodium by immersion in a rhodium sulfate solution $(Rh_2(SO_4)_3(aq))$. Provided with a current of 2.0 A, how long must a 3.0 g white gold broach be immersed to plate 3.0×10^{-5} g of rhodium? (Faraday's constant = 96,500 C/mol e^-)

A) 0.0009 s
B) 0.0098 s
C) 0.042 s
D) 0.56 s

7. A galvanic cell is constructed from two half-cells of platinum and iron. The half-reactions for these two elements are provided as follows:

$$Pt^{2+}(aq) + 2e^- \rightarrow Pt \text{ (s)} \qquad E^\circ = +1.20 \text{ V}$$
$$Fe^{3+}(aq) + 3e^- \rightarrow Fe \text{ (s)} \qquad E^\circ = -0.036 \text{ V}$$

Which of the following statements is true about the galvanic cell?

A) $E^\circ = 1.164$ V, and Pt^{2+} is the reducing agent
B) $E^\circ = 1.164$ V, and Fe^{3+} is the reducing agent.
C) $E^\circ = 1.236$ V, and Pt^{2+} is the oxidizing agent.
D) $E^\circ = 1.236$ V, and Fe^{3+} is the oxidizing agent.

8. An electrochemical cell is constructed using two inert electrodes in one chamber with an inert electrolyte. The binary compound ICl is dissolved in the electrolyte, current is applied, and I_2 and Cl_2 are produced. Which of the following statements is true?

A) Cl_2 was produced by reduction at the cathode.
B) I_2 was produced by oxidation at the cathode.
C) Cl_2 was produced by oxidation at the cathode.
D) I_2 was produced by reduction at the cathode.

CHAPTER 12 PRACTICE PASSAGE

A student follows the schematic below and sets up the following electrochemical cell at room temperature.

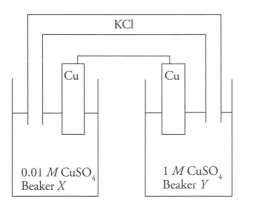

Figure 1   Schematic of an experimental electrochemical cell

The student fills Beaker X with a 0.01 M solution of $CuSO_4$ and Beaker Y with a 1 M solution of $CuSO_4$. Two copper plates serve as electrodes and a $KCl(aq)$ salt bridge is used. Because of the nonstandard conditions, the student uses the Nernst equation to calculate the expected potential of the cell:

$$E = E° - \frac{RT}{nF} \ln Q$$

where $E°$ is the standard cell voltage, R is the universal gas constant, T is the absolute temperature, n is the number of electron moles, F is Faraday's constant, and Q is the reaction quotient. Substituting in the constant variables and converting the natural logarithm, the student obtains the following formula:

$$E = E° - \frac{0.0592}{n} \log Q \text{ at } 25° \text{ C}$$

After setting up the half-cells, the student connects the two electrodes via a voltmeter and measures the initial cell potential.

Table 1   Standard reduction potentials for copper ions

Half-Reaction	$E°$ (V)
$Cu^+ + e^- \rightarrow Cu(s)$	+ 0.52
$Cu^{2+} + 2e^- \rightarrow Cu(s)$	+ 0.34

1. What is the standard cell voltage, $E°$, of the cell used in the experiment?

   A)   + 0.52 V
   B)   + 0.34 V
   C)   + 0.18 V
   D)   0 V

2. Which of the following correctly describes the relationship between the movement of electrons and K^+ ions?

   A) K^+ ions and electrons both travel towards Beaker X.
   B) K^+ ions travel towards Beaker X and electrons travel towards Beaker Y.
   C) K^+ ions travel towards Beaker Y and electrons travel towards Beaker X.
   D) K^+ ions and electrons both travel towards Beaker Y.

3. Which of the following substances has the atom with the greatest oxidation state?

   A) CH_2F_2
   B) K_2O
   C) $S_4O_6^{2-}$
   D) Fe_2O_3

4. Which of the following best describes the cell used in the experiment?

   A)   Beaker X contains the cathode that is negatively charged.
   B)   Beaker Y contains the cathode that is negatively charged.
   C)   Beaker X contains the anode that is negatively charged.
   D)   Beaker Y contains the anode that is negatively charged.

5. What is the expected potential of the cell at the start of the experiment?

   A)   +0.118 V
   B)   +0.059 V
   C)   −0.118 V
   D)   −0.059 V

SOLUTIONS TO CHAPTER 12 FREESTANDING PRACTICE QUESTIONS

1. **B**   Increasing reagent quantity has no effect on voltage (Item I is incorrect, eliminating choices A and C), and placing batteries in parallel would leave the voltage unchanged (Item II is incorrect, eliminating choice D). Oxidation of zinc takes place at the anode, and sodium is a better reducing agent than zinc due to its lower ionization energy and tendency to give up an electron (Item III would result in an increase in voltage; the correct answer is choice B).

2. **D**   *Oxidant* and *reductant* are synonymous with *oxidizing agent* and *reducing agent*, respectively. Choices A and B are saying the same thing, so both can be eliminated. To compare the relative strengths of the ions as oxidizing agents, reverse the half reaction for Fe so that it reads as a reduction:

$$Pb^{2+} + 2e^- \rightarrow Pb(s) \quad E° = -0.13 \text{ V}$$

$$Fe^{2+} + 2e^- \rightarrow Fe(s) \quad E° = -0.45 \text{ V}$$

   Note that the sign of $E°$ is reversed in this process. Pb^{2+} has a more positive reduction potential than Fe^{2+}, making it the better oxidant.

3. **D**   This question is asking about two factors (a two by two question): $\Delta G°$ and $E°$, which are related by $\Delta G° = -nFE°$. For any spontaneous reaction, the change in Gibbs free energy ($\Delta G°$) is always less than 0 (eliminate choices A and C). As shown in the equation above, the standard reduction potential ($E°$) must be positive when $\Delta G°$ is negative, so eliminate choice B.

4. **B**   A large, positive reduction potential indicates a strong tendency to be reduced, and hence ability to act as an oxidizing agent. The question states that high-valent metals act as strong oxidizing agents. Examining the oxidation states of the metals in question, we see that Fe = +3, Os = +8, Zn = +2, and W = 0. Therefore, since Os bears the largest positive oxidation state, we know that it is the strongest oxidizing agent.

5. **C**   The anode is always the site of oxidation and the cathode is always the site of reduction; therefore, electrons always flow from the anode (oxidation) to the cathode (reduction) regardless of the kind of cell (choices A and D are wrong). In a galvanic cell, a spontaneous reaction liberates electrons and they flow freely to the positive electrode, which in this case would be the cathode. However, in an electrolytic cell the current is forcing the electrons to flow where they don't want to go: the negative electrode. In this case the cathode would be the negative electrode (choice B is wrong).

6. **C** Since current (I) = charge(Q) / time(t) we can set up and solve the following equation keeping in mind that the rhodium reduction in question is $Rh^{3+} + 3e^- \rightarrow Rh(s)$.

$$t = \frac{Q}{I} = \frac{(3 \times 10^{-5}\,g)\left(\dfrac{1\,mol\,Rh}{102.9\,g}\right)\left(\dfrac{3\,mol\,e^-}{1\,mol\,Rh}\right)\left(\dfrac{9.65 \times 10^4\,C}{1\,mol\,e^-}\right)}{2.0\,A}$$

$$t \approx \frac{(3 \times 10^{-5}\,g)\left(\dfrac{1\,mol\,Rh}{100\,g}\right)\left(\dfrac{3\,mol\,e^-}{1\,mol\,Rh}\right)\left(\dfrac{1.0 \times 10^5\,C}{1\,mol\,e^-}\right)}{2.0\,A} \approx \frac{9 \times 10^{-2}\,C}{2.0\,A} \approx 0.045\,s$$

7. **C** The half-reaction with the *less positive* reduction potential (in this case, $Fe^{3+}(aq) + 3e \rightarrow$ Fe(s)) should be reversed in order to combine the half-reactions to obtain an $E^0 > 0$ and create a galvanic cell. When the Fe half-reaction is reversed, the sign of the potential must be reversed. Combining the two half-reactions then gives: $3\,Pt^{2+}(aq) + 2\,Fe(s) \rightarrow 2\,Fe^{3+}(aq) + 3\,Pt(s)$ with an $E^0 = 1.236$ V (eliminate choices A and B). Since Fe^{3+} is the product of the reaction, it cannot be the oxidizing agent (eliminate choice D). However, Pt^{2+} is reduced (it gains electrons from the Fe that is oxidized), so it is therefore the oxidizing agent.

8. **D** In the compound ICl, I has an +1 oxidation state, and Cl has a -1 oxidation state owing to the greater electronegativity of Cl. Therefore, production of Cl_2 must be an oxidation, and production of I_2 must be a reduction eliminating choices A and B. Moreover, reduction always takes place at the cathode, eliminating choice C.

SOLUTIONS TO CHAPTER 12 PRACTICE PASSAGE

1. **D** The setup shown is an example of a concentration cell. The difference in concentration will produce an electrical current, until the concentrations in both half-cells become equal. The standard cell voltage for this cell (and all concentration cells) is 0, because reciprocal redox reactions are occurring.

2. **D** No matter the type of cell, electrons always flow from anode to cathode. Also, oxidation always occurs at the anode and reduction always occurs at the cathode. In the concentration cell in the passage, $[Cu^{2+}]$ will increase in Beaker X and decrease in Beaker Y until they equalize. Therefore, oxidation occurs in Beaker X and reduction occurs in Beaker Y. Electrons flow from X to Y, and K^+ ions follow the electrons to minimize the charge build-up in Beaker Y.

3. D   Assigning oxidation states yields:

$$CH_2F_2: F = -1, H = 0, C = -2;$$

$$K_2O: K = +1, O = -2;$$

$$S_4O_6^{2-}: O = -2, S = \text{average of } +2.5;$$

$$Fe_2O_3: O = -2, Fe = +3;$$

Since +3 is the greatest number, choice D is the best answer.

4. C   Electrons always travel from anode to cathode. Loss of electrons, or oxidation, always occurs at the anode and gain of electrons, or reduction, always occurs at the cathode. A concentration cell is spontaneous, so electrons will spontaneously flow to a positive charge. Therefore, the cathode must be positively charged, eliminating choices A and B. Since $[Cu^{2+}]$ will increase in X and decrease in Y, X is the site of oxidation, or anode.

5. B   A concentration cell is spontaneous, eliminating the negative values of potential in choices C and D. The net "reaction" of the concentration cell in the passage is:

$$Cu^{2+}_{1\,M} \rightarrow Cu^{2+}_{0.1\,M}$$

Therefore, the reaction quotient is:

$$Q = \frac{[0.01]}{[1]} = \frac{1}{100}$$

Copper is reacting between the Cu and Cu(II) state, so $n = 2$. Substitute these quantities into the Nernst equation to solve for potential:

$$E = E^\circ - \frac{0.0592}{n} \log Q = 0 - \frac{0.0592}{2} \log \frac{1}{100} = 0.059\,V$$

Glossary

absolute zero
The temperature (–273.15°C or 0 K) at which the volume and pressure of an ideal gas extrapolate to zero according to the ideal gas law. [Section 6.4]

acid
See *Arrhenius acid*, *Brønsted-Lowry acid*, and *Lewis acid*. [Section 11.1]

acid-base indicator
A weak acid and conjugate base pair, such as litmus or phenolphthalein, that changes color with changes in solution pH.

acid-dissociation constant (K_a)
A measure of the extent of dissociation of an acid, HA. K_a is defined as $K_a = [H_3O^+][A^-]/[HA]$. [Section 11.3]

activation energy, E_a
The energy required by the reactants in a chemical reaction to reach a transition state from which the products of the reaction can form. [Section 6.6]

alkali metal
One of the metal elements in Group IA (Li, Na, K, Rb, Cs, and Fr). [Section 4.7]

alkaline earth metal
One of the metal elements in Group IIA (Be, Mg, Ca, Sr, Ba, and Ra). [Section 4.7]

allotropes
Forms of a pure element with different structures and therefore different chemical and physical properties, such as O_2 and O_3 or carbon$_{(diamond)}$ and carbon$_{(graphite)}$. [Section 6.6]

alloy
A blend of two or more metallic elements. Bronze, for example, is an alloy of copper and tin. [Section 10.4]

alpha (α) particle
A positively charged particle consisting of two protons and two neutrons emitted during alpha decay. An alpha particle is identical to a helium-4 nucleus. [Section 4.4]

amphoteric
An ion or molecule, such as H_2O or HCO_3^-, that can act as either a Brønsted-Lowry acid or base. [Section 11.3]

anhydrous
A substance that is devoid of water. Used, for example, to differentiate between liquid (anhydrous) ammonia at temperatures below its boiling point (–33°C) and solutions of ammonia dissolved in water.

anion
A negatively charged ion, such as F⁻. [Section 4.3]

anode
The site of oxidation in a galvanic or electrolytic cell. Also, the electrode towards which anions flow through a salt bridge. [Section 12.2]

aqueous
Solutions of substances where water is the primary solvent. [Section 10.4]

Arrhenius acid
A compound that dissociates when it dissolves in water to give the H⁺ ion. [Section 11.1]

Arrhenius base
A compound that dissociates when it dissolves in water to give the OH⁻ ion. [Section 11.1]

Arrhenius equation
The equation for the rate constant (k) of a chemical reaction, in terms of the temperature (T), activation energy (E_a), and collision frequency/steric orientation factor (A): $k = Ae^{-E_a/RT}$. [Section 9.4]

atomic mass unit (amu, u)
The unit of mass most convenient for individual subatomic particles, atoms, and molecules. [Section 3.5]

atomic number (Z)
The number of protons in the nucleus of an atom. [Section 4.1]

atomic orbital
A region in space where electrons of an atom are most probably found. [**Section 5.2**]

atomic radius
The size of an atom equal to the volume of space carved out by the outermost (valence) electrons. [**Section 4.8**]

atomic weight
The weighted average of the atomic masses of the different isotopes of an element. A single ^{12}C atom, for example, has a mass of 12 amu, but naturally occurring carbon also contains 1.1% ^{13}C. The atomic weight of carbon is therefore 12.011 amu. [**Section 3.5**]

Aufbau principle
The principle that atomic orbitals are filled one at a time, starting with the orbital that has the lowest energy and then filling upwards. [**Section 4.6**]

Avogadro's number
The number of items that make up one mole, approximately 6.02×10^{23}. [**Section 3.6**]

Avogadro's hypothesis
The hypothesis that equal volumes of different gases at the same temperature and pressure contain the same number of particles. [**Section 8.2**]

base
See *Arrhenius base, Brønsted-Lowry base,* and *Lewis base.* [**Section 11.1**]

base-dissociation constant (K_b)
A measure of the extent of dissociation of a base, B: $K_b = [HB^+][OH^-]/[B]$. [**Section 11.3**]

battery
A set of electrochemical cells connected in series or parallel. [**Section 12.6**]

beta (β) decay
A nuclear reaction in which an electron (e^-) or positron (β^+) is absorbed by or emitted from the nucleus of an atom. [**Section 4.4**]

beta (β) particle
An electron or a positron. [**Section 4.4**]

bimolecular
A step in a chemical reaction in which two molecules collide to form products.

Bohr model
A model of the distribution of electrons in an atom based on the assumption that the electron in a hydrogen atom is in one of a limited number of circular orbits. [**Section 4.5**]

Bohr atom
An atom or ion that has just one electron such as H, He^+, Li^{2+}, etc. [**Section 4.5**]

boiling point
The temperature at which the vapor pressure of a liquid is equal to the external or atmospheric pressure. [**Section 5.8**]

bond-dissociation energy/enthalpy
The energy needed to homolytically break an X—Y bond to give X and Y atoms in the gas phase. [**Section 5.2**]

bonding electrons
A pair of electrons, always the outermost (valence) electrons, used to form a covalent bond between adjacent atoms. [**Section 5.1**]

Boyle's law
A statement of the relationship between the pressure and volume of a constant amount of gas at constant temperatures: $P \propto 1/V$. [**Section 8.2**]

Brønsted-Lowry acid
Any molecule or ion that can donate an H^+ (proton) to a base. [**Section 11.1**]

Brønsted-Lowry base
Any molecule or ion that can accept an H^+ (proton) from an acid. [**Section 11.1**]

buffer
A mixture of a weak acid (HA) and its conjugate base (A^-), which should be present in roughly equal amounts. Buffers resist a change in the pH of a solution according to Le Châtelier's principle when small amounts of acid or base are added. [**Section 11.8**]

buffer capacity
The amount of acid or base a buffer solution can absorb without significant changes in pH. [**Section 11.8**]

calorie
The heat needed to raise the temperature of 1 gram of water by 1°C. [**Section 7.2**]

calorimeter
An insulated apparatus used to measure the heat absorbed/released in a chemical reaction.

catalyst
A substance that increases the rate of a chemical reaction without being consumed in the reaction. A substance that lowers the activation energy for a chemical reaction by providing an alternate pathway for the reaction. [**Section 9.3**]

cathode
The site of reduction in a galvanic or electrolytic cell. Also, the electrode in an electrochemical cell towards which cations flow through a salt bridge. [**Section 12.2**]

cation
A positively charged ion, such as Na^+. [**Section 4.3**]

cell potential
A measure of the driving force behind an electrochemical reaction, reported in volts. [**Section 12.3**]

Charles's law
A statement of the relationship between the temperature and volume of a constant amount of gas at constant pressure: $V \propto T$. [**Section 8.3**]

collision theory model
A model used to explain the rates of chemical reactions, which assumes that molecules must collide in order to react. [**Section 9.2**]

common-ion effect
The decrease in the solubility of a salt that occurs when the salt is dissolved in a solution that contains another source of one of its ions. Just another form of Le Châtelier's principle. [**Section 10.6**]

complex ion
An ion in which a ligand is bound to a metal via a coordinate covalent bond. An ion formed when a Lewis acid such as the Co^{2+} ion reacts with a Lewis base such as NH_3 to form an acid-base complex such as the $Co(NH_3)_4^{2+}$ ion. [**Section 10.7**]

compound
A substance with a constant composition that contains two or more elements.

concentration
A measure of the ratio of the amount of solute in a solution to the amount of either solvent or solution. Frequently expressed as molarity (units of moles of solute per liter of solution). [**Section 3.8**]

concentration cell
A type of electrochemical cell that has identical reactants in each half reaction, but at different concentrations, thus driving a weak electrical current. [**Section 12.4**]

conjugate acid-base pair
Two substances related by the gain or loss of a proton. An acid (such as HBr) and its conjugate base (Br^-), or a base (such as NH_3) and its conjugate acid (NH_4^+) are examples of conjugate acid-base pairs. [**Section 11.3**]

coordinate covalent bond
A covalent bond formed as a result of a Lewis acid-base reaction, most often formed between a metal atom and a nonmetal atom. [Section 5.3]

coordination compound
A compound in which one or more ligands are coordinated to a metal atom. [Section 5.3]

corrosion
A process in which a metal is destroyed by a chemical reaction. When the metal is iron, the process is called rusting.

covalent bond
A bond between two atoms formed by the sharing of at least one pair of electrons. [Section 5.3]

covalent compound
A compound, such as water (H_2O), composed of neutral molecules in which the atoms are held together by covalent bonds. [Section 5.3]

critical point
The temperature and pressure at which two phases of a substance that are in equilibrium (usually the gas and liquid phases) become identical and form a single phase. [Section 7.4]

crystal
A three-dimensional solid formed by regular repetition of the packing of atoms, ions, or molecules. [Section 5.8]

Dalton's law of partial pressures
A statement of the relationship between the total pressure of a mixture of gases and the partial pressures of the individual components:
$P_{total} = p_1 + p_2 + p_3 + \ldots$ [Section 8.4]

daughter nucleus
The product nucleus after a nuclear reaction. [Section 4.4]

density
The mass of a sample divided by its volume. [Section 3.2]

deposition
A process in which a gas goes directly to the solid state without passing through an intermediate liquid state. [Section 7.1]

diamagnetic
A substance in which the electrons are all paired. [Section 4.6]

dilution
The process by which more solvent is added to decrease the concentration of a solution.

dimer
A compound (such as B_2H_6) produced by combining two smaller identical molecules (such as BH_3).

dipole
Anything with two equal but opposite electrical charges, such as the positive and negative ends of a polar bond or molecule. [Section 5.6]

diprotic acid
An acid, such as H_2SO_4, that can lose two H^+.

diprotic base
A base, such as the O^{2-} ion, that can accept two H^+.

dissolution
The process in which a bulk solid or liquid breaks up into individual molecules or ions and diffuses throughout a solvent. [Section 10.4]

ductile
Capable of being drawn into thin sheets or wires without breaking; a property of metals. [Section 5.8]

effusion
The process by which a gas escapes through a pinhole into a region of lower pressure. [Section 8.5]

elastic collision
A collision in which no kinetic energy is lost. [Section 8.1]

electrolyte
A substance that increases the electrical conductivity of water by dissociating into ions. [Section 10.1]

electrolysis
A process in which an electric current is used to drive a nonspontaneous chemical reaction. [Section 12.6]

electrolytic cell
A nonspontaneous electric cell in which electrolysis is done. [Section 12.6]

electron
A subatomic particle with a mass of only about 0.0005 amu and a charge of $-1e$ that surrounds the nucleus of an atom. [Section 4.1]

electron affinity
The energy given off when a neutral atom in the gas phase picks up an electron to form a negatively charged ion. [Section 4.8]

electron capture
A type of beta decay where the nucleus of an atom captures an electron and converts a nuclear proton into a neutron. [Section 4.4]

electron configuration
The arrangement of electrons in atomic orbitals; for example, $1s^2 2s^2 2p^3$. [Section 4.6]

electronegativity
The tendency of an atom to draw or polarize bonding electrons toward itself. [Section 4.8]

element
A substance that cannot be decomposed into a simpler substance by a chemical reaction. A substance composed of only one kind of atom. [Section 3.5]

empirical formula
The formula for a compound in which the number of atoms of each element in the compound are represented by the lowest whole number ratio. [Section 3.4]

endergonic
A process that leads to an increase in the free energy of a system and is therefore not spontaneous: ΔG_{rxn} is positive. [Section 6.6]

endothermic
A chemical reaction that absorbs heat from the surroundings: ΔH_{rxn} is positive. [Section 6.2]

endpoint
The point at which the indicator of an acid-base titration changes color.

enthalpy (H)
The total potential energy in a substance due to intermolecular forces and covalent bonds. [Section 6.2]

enthalpy of reaction (ΔH_{rxn})
The change in the enthalpy that occurs during a chemical reaction. The difference between the sum of the enthalpies of the products and the reactants. [Section 6.2]

entropy (S)
A measure of the disorder in a system. Increasing disorder yields a positive ΔS. [Section 6.4]

equilibrium (dynamic)
The point at which there is no longer a change in the concentrations of the reactants and the products of a chemical reaction. The point at which the rates of the forward and reverse reactions are equal: $\Delta G_{rxn} = 0$. [Section 10.4]

equilibrium constant (K_{eq})
The product of the concentrations (or partial pressures) of the products of a reaction at equilibrium divided by the product of the concentrations (or partial pressures) of the reactants. [Section 10.1]

equilibrium expression
The expression used to calculate the equilibrium constant for a reaction that takes the form [products]/[reactants]. [Section 10.1]

equivalence point
The point in an acid-base titration at which the number of moles of H_3O^+ in solution equals the number of moles of OH^- in solution. [**Section 11.10**]

excited state configuration
One of an infinite number of electron configurations of an energized atom where at least one electron occupies an orbital of higher energy than that dictated by Hund's rule and/or the Aufbau principle. [**Section 4.5**]

exergonic
A process that leads to a decrease in the free energy of the system and is therefore spontaneous: ΔG_{rxn} is negative. [**Section 6.6**]

exothermic
A chemical reaction that releases energy to the surroundings: ΔH_{rxn} is negative. [**Section 6.2**]

family
A vertical column of elements in the periodic table, such as the elements Li, Na, K, etc. [**Section 4.6**]

Faraday's law of electrolysis
A statement of the relationship between the amount of electric current that passes through an electrolytic cell and the amount of product formed during electrolysis. The amount of chemical change is proportional to the amount of electric current that flows through the cell. [**Section 12.7**]

first ionization energy
The energy needed to remove the valence electron from a neutral atom in the gas phase. [**Section 4.8**]

first law of thermodynamics
The total energy in the universe is conserved: energy is neither created nor destroyed, but may change from one form to another. [**Section 6.1**]

first-order reaction
A reaction in which the rate is proportional to the concentration of a single reactant raised to the first power: rate = k[A]. [**Section 9.4**]

formal charge
The theoretical charge on an atom in a molecule, calculated by $V - \frac{1}{2}B - L$, where V is the number of valence electrons, B is the number of bonding electrons, and L is the number of lone-pair electrons. [**Section 5.1**]

free energy, Gibbs (G)
The energy associated with a chemical reaction that can be used to do work. The change in free energy of a system is calculated by the formula $\Delta G = \Delta H - T\Delta S$, where G is the free energy, H is enthalpy, T is temperature (in kelvins), and S is entropy. [**Section 6.5**]

free radical
An atom or molecule that contains an unpaired electron. [**Section 5.2**]

freezing point
The temperature at which the solid and liquid phases of a substance are in equilibrium. [**Section 7.1**]

fusion
The melting of a solid to form a liquid. [**Section 7.1**]

galvanic cell
An electrochemical cell that uses a spontaneous chemical reaction to do work. Synonymous with *voltaic cell*. [**Section 12.2**]

gamma ray (γ)
A high energy, short wavelength form of electromagnetic radiation emitted by the nucleus of an atom that carries off some of the energy generated in a nuclear reaction. [**Section 4.4**]

Gibbs free energy
See *free energy*. [**Section 6.5**]

Graham's law
The relationship between the rate at which a gas diffuses or effuses and its molecular weight: rate $\propto 1/(MW)^{1/2}$. [**Section 8.5**]

ground state configuration
The most stable arrangement of electrons in an atom that satisfies Hund's rule and the Aufbau principle. [**Section 4.5**]

group
A vertical column, or family, of elements in the periodic table. [**Section 4.7**]

half-life
The time required for the amount of a decaying substance to decrease to half its initial value. [**Section 4.4**]

halogen
Elements of Group VIIA: F, Cl, Br, I, and At. [**Section 4.7**]

heat (q)
Thermal energy in transit from a hotter system to a colder one. [**Section 6.1**]

heat of fusion
The heat that must be absorbed to melt a unit quantity of a solid. [**Section 7.2**]

heat of reaction
The change in the enthalpy of the system that occurs when a reaction is run at constant pressure. Synonymous with *enthalpy of reaction*, ΔH_{rxn}. [**Section 6.2**]

heat of vaporization
The heat that must be absorbed to boil a unit quantity of a liquid. [**Section 7.2**]

heat capacity
The amount of heat required to raise the temperature of a given amount of a substance by one degree. Not to be confused with *specific heat*. Heat capacity is typically the product of mass and specific heat. [**Section 7.3**]

Hess's law
The heat given off or absorbed in a chemical reaction does not depend on whether the reaction occurs in a single step or in many steps. [**Section 6.3**]

homonuclear diatomic molecule
A molecule, such as O_2 or F_2, that contains two atoms of the same element.

Hund's rule
Rule for placing electrons in equal-energy orbitals, which states that electrons are added with parallel spins until each of the orbitals has one electron, before a second electron is placed in a given orbital. [**Section 4.6**]

hybrid orbitals
Orbitals formed by mixing two or more atomic orbitals. [**Section 5.5**]

hybridization
A process in which things are mixed. A resonance hybrid is a mixture, or average, of two or more Lewis structures. Hybrid orbitals are formed by mixing two or more atomic orbitals. [**Section 5.5**]

hydride
The species H^-. [**Section 5.4**]

hydrogen bonding
A strong dipole-dipole interaction that occurs between a hydrogen atom covalently bonded to an F, O, or N that electrostatically interacts with a lone pair of electrons on another F, O, or N atom. [**Section 5.7**]

hydrophilic
To be attracted or compatible with water (for example, ions that are soluble in water).

hydrophobic
To be incompatible with water (for example, lipids insoluble in water).

ideal gas
A gas that obeys all the postulates of the kinetic-molecule theory and has properties that can be predicted by the ideal gas law. [**Section 8.1**]

ideal gas law
The relationship between the pressure, volume, temperature, and amount of an ideal gas: $PV = nRT$. [**Section 8.2**]

immiscible
Liquids, such as oil and water, that do not dissolve in one another.

indicator
See *acid-base indicator*. [**Section 11.9**]

induced dipole
A short-lived separation of charge, or dipole, of a nonpolar atom or molecule caused by the electrostatic influence of a nearby polar atom or ion. [**Section 5.7**]

inert
Unreactive. Used to describe compounds that do not undergo chemical reactions. [**Section 4.7**]

insoluble
Used to describe a substance that does not noticeably dissolve in a solvent. [**Section 10.4**]

intermolecular forces
Attractive electrostatic forces, the strength of which determine a compound's phase, vapor pressure, melting point, boiling point, solubility, and viscosity. From strongest to weakest, the main categories of intermolecular forces are: *ionic*, *dipole-dipole* (with H bonds the strongest), and *London dispersion forces*. [**Section 5.7**]

intramolecular bonds
Synonym for covalent bonds. There are three primary types: normal covalent bonds, metallic covalent bonds, and coordinate covalent bonds. [**Section 7.1**]

ion product (Q_{sp})
The product of the concentrations of the ions in a solution at any moment. [**Section 10.5**]

ion-product constant of water (K_w)
The product of the equilibrium concentration of the H_3O^+ and OH^- ions in an aqueous solution at $25°C$: $K_w = 1.0 \times 10^{-14}$. [**Section 11.4**]

ionic bond
Misappropriation of the term *bond*. Simply the strong electrostatic attraction between two oppositely charged ions; there is no electron sharing. [**Section 5.3**]

ionic compound
A compound made up of ions (synonymous with *salt*). [**Section 3.5**]

ionizability factor (i)
The number of individual particles formed when an individual solute dissolves. Synonymous with *van't Hoff factor*. [**Section 10.4**]

ionization
A process in which an ion is created from a neutral atom or molecule by adding or removing one or more electrons. [**Section 4.8**]

ionization energy
See *first ionization energy*. [**Section 4.8**]

isoelectronic
Atoms or ions that have the same number of electrons and therefore the same electron configuration, such as O^{2-}, F^-, Ne, and Na^+. [**Section 4.6**]

isotopes
Nuclides of the same element, but with differing numbers of neutrons, such as ^{12}C, ^{13}C, and ^{14}C. Isotopes have nearly identical chemical properties. [**Section 4.2**]

joule
A unit of measurement for both heat and work in the SI system. 1 J = 4.184 cal. [**Section 4.2**]

kinetic energy
The energy associated with motion. The kinetic energy of an object is equal to one-half the product of its mass and the square of its speed: $KE = \frac{1}{2}mv^2$. [**Section 5.8**]

kinetic-molecular theory
The theory that states heat is associated with the thermal motion of particles, taking into account the important assumptions that individual gas molecules take up no volume and collisions between gas molecules are perfectly elastic. [**Section 8.1**]

Le Châtelier's principle
A principle that describes the effect of changes in the temperature, pressure, or concentration of one of the reactants or products of a reaction at equilibrium. It states that when a system at equilibrium is subjected to a stress, it will shift in the direction that minimizes the effect of this stress. [**Section 10.3**]

Lewis acid
An atom or molecule that accepts a pair of electrons to form a new coordinate covalent bond. Almost always a metal atom, positively charged ion, or both. [**Section 5.3**]

Lewis base
An atom or molecule that donates a pair of electrons to form a new coordinate covalent bond. Almost always a nonmetal with a pair of nonbonding electrons. Synonymous with *ligand* and *chelator*. [**Section 5.3**]

ligand
See *Lewis base*. [**Section 5.3**]

limiting reagent
The reactant in a chemical reaction that is exhausted first, thus limiting the amount of product that can be formed. [**Section 3.11**]

London dispersion forces
Intermolecular forces that arise from interactions between an instantaneous dipole/induced dipole pair. Typically, these are the weakest of all intermolecular forces. However LDFs are additive, and nonpolar molecules with large, flat surface areas can experience moderate LDFs. [**Section 5.7**]

malleable
Something that can be hammered, pounded, or pressed into different shapes without breaking (a common property of metals). [**Section 5.8**]

mass number (A)
The total number of protons and neutrons in the nucleus of an atom. [**Section 4.1**]

melting point
The temperature at which the solid and liquid phases of a substance are in equilibrium at a particular external pressure. [**Section 5.7**]

metal
An element that is solid, has a metallic luster, is malleable and ductile, and conducts both heat and electricity. [**Section 3.9**]

metalloid
An element with properties that fall between the extremes of metals and nonmetals. [**Section 4.7**]

mixture
A substance that contains two or more elements or compounds that retain their chemical identities and can be separated by a physical process. For example, the mixture of N_2 and O_2 in the atmosphere. [**Section 3.8**]

molarity (M)
The number of moles of a solute in a solution divided by the volume of the solution in liters. [**Section 3.1**]

mole
6.02×10^{23} of anything. [**Section 3.6**]

mole fraction (X)
The fraction of the total number of moles in a mixture due to one component of the mixture. The mole fraction of a solute, for example, is the number of moles of solute divided by the total number of moles of solute plus solvent. [Section 3.8]

mole ratio
The ratio of the moles of one reactant or product to the moles of another reactant of product in the balanced equation for a chemical reaction.

molecular formula
The formula representing the number and type of constituent atoms in a compound. [Section 3.3]

molecular geometry
The arrangement of atoms surrounding a central atom of a small molecule. Molecular geometry (or the shape of a molecule) and orbital geometry are identical only when the central atom possesses no lone pairs of electrons. [Section 5.4]

molecular weight
The weight of the molecular formula, calculated from a table of atomic weights. Note that atomic weights are a weighted average of masses of isotopes as they occur in nature. [Section 5.7]

molecule
The smallest particle that has any of the chemical or physical properties of a compound. [Section 3.3]

monoprotic acid (HA)
An acid, such as HF or HOCl, that can lose only one H^+.

negative electrode
The electrode in an electrochemical cell that carries a negative charge. In a galvanic cell, it is the anode; in an electrolytic cell, it is the cathode.

Nernst equation
Used to calculate or track the voltage of an electrochemical cell under *nonstandard* conditions: $E = E° - (0.06/n) \log Q$. [Section 12.4]

network solid
A solid, such as diamond, in which every atom is covalently bonded to its nearest neighbors to form an extended array of atoms rather than individual molecules. [Section 5.8]

neutron
A subatomic particle with a mass of about 1 amu and no charge. [Section 4.1]

noble gases
The elements in the last column of the periodic table that are chemically unreactive. [Section 4.6]

nonbonding electrons
Electrons in the valence shell of an atom that are not used to form covalent bonds. [Section 5.1]

nonmetal
An element that lacks the properties generally associated with metals. These elements are found in the upper right of the periodic table. [Section 4.7]

nonpolar
Used to describe a compound that has a homogenous electron distribution and thus does not carry a permanent dipole moment. [Section 5.3]

nonspontaneous
A reaction in which the products are not favored, implying that the reverse reaction would be favored: ΔG_{rxn} is positive (and E_{cell} is negative). [Section 2.6]

nucleon
Generic term for a proton or neutron. [Section 4.1]

nuclide
The generic term for any particular isotope of an element, such as the ^{13}C nuclide.

octet rule
The tendency of main-group elements to react in order to possess eight valence-shell electrons in their compounds.

orbital geometry
The arrangement of electron clouds surrounding a central atom of a small molecule. Orbital geometry is a consequence of hybridization. Not to be confused with *shape,* or *molecular geometry.* [Section 5.4]

orbitals
Regions in space where electrons have a high probability of existing. [Section 4.5]

order
Used to describe the relationship between the rate of a step in a chemical reaction and the concentration of one of the reactants consumed in that step. Essentially just the value of the exponent found in a reactant term in the rate law. [Section 9.4]

oxidation
A process in which an atom, ion, or molecule loses one or more electrons. [Section 3.13]

oxidation number
Synonymous with *oxidation state.* It is the hypothetical charge that would be present on each atom if a molecule was shattered into its individual constituent atoms with bonding electrons ending up with the atom of the bond having the higher electronegativity. [Section 3.13]

oxidation-reduction reaction
A chemical reaction involving the exchange of electrons such that oxidation numbers of reactants change. [Section 12.1]

oxidizing agent / oxidant
An atom, ion, or molecule that undergoes reduction by gaining electrons, thereby oxidizing something else. [Section 4.7]

pH
A measure of acidity ranging from about –1.5 to 15.5 in aqueous media, defined as $-\log[H_3O^+]$. [Section 11.5]

pOH
The complement of pH, defined as $-\log[OH^-]$. [Section 11.5]

paramagnetic
A compound that contains one or more unpaired electrons and is attracted into a magnetic field. [Section 4.6]

parent nucleus
The initial nucleus prior to a nuclear reaction. [Section 4.4]

partial pressure
The fraction of the total pressure of a mixture of gases that is due to one component of the mixture. As molarity is the primary way of expressing the amount of solute in a solution, so too is partial pressure the primary way to report the quantity of a gas in a mixture of gases. [Section 8.4]

Pauli exclusion principle
The maximum number of electrons in any given orbital is two, and they must have the opposite spin. [Section 4.6]

period
A horizontal row in the periodic table. [Section 4.6]

polar covalent bond
A covalent bond between atoms with differing electronegativities such that electrons spend more time in the vicinity of one atom than the other.

polar
Used to describe a molecule that has a dipole moment because it consists of a positive pole and a negative pole. [**Section 5.3**]

polyatomic ion
An ion that contains more than one atom, such as CO_3^{2-} or SO_4^{2-}.

polyprotic acid
An acid, such as H_2SO_4 or H_3PO_4, that can lose more than one H^+. [**Section 11.4**]

polyprotic base
A base, such as the PO_4^{3-} ion, that can accept more than one H^+.

positive electrode
The electrode in an electrochemical cell that carries a positive charge. In a galvanic cell, it is the cathode; in an electrolytic cell, it is the anode.

positron (β')
The antiparticle of the electron. A positron has the same mass as an electron but is positively charged. Contact between an electron and positron results in instant annihilation and emission of two high energy gamma rays. [**Section 4.4**]

positron emission
A mode of beta decay where a positron is emitted as a consequence of the conversion of a nuclear proton to a neutron. [**Section 4.4**]

potential
A measure of the driving force behind an electrochemical reaction that is reported in units of volts. [**Section 12.3**]

precipitation
A process where dissolved ions combine to form a solid salt in solution. [**Section 10.4**]

precision
A measure of the extent to which individual measurements of the same phenomenon agree.

pressure
The force exerted perpendicular to a surface divided by the area of the surface. [**Section 5.7**]

proton
A subatomic particle that has a charge of $+1e$ and a mass of about 1 amu. (Synonymous with H^+.) [**Section 4.1**]

quantized
A property or quality that appears only in certain discrete amounts, such as electric charge. [**Section 4.5**]

radioactivity
The spontaneous disintegration of an unstable nuclide by a first-order rate law. Synonymous with *nuclear decay*. [**Section 4.4**]

rate of reaction
The change in the concentration of a compound divided by the amount of time necessary for this change to occur: rate = $\Delta[X]/\Delta t$. [**Section 9.1**]

rate constant (k)
The proportionality constant in the equation that describes the relationship between the rate of a step in a chemical reaction and the product of the concentrations of the reactants consumed in that step. [**Section 9.4**]

rate law
An equation that describes how the rate of a chemical reaction depends on the concentrations of the reactants consumed in that reaction, along with the rate constant that takes into account temperature, activation energy, and collision frequency / steric effects. [**Section 9.4**]

rate-determining step
The slowest step in a chemical reaction. [**Section 9.1**]

reaction quotient (Q)
The quotient obtained when the concentrations (or partial pressures) of the products of a reaction are multiplied and the result is divided by the product of the concentrations (or partial pressures) of the reactants. Basically, putting nonequilibrium values into an equilibrium expression yields a reaction quotient instead of the equilibrium constant. [**Section 10.2**]

real gas
A gas that deviates from the behavior predicted by the ideal gas law. Real gases differ from the expected behavior of an ideal gas (e.g., lower V and P) for two reasons: (1) the forces of attraction between the particles in a gas are not zero and (2) the volume of the particles in a gas is not zero. [**Section 8.3**]

redox
An abbreviation for oxidation-reduction. [**Section 12.1**]

reducing agent / reductant
An atom, ion, or molecule that is oxidized by giving up electrons, thereby reducing something else. [**Section 12.1**]

reduction
A process in which an atom, ion, or molecule gains one or more electrons. [**Section 12.1**]

resonance structures
Two or more Lewis dot structures that differ only by the placement of electrons in the molecule. Taken together as an average (a resonance hybrid), they best approximate the electron distribution and types of bonds in the molecule better than any one structure can alone. [**Section 5.1**]

salt
Synonymous with *ionic compound*. [**Section 5.8**]

salt bridge
An ion-rich junction between the anodic and cathodic chambers of an electrochemical cell that prevents charge separation that would otherwise stop the cell from functioning. Anions always migrate toward the anode, and cations always migrate toward the cathode of any cell. [**Section 12.2**]

saturated solution
A solution that contains as much solute as possible. [**Section 10.4**]

second ionization energy
The energy needed to remove an electron from a +1 cation in the gas phase. [**Section 4.8**]

second law of thermodynamics
Processes that increase the entropy in the universe are spontaneous. [**Section 6.4**]

second-order reaction
A reaction in which rate is proportional to the concentration of a single reactant raised to the second power: rate = $k[A]^2$, or two reactants each raised to the first power: rate = $k[A][B]$.

shielding
The masking and weakening of the electrostatic attraction between the nucleus and outer electrons by inner electrons. [**Section 4.8**]

solubility
The ratio of the maximum amount of solute to the volume of solvent in which this solute can dissolve. Often expressed in units of grams of solute per 100 g of water, or in moles of solid per liter of solution. [**Section 10.4**]

solubility equilibria
Equilibria that exist in a saturated solution, in which additional solid dissolves at the same rate that particles of solution come together to precipitate more solid.

solubility product (K_{sp})
The product of the equilibrium concentrations of the ions in a saturated solution of a salt. [Section 10.1]

solute
The substance that dissolves in a solvent to form a solution. [Section 10.4]

solution
A homogeneous mixture of one or more solutes dissolved in a solvent. [Section 10.4]

solvent
The substance in which a solute dissolves. [Section 10.4]

specific heat
The amount of heat required to raise the temperature of 1 g of a substance by 1°C (or 1 K). (Do not confuse with *heat capacity*). [Section 7.2]

spontaneous reaction
A reaction in which the products are favored: ΔG_{rxn} is negative (and E_{cell} is positive). [Section 6.5]

standard cell potential
The potential, $E°_{cell}$, of a cell measured under standard-state conditions.

standard heat of formation ($\Delta H_f°$)
The change in the enthalpy that occurs during a chemical reaction that leads to the formation of one mole of a compound from its elements in their standard states at standard conditions. [Section 6.3]

standard state/condition
State in which $T = 298$ K (25°C), $P = 1$ atm, and all concentrations are 1 M. Not to be confused with STP. [Section 6.3]

standard temperature and pressure (STP)
State in which $T = 273$ K (0°C) and $P = 1$ atm. Generally used when referring to gases. Not to be confused with *standard state* or *standard conditions*. [Section 6.3]

state
1. One of the three states of matter: gas, liquid, or solid.

2. A set of physical properties that describe a system. [Section 3.12]

state function
A quantity whose value depends only on the state of the system and not its history; X is a state function, if and only if, the value of ΔX does not depend on the path used to go from the initial to the final state of the system. [Section 6.3]

stoichiometry
The study of the quantitative relationships between the reactants and the products of a balanced chemical reaction. [Section 3.10]

strong acid
An acid that dissociates completely in water. [Section 11.3]

strong base
A base that dissociates completely in water. [Section 11.3]

sublimation
The process in which a solid goes directly to the gas phase without passing through an intermediate liquid state. [Section 6.4]

supercooled liquid
A substance that is a liquid even though its temperature is below its freezing point.

supercritical fluid
A substance that displays properties of both a liquid and a gas and exists under conditions of high temperature and pressure. If a substance is in this state—where the liquid and gas phases are no longer distinct—no amount of increased pressure can force the substance back into its liquid phase. [Section 7.4]

surface tension
The perpendicular force per unit length of liquid surface that acts to reduce the surface area of a liquid, resulting from intermolecular forces below the surface.

surroundings
In thermodynamics, the part of the universe not included in the system. [Section 6.1]

system
In thermodynamics, that small portion of the universe in which we are interested at the moment. [Section 6.1]

thermal conductor
A substance or object that readily conducts heat (metals, for example).

thermal insulator
An object, such as a blanket or a fur coat, that tends to slow down the rate at which heat is transferred from one object to another.

titrant
The strong acid or base reagent added to the unknown solution in a titration experiment. [Section 11.10]

titration
A technique used to determine the concentration and/or the chemical identity of a solute in a solution. [Section 11.10]

torr
A unit of pressure equal to the pressure exerted by a column of mercury 1 millimeter tall. By definition, 1 torr = 1 mm Hg. [Section 8.1]

transition metal
Metals in the block of elements that serve as a transition between the two columns on the left side of the table, where s orbitals are filled, and the six columns on the right, where p orbitals are filled. [Section 3.13]

triple point
The unique pressure and temperature at which the three phases of a substance (gas, liquid, and solid) can all coexist in equilibrium. [Section 7.4]

unimolecular
Describes a step in a reaction mechanism in which only one reactant molecule is present. [Section 9.4]

valence electrons
Electrons in the outermost or highest-energy level or shell of an atom. The electrons that are gained, shared, or lost in a chemical reaction. [Section 3.13]

van der Waals equation
An equation that accounts for deviations from ideal behavior in gaseous systems due to interactions between gas particles and particle volume. [Section 8.3]

van't Hoff factor (*i*)
See *ionizability factor*. [Section 10.4]

vapor pressure
The partial pressure of the gas molecules over the surface of a liquid that originate from the surface of a liquid. [Section 5.7]

voltaic cell
An electrochemical cell in which a spontaneous chemical reaction is used to create electricity. Synonymous with *galvanic cell*. [Section 12.2]

volatile
The physical characteristic of having a high vapor pressure at standard conditions. [Section 5.7]

VSEPR theory
A model in which the repulsion between pairs of valence electrons is used to predict the shape of a molecule. [**Section 5.4**]

weak acid
An acid that only partially dissociates in water. [**Section 11.3**]

weak base
A base that only partially dissociates in water. [**Section 11.3**]

zero-order reaction
A reaction in which rate is not proportional to the concentration of any of the reactants.

MCAT G-Chem
Formula Sheet

Stoichiometry

Avogadro's number: $N_A = 6.02 \times 10^{23}$

$$\text{\# moles} = \frac{\text{mass in grams}}{\text{MW}}$$

$$\text{\% composition by mass of } X = \frac{\text{mass of X}}{\text{mass of molecule}} \times 100\%$$

$$\text{Mole fraction: } X_S = \frac{\text{moles of S}}{\text{total moles}}$$

$$\text{Molarity : } M = \frac{\text{moles of solute}}{\text{L of solution}}$$

Nuclear and Atomic Chemistry

N_A amu (u) = 1 gram

$E_{photon} = hf = hc \,/\, \lambda$

electron energy: $E_n = \dfrac{(-2.178 \times 10^{-18}\,\text{J})}{n^2}$ for any 1-electron (Bohr) atom

Z = # of protons = atomic number, N = # of neutrons

$A = Z + N$ = mass number

Decay	Description	ΔZ	ΔN	ΔA
α	eject $\alpha = {}_2^4\text{He}$	-2	-2	-4
β^-	$n \rightarrow p + e^-$	+1	-1	0
β^+	$p \rightarrow n + e^+$	-1	+1	0
EC	$p + e^- \rightarrow n$	-1	+1	0
γ	$X^* \rightarrow X + \gamma$	0	0	0

Bonding and Intermolecular Forces

formal charge: $FC = V - (\frac{1}{2}B + L)$

V = (# of valence e^- s)

B = (# of bonding e^- s)

L = (# of lone-pair e^- s)

VSEPR Theory

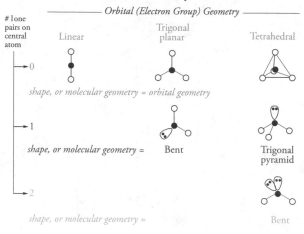

intermolecular forces (D=dipole, I=induced, i=instantaneous):

ion–ion > ion–D > H-bonds > D–D > D–ID > iD–ID (London dispersion)

Periodic Trends

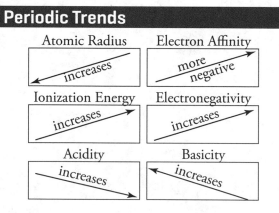

electronegativity of some common atoms:

$F > O > (N \approx Cl) > Br > (I \approx S \approx C) > H$

Thermodynamics

T (in K) $= T_{°C} + 273$, 1 cal ≈ 4.2 J, $q =$ heat

$q = mc\Delta T = C\Delta T$ (if no phase changes)

$q = n\Delta H_{phase\ change}$ ($\Delta T = 0$ during phase change)

enthalpy change: $\Delta H =$ heat of rxn at const P

$\Delta H < 0 \Leftrightarrow$ exothermic, $\Delta H > 0 \Leftrightarrow$ endothermic

standard state: 1 M, 25°C, 1 atm

$\Delta H^{\circ}_{rxn} = \sum n\Delta H^{\circ}_{f,products} - \sum n\Delta H^{\circ}_{f,reactants}$

Laws of Thermodynamics ($E =$ energy, $S =$ entropy):

1) $E_{universe}$ is constant. $\Delta E_{system} = Q - W$.

2) Spontaneous rxn $\Rightarrow \Delta S_{universe} > 0$

3) $S = 0$ for pure crystal at $T = 0$ K

Gibbs Free Energy: $\Delta G = \Delta H - T\Delta S$ [const.T]

$\Delta G < 0 \Leftrightarrow$ forward reaction is spontaneous

$\Delta G = 0 \Leftrightarrow$ at equilibrium

$\Delta G > 0 \Leftrightarrow$ reverse reaction is spontaneous

$$\Delta G^{\circ} = -RT \ln K \approx -2.3RT \log K$$

Gases

STP:

$T = 0\ °C = 273$ K, $P = 1$ atm $= 760$ torr $= 760$ mmHg

Avogadro's Law: $V \propto n$

$$V_{at\ STP} = n(22.4\ L)$$

Boyle's Law: $V \propto 1/P$ (at constant T)

Charles's Law: $V \propto T$ (at constant P)

Combined: $P_1 V_1 / T_1 = P_2 V_2 / T_2$

Ideal-Gas Law: $PV = nRT$

van der Waals: $\left(P + \dfrac{an^2}{V^2} \right)(V - nb) = nRT$

Dalton's law of partial pressures: $P_{tot} = \sum p_i$

Graham's law of effusion:

$$v_{2,rms} = v_{1,rms} \sqrt{\frac{m_1}{m_2}} \Rightarrow \frac{\text{rate of effusion of gas 2}}{\text{rate of effusion of gas 1}} = \sqrt{\frac{m_1}{m_2}}$$

Kinetics

Concentration rate =

$$-\frac{\Delta[\text{reactant}]}{\text{time}} \quad \text{or} \quad +\frac{\Delta[\text{product}]}{\text{time}}$$

Reaction rate =

$$-\frac{1}{\text{coeff}} \frac{\Delta[\text{reactant}]}{\text{time}} \quad \text{or} \quad +\frac{1}{\text{coeff}} \frac{\Delta[\text{product}]}{\text{time}}$$

Rate law for rate-determining step:

$$\text{rate} = k[\text{reactant}_1]^{\text{coeff}_1}\ldots$$

Arrhenius equation: $k = Ae^{-Ea/RT}$

Equilibrium

For generic balanced reaction

$a\text{A} + b\text{B} \rightleftharpoons c\text{C} + d\text{D}$,

equilibrium constant: $K_{eq} = \dfrac{[\text{C}]^c_{at\ eq}[\text{D}]^d_{at\ eq}}{[\text{A}]^a_{at\ eq}[\text{B}]^b_{at\ eq}}$ (excluding pure solids and liquids)

(gas rxns use partial pressures in K_p expression)

K_{eq} is a constant at a given temperature

$K_{eq} < 1 \Leftrightarrow$ equilibrium favors reactants

$K_{eq} > 1 \Leftrightarrow$ equilibrium favors products

Reaction quotient: $Q = \dfrac{[\text{C}]^c[\text{D}]^d}{[\text{A}]^a[\text{B}]^b}$

Le Châtelier's Principle

$Q < K_{eq} \Leftrightarrow$ rxn proceeds forward

$Q = K_{eq} \Leftrightarrow$ rxn at equilibrium

$Q > K_{eq} \Leftrightarrow$ rxn proceeds in reverse

Acids and Bases

$pH = -\log[H^+] = -\log[H_3O^+]$

$pOH = -\log[OH^-]$

$K_w = [H^+][OH^-] = 1 \times 10^{-14}$ at 25 °C

$pH + pOH = 14$ at 25 °C

$K_a = \dfrac{[H^+][A^-]}{[HA]}$

$pK_a = -\log K_a$

$K_b = \dfrac{[OH^-][HB^+]}{[B]}$

$pK_b = -\log K_b$

$K_a K_b = K_w$ = ion-product constant for water

Henderson-Hasselbalch equations:

$pH = pK_a + \log \dfrac{[\text{conjugate base}]}{[\text{weak acid}]}$

$\quad = pK_a - \log \dfrac{[\text{weak acid}]}{[\text{conjugate base}]}$

$pOH = pK_b + \log \dfrac{[\text{conjugate acid}]}{[\text{weak base}]}$

$\quad = pK_b - \log \dfrac{[\text{weak base}]}{[\text{conjugate acid}]}$

acid-base neutralization:

$$a \times [A] \times V_A = b \times [B] \times V_B$$

Redox and Electrochemistry

Rules for determining oxidation state (*OS*):[*]

1) *OS* of pure element = 0
2) sum of *OS*'s = 0 in neutral molecule
   sum of *OS*'s = charge on ion
3) Group 1 metals: *OS* = +1
   Group 2 metals: *OS* = +2
4) *OS* of F = −1
5) *OS* of H = +1
6) *OS* of O = −2
7) *OS* of halogens = −1 of O family = −2

If one rule contradicts another, rule higher in list takes precedence.

F = faraday = 96,500 C/mol e^-

$\Delta G = -nFE_{cell}$

$E_{cell} > 0 \Leftrightarrow$ spontaneous

$E_{cell} < 0 \Leftrightarrow$ reverse rxn is spontaneous

Nernst equation: $E = E° - \dfrac{0.06}{n} \log Q$

Faraday's Law of Electrolysis:

The amount of chemical charge is proportional to the amount of electricity that flows through the cell.

---

[*] These rules work 99 percent of the time.

MCAT Math for General Chemistry

PREFACE

The MCAT is primarily a conceptual exam, with little actual mathematical computation. Any math that is on the MCAT is fundamental: just arithmetic, algebra, and trigonometry (and there is virtually no trigonometry in General Chemistry). There is absolutely no calculus. The purpose of this section of the book is to go over some math topics (as they pertain to General Chemistry) with which you may feel a little rusty[1].

This text is intended for reference and self-study. Therefore, there are lots of examples, all completely solved. Practice working through these examples and master the fundamentals!

---

[1]   For a complete discussion of all the math found on the MCAT, see our book *MCAT Physics and Math Review*.

Chapter 13
Arithmetic, Algebra, and Graphs

13.1 THE IMPORTANCE OF APPROXIMATION

Since you aren't allowed to use a calculator on the MCAT, you need to practice doing arithmetic calculations by hand again. Fortunately, the amount of calculation you'll have to do is small, and you'll also be able to approximate. For example, let's say you were faced with performing the following calculation:

$$
\begin{array}{r}
23.6 \\
\times\ 72.5 \\
\hline
1180 \\
472 \\
1652 \\
\hline
1711.00
\end{array}
$$

Your first inclination would be to reach for your calculator, but…you don't have one available. Now what? Realize that on the Chemical and Physical Foundations of Biological Systems section of the MCAT, you have roughly a minute and twenty-five seconds per question, so there simply cannot be questions requiring lengthy, complicated computation. Instead, we'll figure out a reasonably accurate (and fast) approximation of the value of the expression above:

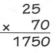

$$
\begin{array}{r}
25 \\
\times\ \ 70 \\
\hline
1750
\end{array}
$$

So, if the answer to an MCAT question was the value of the expression above, and the four answer choices were, say, 1324, 1617, 1711, and 1856, we'd know right away that the answer is 1711. The choices are far enough apart that even with our approximations, we were still able to tell which choice was the correct one. Just as importantly, we didn't waste time trying to be more precise; it was unnecessary, and it would have decreased the amount of time we had to spend on other questions.

If you find yourself writing out lengthy calculations on your scratch paper when you're working through MCAT questions that contain some mathematical calculation, it's important that you recognize that you're not using your time efficiently. Say to yourself, "I'm wasting valuable time trying to get a precise answer, when I don't need to be precise."

Try this one: What's 1583 divided by 32.1? (You have five seconds. Go.)

For the previous practice exercise, you should have written (or done in your head): $\frac{1500}{30} = 50$

13.2 SCIENTIFIC NOTATION, EXPONENTS, AND RADICALS

It's well known that very large or very small numbers can be handled more easily when they're written in **scientific notation**, that is, in the form $\pm\, m \times 10^n$, where $1 \leq m < 10$ and n is an integer. For example:

$$602,000,000,000,000,000,000,000 = 6.02 \times 10^{23}$$
$$-35,000,000,000 = -3.5 \times 10^{10}$$
$$0.000000004 = 4 \times 10^{-9}$$

Quantities like these come up all the time in physical problems, so you must be able to work with them confidently. Since a power of ten (the term 10^n) is part of every number written in scientific notation, the most important rules for dealing with such expressions are the Laws of Exponents:

Laws of Exponents		
		Illustration (with b = 10 or a power of 10)
Law 1	$b^p \times b^q = b^{p+q}$	$10^5 \times 10^{-9} = 10^{5+(-9)} = 10^{-4}$
Law 2	$b^p/b^q = b^{p-q}$	$10^5/10^{-9} = 10^{5-(-9)} = 10^{14}$
Law 3	$(b^p)^q = b^{pq}$	$(10^{-3})^2 = 10^{(-3)(2)} = 10^{-6}$
Law 4	$b^0 = 1$ (if $b \neq 0$)	$10^0 = 1$
Law 5	$b^{-p} = 1/b^p$	$10^{-7} = 1/10^7$
Law 6	$(ab)^p = a^p b^p$	$(2 \times 10^4)^3 = 2^3 \times (10^4)^3 = 8 \times 10^{12}$
Law 7	$(a/b)^p = a^p/b^p$	$[(3 \times 10^{-6})/10^2]^2 = (3 \times 10^{-6})^2/(10^2)^2 = 9 \times 10^{-16}$

Example 13-1: Simplify each of the following expressions, writing your answer in scientific notation:

a) $(4 \times 10^{-3})(5 \times 10^9)$
b) $(4 \times 10^{-3})/(5 \times 10^9)$
c) $(3 \times 10^{-4})^3$
d) $[(1 \times 10^{-2})/(5 \times 10^{-7})]^2$

Solution:

a) $(4 \times 10^{-3})(5 \times 10^9) = (4)(5) \times 10^{-3+9} = 20 \times 10^6 = 2 \times 10^7$
b) $(4 \times 10^{-3})/(5 \times 10^9) = (4/5) \times 10^{-3-9} = 0.8 \times 10^{-12} = 8 \times 10^{-13}$
c) $(3 \times 10^{-4})^3 = 3^3 \times (10^{-4})^3 = 27 \times 10^{-12} = 2.7 \times 10^{-11}$
d) $[(1 \times 10^{-2})/(5 \times 10^{-7})]^2 = (1 \times 10^{-2})^2/(5 \times 10^{-7})^2 = (1 \times 10^{-4})/(25 \times 10^{-14}) = (1/25) \times 10^{-4-(-14)}$
    $= (4/100) \times 10^{10} = 4 \times 10^8$

Another important skill involving numbers written in scientific notation involves changing the power of 10 (and compensating for this change so as not to affect the original number). The approximation carried out in the very first example in this chapter is a good example of this. To find the square root of 5×10^{-7}, it is much easier to first rewrite this number as 50×10^{-8}, because then the square root is easy:

$$\sqrt{50 \times 10^{-8}} = \sqrt{50} \times \sqrt{10^{-8}} \approx 7 \times 10^{-4}$$

Other examples of this procedure are found in Example 13-1 above; for instance,

$$20 \times 10^6 = 2 \times 10^7$$

$$0.8 \times 10^{-12} = 8 \times 10^{-13}$$

$$27 \times 10^{-12} = 2.7 \times 10^{-11}$$

In writing $\sqrt{50 \times 10^{-8}} = \sqrt{50} \times \sqrt{10^{-8}} \approx 7 \times 10^{-4}$, I used a familiar law of square roots, that the square root of a product is equal to the product of the square roots. Here's a short list of rules for dealing with radicals:

Laws of Radicals		
		Illustration
Law 1	$\sqrt{ab} = \sqrt{a} \cdot \sqrt{b}$	$\sqrt{9 \times 10^{12}} = \sqrt{9} \times \sqrt{10^{12}} = 3 \times 10^6$
Law 2	$\sqrt{a/b} = \sqrt{a} / \sqrt{b}$	$\sqrt{(4 \times 10^{-6})/10^{-18}} = \sqrt{(4 \times 10^{-6})} / \sqrt{10^{-18}} =$ $(2 \times 10^{-3})/10^{-9} = 2 \times 10^6$
Law 3	$\sqrt[q]{a^p} = a^{p/q}$	$\sqrt[3]{(8 \times 10^6)^2} = (8 \times 10^6)^{2/3} = 8^{2/3} \times 10^{(6)(2/3)} = 4 \times 10^4$

A couple of remarks about this list: First, Laws 1 and 2 illustrate how to handle square roots, which are the most common. However, the same laws are true even if the index of the root is not 2. [The **index** of a root (or radical) is the number that indicates the root that's to be taken; it's indicated by the little q in front of the radical sign in Law 3. Cube roots are index 3 and written $\sqrt[3]{}$; fourth roots are index 4 and written $\sqrt[4]{}$; and square roots are index 2 and written $\sqrt[2]{}$, although we hardly ever write the little 2.] Second, Law 3 provides the link between exponents and radicals.

Example 13-2: Approximate each of the following expressions, writing your answer in scientific notation:

a) $\sqrt{3.5 \times 10^9}$

b) $\sqrt{8 \times 10^{-11}}$

c) $\sqrt{\dfrac{1.5 \times 10^{-5}}{2.5 \times 10^{-17}}}$

Solution:

a) $\sqrt{3.5 \times 10^9} = \sqrt{35 \times 10^8} = \sqrt{35} \times \sqrt{10^8} \approx \sqrt{36} \times \sqrt{10^8} = 6 \times 10^4$

b) $\sqrt{8 \times 10^{-11}} = \sqrt{80 \times 10^{-12}} = \sqrt{80} \times \sqrt{10^{-12}} \approx \sqrt{81} \times \sqrt{10^{-12}} = 9 \times 10^{-6}$

c) $\sqrt{\dfrac{1.5 \times 10^{-5}}{2.5 \times 10^{-17}}} = \dfrac{\sqrt{1.5 \times 10^{-5}}}{\sqrt{2.5 \times 10^{-17}}} = \dfrac{\sqrt{15 \times 10^{-6}}}{\sqrt{25 \times 10^{-18}}} \approx \dfrac{\sqrt{16} \times \sqrt{10^{-6}}}{\sqrt{25} \times \sqrt{10^{-18}}} = \dfrac{4 \times 10^{-3}}{5 \times 10^{-9}} = 0.8 \times 10^6 = 8 \times 10^5$

Example 13-3: Approximate each of the following expressions, writing your answer in scientific notation:

a) The mass (in grams) of 4.7×10^{24} molecules of CCl_4:
$$\frac{(4.7 \times 10^{24})(153.8)}{6.02 \times 10^{23}}$$

b) The electrostatic force (in newtons) between the proton and electron in the ground state of hydrogen:
$$\frac{(8.99 \times 10^9)(1.6 \times 10^{-19})^2}{(5.3 \times 10^{-11})^2}$$

Solution:

a) $$\frac{(4.7 \times 10^{24})(153.8)}{6.02 \times 10^{23}} \approx \frac{5(150)}{6} \times 10^{24-23} = 5(25) \times 10 = 1.25 \times 10^3$$

b) $$\frac{(8.99 \times 10^9)(1.6 \times 10^{-19})^2}{(5.3 \times 10^{-11})^2} \approx \frac{9(1.6)^2 \times 10^{9+(-19)(2)}}{(5.3)^2 \times 10^{(-11)(2)}} \approx \frac{(9)3 \times 10^{-29}}{27 \times 10^{-22}} = 1 \times 10^{-7}$$

13.3 FRACTIONS, RATIOS, AND PERCENTS

A **fraction** indicates a division; for example, 3/4 means 3 divided by 4. The number above (or to the left of) the fraction bar is the numerator, and the number below (or to the right) of the fraction bar is called the denominator.

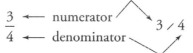

$$\frac{3}{4} \quad \begin{matrix} \leftarrow \text{numerator} \\ \leftarrow \text{denominator} \end{matrix} \qquad 3 \diagup 4$$

Our quick review of the basic arithmetic operations on fractions begins with the simplest rule: the one for multiplication:

$$\frac{a}{b} \times \frac{c}{d} = \frac{ac}{bd}$$

In words, just multiply the numerators and then, separately, multiply the denominators.

Example 13-4: What is 4/9 times 2/5?

Solution:

$$\frac{4}{9} \times \frac{2}{5} = \frac{4 \times 2}{9 \times 5} = \frac{8}{45}$$

The rule for dividing fractions is based on the reciprocal. If $a \neq 0$, then the **reciprocal** of a/b is simply b/a; that is, to form the reciprocal of a fraction, just flip it over. For example, the reciprocal of 3/4 is 4/3; the reciprocal of −2/5 is −5/2; the reciprocal of 3 is 1/3; and the reciprocal of −1/4 is −4. (The number 0 has no reciprocal.) As a result of this definition, we have the following basic fact: The product of any number and its reciprocal is 1.

Example 13-5: Find the reciprocal of each of these numbers:

   a)   2.25
   b) 5×10^{-4}
   c) 4×10^{5}

Solution:

   a)   2.25 is equal to 2 + (1/4), which is 9/4. The reciprocal of 9/4 is 4/9.

   b) $\dfrac{1}{5 \times 10^{-4}} = \dfrac{1}{5} \times \dfrac{1}{10^{-4}} = 0.2 \times 10^{4} = 2 \times 10^{3}$

   c) $\dfrac{1}{4 \times 10^{5}} = \dfrac{1}{4} \times \dfrac{1}{10^{5}} = 0.25 \times 10^{-5} = 2.5 \times 10^{-6}$

Now, in words, the rule for dividing fractions reads: *multiply by the reciprocal of the divisor.* That is, flip over whatever you're dividing by, and then multiply:

$$\frac{a}{b} \div \frac{c}{d} = \frac{a}{b} \times \frac{d}{c}$$

Example 13-6: What is 4/9 divided by 2/5?

Solution:

$$\frac{4}{9} \div \frac{2}{5} = \frac{4}{9} \times \frac{5}{2} = \frac{4 \times 5}{9 \times 2} = \frac{20}{18} = \frac{10}{9}$$

Finally, we turn to addition and subtraction. In elementary and junior high school, you were probably taught to find a common denominator (preferably, the *least* common denominator, known as the LCD), rewrite each fraction in terms of this common denominator, then add or subtract the numerators. If a common denominator is easy to spot, this may well be the fastest way to add or subtract fractions:

$$\frac{1}{2} + \frac{3}{4} = \frac{2}{4} + \frac{3}{4} = \frac{2+3}{4} = \frac{5}{4}$$

However, it's now time to learn the grown-up way to add or subtract fractions:

$$\frac{a}{b} \otimes \frac{c}{d} = \frac{ad+bc}{bd} \qquad \frac{a}{b} \otimes \frac{c}{d} = \frac{ad-bc}{bd}$$

$$\frac{a}{b} + \frac{c}{d} = \frac{ad+bc}{bd} \qquad \frac{a}{b} - \frac{c}{d} = \frac{ad-bc}{bd}$$

Here's what the arrows in the top line represent: "Multiply *up* (*d* times *a* gives *ad*), multiply *up* again (*b* times *c* gives *bc*), do the adding or subtracting of these products, and place the result over the product of the denominators (bd)." The length of this last sentence hides the simplicity of the rule, but it describes the recipe to follow. For example,

$$\frac{4}{9} + \frac{2}{5} = \frac{20+18}{45} = \frac{38}{45} \qquad \frac{4}{9} - \frac{2}{5} = \frac{20-18}{45} = \frac{2}{45}$$

Example 13-7:

a) Approximate the sum $\dfrac{1}{2.4\times10^5} + \dfrac{1}{6\times10^4}$

b) What is the reciprocal of this sum?

c) Simplify: $\dfrac{1}{2\times10^{-8}} - \dfrac{2}{5\times10^{-7}}$

Solution:

a) Using the rule illustrated above, we find that

$$\frac{1}{2.4\times10^5} + \frac{1}{6\times10^4} = \frac{(6\times10^4)+(2.4\times10^5)}{(2.4\times10^5)(6\times10^4)} = \frac{(6\times10^4)+(24\times10^4)}{(2.4\times10^5)(6\times10^4)} = \frac{(6+24)\times10^4}{(2.4)(6)\times10^{5+4}} \approx \frac{30\times10^4}{15\times10^9} = 2\times10^{-5}$$

b) The reciprocal of this result is $\dfrac{1}{2\times10^{-5}} = \dfrac{1}{2}\times\dfrac{1}{10^{-5}} = 0.5\times10^5 = 5\times10^4$.

c)

$$\frac{1}{2\times10^{-8}} - \frac{2}{5\times10^{-7}} = \frac{(5\times10^{-7})-(2\times10^{-8})(2)}{(2\times10^{-8})(5\times10^{-7})} = \frac{(50\times10^{-8})-(4\times10^{-8})}{(2)(5)\times10^{-8+(-7)}} = \frac{(50-4)\times10^{-8}}{10\times10^{-15}} = 46\times10^6$$
$$= 4.6\times10^7$$

Let's now move on to ratios. A **ratio** is simply another way of saying *fraction*. For example, the ratio of 3 to 4, written 3:4, is equal to the fraction 3/4. Here's an illustration using isotopes of chlorine: The statement *the ratio of ^{35}Cl to ^{37}Cl is 3:1* means that there are 3/1 = 3 times as many ^{35}Cl atoms as there are ^{37}Cl atoms.

A particularly useful way to interpret a ratio is in terms of parts of a total. A ratio of $a:b$ means that there are $a + b$ total parts, with a of them being of the first type and b of the second type. Therefore, *the ratio of ^{35}Cl to ^{37}Cl is 3:1* means that if we could take all ^{35}Cl and ^{37}Cl atoms, we could partition all them into 3 + 1 = 4 equal parts such that 3 of these parts will all be ^{35}Cl atoms, and the remaining 1 part will all be ^{37}Cl atoms. We can now restate the original ratio as a ratio of these parts to the total. Since ^{35}Cl atoms account for 3 parts out of the 4 total, the ratio of ^{35}Cl atoms to all Cl atoms is 3:4; that is, 3/4 of all Cl atoms are ^{35}Cl atoms. Similarly, the ratio of ^{37}Cl atoms to all Cl atoms is 1:4, which means that 1/4 of all Cl atoms are ^{37}Cl atoms.

Example 13-8: The formula for the compound TNT (trinitrotoluene) is $C_7H_5N_3O_6$.

a) What fraction of the atoms in this compound are nitrogen atoms?
b) If the molar masses of C, H, N, and O are 12 g, 1 g, 14 g, and 16 g, respectively, what is the ratio of the mass of all the nitrogens to the total mass?

Solution:

a) There are a total of $7 + 5 + 3 + 6 = 21$ atoms per molecule. The ratio of N atoms to the total is 3:21, or, more simply, 1:7. Therefore, 1/7 of the atoms in this compound are nitrogen atoms.

b) The desired ratio of masses is calculated like this:

$$\frac{\text{mass of all N atoms}}{\text{total mass of molecule}} = \frac{3(14)}{7(12)+5(1)+3(14)+6(16)} = \frac{42}{227} \approx \frac{40}{220} = \frac{2}{11}$$

Example 13-9: In a simple hydrocarbon (molecular formula C_xH_y), the ratio of C atoms to H atoms is 5:4, and the total number of atoms in the molecule is 18. Find x and y.

Solution: Since the ratio of C atoms to H atoms is 5:4, there are 5 parts C atoms and 4 parts H atoms, for a total of 9 equal parts. These 9 equal parts account for 18 total atoms, so each part must contain 2 atoms. Thus, C (which has 5 parts) has $5 \times 2 = 10$ atoms, and H (which has 4 parts) has $4 \times 2 = 8$ atoms. Therefore, $x = 10$ and $y = 8$.

Example 13-10: The ratio of O atoms to C atoms in each molecule of triethylene glycol is 2:3, and the ratio of O atoms to the total number of C atoms and H atoms is 1:5. If there are 24 atoms (C, H, and O only) per molecule, find the formula for this compound.

Solution: The ratio of O to C atoms is 2:3, which tells us there are 2 parts O atoms and 3 parts C atoms, for a total of 5 parts C and O. Since the ratio of O to (C *and* H) atoms is 1:5, there are 5 times as many C and H atoms as there are O atoms. But, we have found that there are 2 parts O atoms, so C and H must account for 5 times as many: 10 parts. And, because there are 3 parts C atoms, there must be $10 - 3 = 7$ parts H atoms. We therefore have $2 + 3 + 7 = 12$ parts total, accounting for 24 atoms, which means 2 atoms per part. So, there must be $2 \times 2 = 4$ O atoms, $3 \times 2 = 6$ C atoms, and $7 \times 2 = 14$ H atoms. The formula is $C_6H_{14}O_4$.

The word **percent**, symbolized by %, is simply an abbreviation for the phrase "out of 100". Therefore, a percentage is represented by a fraction whose denominator is 100. For example, 60% means 60/100, or 60 out of 100. The three main question types involving percents are as follows:

1) What is y % of z?
2) x is what percent of z?
3) x is y % of what?

Fortunately, all three question types fit into a single form and can all be answered by one equation. Translating the statement *x is y % of z* into an algebraic equation, we get

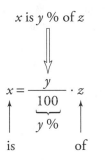

So, if you know any two of the three quantities x, y, and z, you can use the equation above to figure out the third.

Example 13-11:

a) What is 25% of 200?
b) 30 is what percent of 150?
c) 400 is 80% of what?

Solution:

a) Solving the equation $x = (25/100) \times 200$, we get $x = 25 \times 2 = 50$.
b) Solving the equation $30 = (y/100) \times 150$, we get $y = (30/150) \times 100 = (1/5) \times 100 = 20$.
c) Solving the equation $400 = (80/100) \times z$, we get $z = (100/80) \times 400 = 100 \times 5 = 500$.

It's also helpful to think of a simple fraction that equals a given percent, which can be used in place of $y/100$ in the equation above. For example, 25% = 1/4, 50% = 1/2, and 75% = 3/4. Other common fractional equivalents are: 20% = 1/5, 40% = 2/5, 60% = 3/5, and 80% = 4/5; 33 1/3% = 1/3 and 66 2/3% = 2/3; and 10n% = n/10 (for example, 10% = 1/10, 30% = 3/10, 70% = 7/10, and 90% = 9/10).

Example 13-12:

a) What is 60% of 35?
b) 12 is 75% of what?
c) What is 70% of 400?

Solution:

a) Since 60% = 3/5, we find that $x = (3/5) \times 35 = 3 \times 7 = 21$.
b) Because 75% = 3/4, we solve the equation $12 = (3/4) \times z$, and find $z = 12 \times (4/3) = 16$.
c) Since 70% = 7/10, we find that $x = (7/10) \times 400 = 7 \times 40 = 280$.

13.3

Example 13-13:

a) What is the result when 50 is increased by 50%?
b) What is the result when 80 is decreased by 40%?

Solution:

a) "Increasing 50 by 50%" means adding (50% of 50) to 50. Since 50% of 50 is 25, increasing 50 by 50% gives us 50 + 25 = 75.
b) "Decreasing 80 by 40%" means subtracting (40% of 80) from 80. Since 40% of 80 is 32, decreasing 80 by 40% gives us 80 − 32 = 48.

Example 13-14:

a) What is 250% of 60?
b) 2400 is what percent of 500?

Solution:

a) Solving the equation $x = (250/100) \times 60$, we get $x = 25 \times 6 = 150$.
b) Solving the equation $2400 = (y/100) \times 500$, we get $2400 = 5y$, so $y = 2400/5 = 480$.

Example 13-15: There are three stable isotopes of magnesium: ^{24}Mg, ^{25}Mg, and ^{26}Mg. The relative abundance of ^{24}Mg is 79%. Consider a sample of natural magnesium containing a total of 8×10^{24} atoms.

a) About how many atoms in the sample are ^{24}Mg atoms?
b) If the number of ^{25}Mg atoms in the sample is 8×10^{23}, what is the relative abundance (as a percentage) of ^{25}Mg?
c) What's the relative abundance of ^{26}Mg?

Solution:

a) Since the question is asking, *What is 79% of 8×10^{24}?*, we have

$$x = \frac{79}{100} \times (8 \times 10^{24}) \approx \frac{80}{100} \times (8 \times 10^{24}) = 6.4 \times 10^{24}$$

b) The question is asking, *8×10^{23} is what percent of 8×10^{24}?*, so we write

$$8 \times 10^{23} = \frac{y}{100} \times (8 \times 10^{24}) \Rightarrow \frac{y}{100} = \frac{8 \times 10^{23}}{8 \times 10^{24}} = \frac{1}{10} \Rightarrow y = 10 \Rightarrow \text{relative abundance} = 10\%$$

c) Assuming that these three isotopes account for all naturally occurring magnesium, the sum of the relative abundance percentages should be 100%. Therefore, we need only solve the equation 79% + 10% + Y% = 100%, from which we find that Y = 11.

Example 13-16: What is the percentage by mass, of carbon in $C_7H_5N_3O_6$? (Given: Molar mass of compound = 227 g.)

A)   26%
B)   37%
C)   49%
D)   62%

Solution: Once the fraction of the total molar mass of the compound that's contributed by carbon is calculated, we obtain a percentage by multiplying this fraction by 100%. Since the molar mass of carbon is 12 g, and the molecule contains 7 C atoms, we have

$$\%C, \text{ by mass } = \frac{7(12)}{227} = \frac{84}{227} \approx \frac{100}{250} = \frac{2}{5} = \frac{2}{5} \times 100\% = 40\%$$

Therefore, choice B is best.

13.4   EQUATIONS AND INEQUALITIES

You may have several questions on the MCAT that require you to solve—or manipulate—an algebraic equation or inequality. Fortunately, these equations and inequalities won't be very complicated.

When manipulating an algebraic equation, there's basically only one rule to remember: *Whatever you do to one side of the equation, you must do to the other side.* (Otherwise, it won't be a valid equation anymore.) For example, if you add 5 to the *left*-hand side, then add 5 to the *right*-hand side; if you multiply the *left*-hand side by 2, then multiply the *right*-hand side by 2, and so forth.

Inequalities are a little more involved. While it's still true that whatever you do to one side of an inequality you must also do the other side, there are a couple of additional rules, both of which involve flipping the inequality sign—that is, changing > to < (or vice versa) or changing ≥ to ≤ (or vice versa).

1)   *If you multiply both sides of an inequality by a negative number, then you must flip the inequality sign.*

> For example, let's say you're given the inequality $-2x > 6$. To solve for x, you'd multiply both sides by $-1/2$. Since this is a negative number, the inequality sign must be flipped: $x < -3$.

2)   *If both sides of an inequality are positive quantities, and you take the reciprocal of both sides, then you must flip the inequality sign.*

> For example, let's say you're given the inequality $2/x \leq 6$, where it's known that x must be positive. To solve for x, you can take the reciprocal of both sides. Upon doing so, the inequality sign must be flipped: $x/2 \geq 1/6$, so $x \geq 1/3$.

Example 13-17:

a) Solve for T: $PV = nRT$
b) Solve for v: $KE = (1/2)mv^2$
c) Solve for x (given that x is positive): $4x^2 = 2.4 \times 10^{-11}$
d) Solve for B: $h = k + \log(B/A)$
e) If $F = q_1 q_2 / r^2$ and r is positive, solve for r in terms of F, q_1, and q_2.
f) Solve for x: $3(2 - x) < 18$
g) Find all positive values of λ that satisfy

$$\frac{2 \times 10^{-25}}{\lambda} \geq 4 \times 10^{-19}$$

Solution:

a) Dividing both sides by nR, we get $T = PV/(nR)$.

b) Multiply both sides $2/m$, then take the square root: $v = \sqrt{\dfrac{2KE}{m}}$.

c) $4x^2 = 2.4 \times 10^{-11} \Rightarrow x^2 = 6 \times 10^{-12} \Rightarrow x = \sqrt{6} \times 10^{-6} \approx 2.5 \times 10^{-6}$

d) $h = k + \log \dfrac{B}{A} \Rightarrow \log \dfrac{B}{A} = h - k \Rightarrow 10^{h-k} = \dfrac{B}{A} \Rightarrow B = 10^{h-k} A$ [see Section 3.2]

e) $F = \dfrac{q_1 q_2}{r^2} \Rightarrow r^2 = \dfrac{q_1 q_2}{F} \Rightarrow r = \sqrt{\dfrac{q_1 q_2}{F}}$

f) $3(2 - x) < 18 \Rightarrow 2 - x < 6 \Rightarrow -x < 4 \Rightarrow x > -4$

g) $\dfrac{2 \times 10^{-25}}{\lambda} \geq 4 \times 10^{-19} \Rightarrow \dfrac{\lambda}{2 \times 10^{-25}} \leq \dfrac{1}{4 \times 10^{-19}} \Rightarrow \lambda \leq \dfrac{2 \times 10^{-25}}{4 \times 10^{-19}} = 0.5 \times 10^{-6} \Rightarrow \lambda \leq 5 \times 10^{-7}$

13.5   THE x-y PLANE, LINES, AND OTHER GRAPHS

The figure below shows the familiar **x-y plane**, which we use to plot data and draw lines and curves showing how one quantity is related to another one:

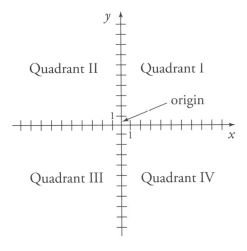

The x-y plane is formed by intersecting two number lines perpendicularly at the origins. The horizontal axis is generically referred to as the **x-axis** (although the quantity measured along this axis might be named by some other letter, such as time, t), and the vertical axis is generically known as the **y-axis**. The axes split the plane into four **quadrants**, which are numbered consecutively in a counterclockwise fashion. Quadrant I is in the upper right and represents all points (x, y) where x and y are both positive; in Quadrant II, x is negative and y is positive; in Quadrant III, x and y are both negative; and in Quadrant IV, x is positive and y is negative.

Suppose that two quantities, x and y, were related by the equation $y = 2x^2$. We would consider x as the **independent variable**, and y as the **dependent variable**, since for each value of x we get a unique value of y (that is, y *depends* uniquely on x). The independent variable is plotted along the horizontal axis, while the dependent variable is plotted long the vertical axis. Constructing a graph of an equation usually consists of plotting specific points (x, y) that satisfy the equation—in this case, examples include $(0, 0)$, $(1, 2)$, $(2, 8)$, $(-1, 2)$, $(-2, 8)$, etc.—and then connecting these points with a line or other smooth curve. The first coordinate of each point—the x coordinate—is known as the **abscissa**, and the second coordinate of each point—the y coordinate—is known as the **ordinate**.

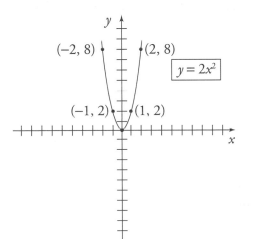

Lines

One of the simplest and most important graphs is the (straight) **line**. A line is determined by its slope—its steepness—and one specific point on the line, such as its intersection with either the *x*- or *y*-axis. The **slope** of a line is defined to be a change in *y* divided by the corresponding change in *x* ("rise over run"). Lines with positive slope rise to the right; those with negative slope fall to the right. And the greater the magnitude (absolute value) of the slope, the steeper the line.

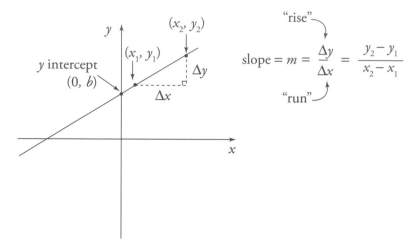

Perhaps the simplest way to write the equation of a line is in terms of its slope and the *y*-coordinate of the point where it crosses the *y*-axis. If the slope is *m* and the *y*-intercept is *b*, the equation of the line can be written in the form

$$y = mx + b$$

The only time this form doesn't work is when the line is vertical, since vertical lines have an undefined slope and such a line either never crosses the *y*-axis (no *b*) or else coincides with the *y*-axis. The equation of every vertical line is simply $x = a$, where *a* is the *x*-intercept.

Example 13-18:

a) Where does the line $y = 3x - 4$ cross the *y*-axis? the *x*-axis? What is its slope?
b) Find the equation of the line that has slope –2 and crosses the *y*-axis at the point (0, 3).
c) Find the equation of the line that has slope 4 and crosses the *y*-axis at the origin.
d) A *linear* function is a function whose graph is a line. Let's say it's known that some quantity *p* is a linear function of *x*. If $p = 50$ when $x = 0$ and $p = 250$ when $x = 20$, find an equation for *p* in terms of *x*. Then use the equation to find the value of *p* when $x = 40$.

Solution:
a) The equation $y = 3x - 4$ matches the form $y = mx + b$ with $m = 3$ and $b = -4$. Therefore, this line has slope 3 and crosses the *y*-axis at the point (0, –4). To find the *x*-intercept, we set *y* equal to 0 and solve for *x*: $0 = 3x - 4$ implies that $x = 4/3$. Therefore, this line crosses the *x*-axis at the point (4/3, 0).
b) We're given $m = -2$ and $b = 3$, so the equation of the line is $y = -2x + 3$.
c) We're given $m = 4$ and $b = 0$, so the equation of the line is $y = 4x$.
d) Since *p* is a linear function of *x*, it must have the form $p = mx + b$ for some values of *m* and *b*. Because $p = 50$ when $x = 0$, we know that $b = 50$, so $p = mx + 50$. Now, since $p = 250$ when $x = 20$, we have $250 = 20m + 50$, so $m = 10$. Thus, $p = 10x + 50$. Finally, plugging in $x = 40$ into this formula, we find that the value of *p* when $x = 40$ is $(10)(40) + 50 = 450$.

Example 13-19: An insulated 50 cm^3 sample of water has an initial temperature of $T_i = 10°C$. If Q calories of heat are added to the sample, the temperature of the water will rise to T, where $T = kQ + T_i$. When the graph of T vs. Q is sketched (with Q measured along the horizontal axis), it's found that the point $(Q, T) = (200, 14)$ lies on the graph.

a) What is the value of k?
b) How much heat is required to bring the water to 20°C?
c) If $Q = 2200$ cal, what will be the value of T?

13.5

Solution:

a) The equation $T = kQ + T_i$ matches the form $y = mx + b$, so k is the slope of the line. To find the slope, we evaluate the *rise-over-run* expression—which in this case is $\Delta T/\Delta Q$—for two points on the line. Using $(Q_1, T_1) = (0, 10)$ and $(Q_2, T_2) = (200, 14)$, we find that

$$k = \text{slope} = \frac{\Delta T}{\Delta Q} = \frac{T_2 - T_1}{Q_2 - Q_1} = \frac{14 - 10}{200 - 0} = \frac{1}{50}$$

b) We set T equal to 20 and solve for Q:

$$T - kQ + T_i \rightarrow T = \frac{1}{50}Q + 10 \Rightarrow 20 = \frac{1}{50}Q + 10 \Rightarrow Q = 500 \text{ (cal)}$$

c) Here we set $Q = 2200$ and evaluate T:

$$T = kQ + T_i \Rightarrow T = \frac{1}{50}Q + 10 \Rightarrow T = \frac{1}{50}(2200) + 10 = 44 + 10 = 54 \text{ (°C)}$$

(*Technical note:* The equation for the temperature of the water, $T = kQ + T_i$, is valid as long as no phase change occurs.)

Besides lines, there are a few other graphs and features you should be familiar with.

The equation $y = kx^2$, where $k \neq 0$, describes the basic **parabola**, one whose turning point (**vertex**) is at the origin. It has a U shape, and opens upward if k is positive and downward if k is negative. The graph of the related equation $y = k(x - a)^2$ is obtained from the basic parabola by shifting it horizontally so that its vertex is at the point $(a, 0)$. The graph of the equation $y = kx^2 + b$ is obtained from the basic parabola by shifting it vertically so that its vertex is at the point $(0, b)$. Finally, the graph of the equation $y = k(x - a)^2 + b$ is obtained from the basic parabola in two shifting steps: First, shift the basic parabola horizontally so that its vertex is at the point $(a, 0)$; next, shift this parabola vertically so that the vertex is at the point (a, b). These parabolas are illustrated below for positive a, b, k, and x:

The equation $y = k/x$, where $k \neq 0$, describes a **hyperbola**. It is the graph of an inverse proportion (see Section 2.2). For small values of x, the values of y are large; and for large values of x, the values of y are small. Notice that the graph of a hyperbola approaches—but never touches—both the x- and y-axes. These lines are therefore called **asymptotes**.

The equation $y = k/x^2$, where $k \neq 0$, has a graph whose shape is similar to a hyperbola but it approaches its asymptotes faster than a hyperbola does (because of the square in the denominator).

The graph of the equation $y = Ae^{-kx}$ (where k is positive) is an **exponential decay curve**. It intersects the y axis at the point $(0, A)$, and, as x increases, the value of y decreases. Here, the x-axis is an asymptote.

The graph of the equation $y = A(1 - e^{-kx})$, where k is positive, contains the origin, and as x increases, the graph rises to approach the horizontal line $y = A$. This line is an asymptote.

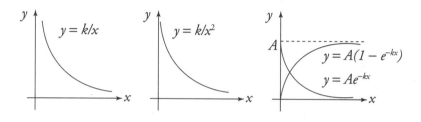

Chapter 14
Proportions

The concept of proportionality is fundamental to analyzing the behavior of many physical phenomena and is a common topic for MCAT questions.

14.1 DIRECT PROPORTIONS

If one quantity is always equal to a constant times another quantity, we say that the two quantities are **proportional** (or **directly proportional**, if emphasis is desired). For example, if k is some nonzero constant and the equation $A = kB$ is always true, then A and B are proportional, and k is called the **proportionality constant**. We express this fact mathematically by using this symbol: $\propto$, which means *is proportional to*. So, if $A = kB$, we'd write $A \propto B$. Of course, if $A = kB$, then $B = (1/k)A$, so we could also say that $B \propto A$.

Here are a few examples:

Example 14-1: Energy is equal to Planck's constant times frequency, $E = hf$. Therefore $E \propto f$.

Example 14-2: The ideal gas law states that $PV = nRT$. If n, V, and R are constant, $P \propto T$.

Example 14-3: The rate law for a chemical reaction that is first order with respect to reactant A is rate = $k[A]$. Assuming k is constant, rate $\propto [A]$.

The most important fact about direct proportions is this:

> *If $A \propto B$, and B is multiplied by a factor of b, then A will also be multiplied by a factor of b.*

After all, if $A = kB$, then $bA = k(bB)$.

Example 14-4: Since the energy of a photon is proportional to its frequency, $E \propto f$, then, if the frequency is doubled, so is the energy. If the frequency is reduced by half, so is the energy. If the frequency is tripled, so is the energy.

Example 14-5: Since the pressure inside a system is proportional to its temperature when volume and the number of moles present are constant, $P \propto T$, when the temperature is quadrupled, the pressure is quadrupled. When the pressure is decreased by a factor of 3, the temperature is also decreased by a factor of 3.

Example 14-6: Since the rate of a first order chemical reaction is proportional to the concentration of reactant A, [rate] $\propto [A]$, if $[A]$ is increased by a factor of 2, the rate also increases by a factor of 2. If $[A]$ is decreased by a factor of 4 (same as multiplying by ¼), the rate of reaction is ¼ of what it was originally.

It's important to notice that the actual numerical value of the proportionality constant was irrelevant in the statements made above. For example, the fact that h is the proportionality constant in the equation $E = hf$ did not affect the conclusions made above. If E and f were some other quantities and E happened to always be equal to $(17,000)f$, we'd still say $E \propto f$, and all the conclusions made in Example 14-4 above would still be correct.

Graphically, proportions are easy to spot. If the horizontal and vertical axes are labeled linearly (as they usually are), then *the graph of a proportion is a straight line through the origin*. Be careful not to make the common mistake of thinking that any straight line is the graph of a proportion. If the line doesn't go through the origin, then it's *not* the graph of a proportion.

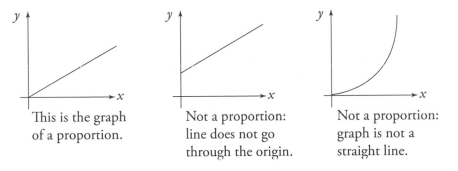

| This is the graph of a proportion. | Not a proportion: line does not go through the origin. | Not a proportion: graph is not a straight line. |

The examples we've seen so far have been the equations $E = hf$, $PV = nRT$, and $rate = k[A]$. Notice that in all of these equations, all the variables are present to the first power. But what about an equation like this: $KE = \frac{1}{2}mv^2$? This equation gives the kinetic energy of an object of mass m moving with speed v. So, if m is constant, KE is proportional to v^2. Now, what if v were multiplied by, say, a factor of 3, what would happen to KE? Because $KE \propto v^2$, if v increases by a factor of 3, then KE will increase by a factor of 3^2, which is 9. (By the way, this does not mean that if we graph KE versus v, we'll get a straight line through the origin. KE is not proportional to v; it's proportional to v^2. If we were to graph KE vs. v^2, *then* we'd get a straight line through the origin.) Here's another example using the same proportion, $KE \propto v^2$: If v were decreased by a factor of 2, then KE would decrease by a factor of $2^2 = 4$.

Here is one more example:

Example 14-7: The reaction quotient Q for a reaction is described by $Q = [A][B]^3$. Therefore, Q is proportional to the concentration of $[B]^3$: $Q \propto [B]^3$. So, for example, if $[B]$ were doubled, Q would increase by a factor $2^3 = 8$.

14.2 INVERSE PROPORTIONS

If one quantity is always equal to a nonzero constant *divided* by another quantity (that is, if $A = k/B$, where k is some constant), we say that the two quantities are **inversely proportional**. Here are two equivalent ways of saying this:

(i) If the product of two quantities is a constant ($AB = k$), then the quantities are inversely proportional.

(ii) If A is proportional to $1/B$ [that is, if $A = k(1/B)$], then A and B are inversely proportional.

In fact, we'll use this final description to symbolize an inverse proportion. That is, if A is inversely proportional to B, then we'll write $A \propto 1/B$. (There's no commonly accepted single symbol for *inversely proportional to*.) Of course, if $A = k/B$, then $B = k/A$, so we could also say that $B \propto 1/A$.

Here are a couple of examples:

Example 14-8: The pressure P and volume V of a sample containing n moles of an ideal gas at a fixed temperature T is given by the equation $PV = nRT$, where R is a constant. Therefore, the pressure is inversely proportional to the volume: $P \propto 1/V$.

Example 14-9: For electromagnetic waves traveling through space, the wavelength λ and frequency f are related by the equation $\lambda f = c$, where c is the speed of light (a universal constant). Therefore, wavelength is inversely proportional to frequency: $\lambda \propto 1/f$.

The most important fact about inverse proportions is this:

> *If $A \propto 1/B$, and B is multiplied by a factor of b, then A will be multiplied by a factor of $1/b$.*

After all, if $A = k/B$, then $(1/b)A = k/(bB)$. Intuitively, if one quantity is *increased* by a factor of b, the other quantity will *decrease* by the same factor, and vice versa.

Example 14-10: Since the pressure of an ideal gas at constant temperature is inversely proportional to the volume, $P \propto 1/V$, then if the volume is doubled, the pressure is reduced by a factor of 2. If the volume is quadrupled, the pressure is reduced by a factor of 4. If the volume is divided by 3 (which is the same as saying it's multiplied by 1/3), then the pressure will increase by a factor of 3.

Example 14-11: Because for electromagnetic waves traveling through space, the wavelength is inversely proportional to frequency, $\lambda \propto 1/f$, if f is increased by a factor of 10, λ will decrease by a factor of 10. If the frequency is decreased by a factor of 2, the wavelength will increase by a factor of 2.

The graph of an inverse proportion is a *hyperbola*. In the graph below, $xy = k$, so x and y are inversely proportional to each other.

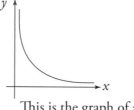

This is the graph of an
inverse proportion.

The examples we've seen so far have been where one quantity is inversely proportional to the first power of another quantity. But what about an equation like this:

$$F = \frac{q_1 q_2}{r^2}$$

This equation gives the electrostatic force between two point charges of magnitude q_1 and q_2 separated by a distance r. So, if q_1 and q_2 are constant, F is inversely proportional to r^2. Now, if r were increased by, say, a factor of 3, what would happen to F? Because $F \propto 1/r^2$, if r increases by a factor of 3, then F will decrease by a factor of 3^2, which is 9. Here's another example using the same proportion, $F \propto 1/r^2$: If r were decreased by a factor of 2, then F would increase by a factor of $2^2 = 4$.

Example 14-12: Graham's law of effusion states that

$$\frac{\text{rate of effusion of Gas 1}}{\text{rate of effusion of Gas 2}} = \sqrt{\frac{m_2}{m_1}},$$

where m_2 is the molecular mass of Gas 2 and m_1 is the molecular mass of Gas 1. Therefore, the rate of effusion of Gas 1 is inversely proportional to the square root of its molecular mass, rate of effusion of Gas 1 $\propto \sqrt{\dfrac{1}{m_1}}$. So, if Gas 1 were changed to a molecule whose mass was 4 times greater, the rate of effusion of Gas 1 would decrease by a factor of 2.

Example 14-13: The kinetic energy of an object of mass m traveling with speed v is given by the formula $KE = mv^2/2$.
   a)   If v is increased by a factor of 6, what happens to KE?
   b)   In order to increase KE by a factor of 6, what must happen to v?

Solution:
   a)   Since $KE \propto v^2$, if v increases by a factor of 6, then KE increases by a factor of $6^2 = 36$.
   b)   Since $KE \propto v^2$, it follows that $\sqrt{KE} \propto v$. So, if KE is to increase by a factor of 6, then v must be increased by a factor of $\sqrt{6}$.

Chapter 15
Logarithms

15.1 THE DEFINITION OF A LOGARITHM

A **logarithm** (or just **log**, for short) is an exponent.

For example, in the equation $2^3 = 8$, 3 is the exponent, so 3 is the logarithm. More precisely, since 3 is the exponent that gives 8 when the base is 2,

$$\underset{\text{base}}{\overset{\text{exponent}}{\text{(logarithm)}}} \quad 2^3 = 8$$

we say that the base-2 log of 8 is 3, symbolized by the equation $\log_2 8 = 3$.

Here's another example: Since $10^2 = 100$, the base-10 log of 100 is 2; that is, $\log_{10} 100 = 2$. The logarithm of a number to a given base is the exponent the base needs to be raised to give the number. What's the log, base 3, of 81? It's the exponent we'd have to raise 3 to in order to give 81. Since $3^4 = 81$, the base-3 log of 81 is 4, which we write as $\log_3 81 = 4$.

The exponent equation $2^3 = 8$ is equivalent to the log equation $\log_2 8 = 3$; the exponent equation $10^2 = 100$ is equivalent to the log equation $\log_{10} 100 = 2$; and the exponent equation $3^4 = 81$ is equivalent to the log equation $\log_3 81 = 4$. For every exponent equation, $b^x = y$, there's a corresponding log equation: $\log_b y = x$, and vice versa. To help make the conversion, use the following mnemonic, called the *two arrows method*:

$$\log_2 8 = 3 \iff 2^3 = 8$$

$$\log_b y = x \iff b^x = y$$

You should read the log equations with the two arrows like this:

$$\log_2 8 = 3 \iff 2 \xrightarrow{\text{to the}} 3 \longrightarrow 8 \iff 2^3 = 8$$

$$\log_b y = x \iff b \xrightarrow{\text{to the}} x \longrightarrow y \iff b^x = y$$

Always remember: The log is the exponent.

15.2 LAWS OF LOGARITHMS

There are only a few rules for dealing with logs that you'll need to know, and they follow directly from the rules for exponents (given earlier, in Chapter 1). After all, logs *are* exponents.

In stating these rules, we will assume that in an equation like $\log_b y = x$, the base b is a positive number that's different from 1, and that y is positive. (Why these restrictions? Well, if b is negative, then not every number has a log. For example, $\log_{-3} 9$ is 2, but what is $\log_{-3} 27$? If b were 0, then only 0 would have a log; and if b were 1, then every number x could equal $\log_1 y$ if $y = 1$, and *no* number x could equal $\log_1 y$ if $y \neq 1$. And why must y be positive? Because if b is a positive number, then b^x [which is y] is always positive, no matter what real value we use for x. Therefore, only positive numbers have logs.)

Laws of Logarithms	
Law 1	The log of a product is the sum of the logs: $\log_b (yz) = \log_b y + \log_b z$
Law 2	The log of a quotient is the difference of the logs: $\log_b (y/z) = \log_b y - \log_b z$
Law 3	The log of (a number to a power) is that power times the log of the number: $\log_b (y^z) = z \log_b y$

We could also add to this list that *the log of 1 is 0*, but this fact just follows from the definition of a log: Since $b^0 = 1$ for any allowed base b, we'll always have $\log_b 1 = 0$.

For the MCAT, the two most important bases are $b = 10$ and $b = e$. Base-10 logs are called **common** logs, and the "10" is often not written at all:

$$\log y \text{ means } \log_{10} y$$

The base-10 log is useful because we use a *decimal* number system, which is based (pun intended) on the number 10. For example, the number 273.15 means $(2 \times 10^2) + (7 \times 10^1) + (3 \times 10^0) + (1 \times 10^{-1}) + (5 \times 10^{-2})$. In physics, the formula for the decibel level of a sound uses the base-10 log. In chemistry, the base-10 log has many uses, such as finding values of the pH, pOH, pK_a, and pK_b.

Base-e logs are known as **natural** logs. Here, e is a particular constant, approximately equal to 2.7. This may seem like a strange number to choose as a base, but it makes calculus run smoothly—which is why it's called the *natural* logarithm—because (and you don't need to know this for the MCAT) the only numerical value of b for which the function $f(x) = b^x$ is its own derivative is $b = e = 2.71828\ldots$. Base-e logs are often used in the mathematical description of physical processes in which the rate of change of some quantity is proportional to the quantity itself; radioactive decay is a typical example. The notation "ln" (the abbreviation, in reverse, for natural logarithm) is often used to mean $\log_e$:

$$\ln y \text{ means } \log_e y$$

The relationship between the base-10 log and the base-e log of a given number can be expressed as $\ln y \approx 2.3 \log y$. For example, if $y = 1000 = 10^3$, then $\ln 1000 \approx 2.3 \log 1000 = 2.3 \times 3 = 6.9$. You may also find it useful to know the following approximate values:

$\log 2 \approx 0.3$	$\ln 2 \approx 0.7$
$\log 3 \approx 0.5$	$\ln 3 \approx 1.1$
$\log 5 \approx 0.7$	$\ln 5 \approx 1.6$

Example 15-1:
a) What is $\log_3 9$?
b) Find $\log_5 (1/25)$.
c) Find $\log_4 8$.
d) What is the value of $\log_{16} 4$?
e) Given that $\log 5 \approx 0.7$, what's $\log 500$?
f) Given that $\log 2 \approx 0.3$, find $\log (2 \times 10^{-6})$.
g) Given that $\log 2 \approx 0.3$ and $\log 3 \times 0.5$, find $\log (6 \times 10^{23})$.

Solution:
a) $\log_3 9 = x$ is the same as $3^x = 9$, from which we see that $x = 2$. So, $\log_3 9 = 2$.
b) $\log_5 (1/25) = x$ is the same as $5^x = 1/25 = 1/5^2 = 5^{-2}$, so $x = -2$. Therefore, $\log_5 (1/25) = -2$.
c) $\log_4 8 = x$ is the same as $4^x = 8$. Since $4^x = (2^2)^x = 2^{2x}$ and $8 = 2^3$, the equation $4^x = 8$ is the same as $2^{2x} = 2^3$, so $2x = 3$, which gives $x = 3/2$. Therefore, $\log_4 8 = 3/2$.
d) $\log_{16} 4 = x$ is the same as $16^x = 4$. To find x, you might notice that the square root of 16 is 4, so $16^{1/2} = 4$, which means $\log_{16} 4 = 1/2$. Alternatively, we can write 16^x as $(4^2)^x = 4^{2x}$ and 4 as 4^1. Therefore, the equation $16^x = 4$ is the same as $4^{2x} = 4^1$, so $2x = 1$, which gives $x = 1/2$.
e) $\log 500 = \log (5 \times 100) = \log 5 + \log 100$, where we used Law 1 in the last step. Since $\log 100 = \log 10^2 = 2$, we find that $\log 500 \approx 0.7 + 2 = 2.7$.
f) $\log (2 \times 10^{-6}) = \log 2 + \log 10^{-6}$, by Law 1. Since $\log 10^{-6} = -6$, we find that $\log (2 \times 10^{-6}) \approx 0.3 + (-6) = -5.7$.
g) $\log (6 \times 10^{23}) = \log 2 + \log 3 + \log 10^{23}$, by Law 1. Since $\log 10^{23} = 23$, we find that $\log (6 \times 10^{23}) \approx 0.3 + 0.5 + 23 = 23.8$.

Example 15-2: In each case, find y.
a) $\log_2 y = 5$
b) $\log_2 y = -3$
c) $\log y = 4$
d) $\log y = 7.5$
e) $\log y = -2.5$
f) $\ln y = 3$

Solution:
a) $\log_2 y = 5$ is the same as $2^5 = y$, so $y = 32$.
b) $\log_2 y = -3$ is the same as $2^{-3} = y$, which gives $y = 1/2^3 = 1/8$.
c) $\log y = 4$ is the same as $10^4 = y$, so $y = 10,000$.
d) $\log y = 7.5$ is the same as $10^{7.5} = y$. We'll rewrite 7.5 as $7 + 0.5$, so $y = 10^{7+(0.5)} = 10^7 \times 10^{0.5}$. Because $10^{0.5} = 10^{1/2} = \sqrt{10}$, which is approximately 3, we find that $y \approx 10^7 \times 3 = 3 \times 10^7$.

e) $\log y = -2.5$ is the same as $10^{-2.5} = y$. We'll rewrite -2.5 as $-3 + 0.5$, so $y = 10^{-3+(0.5)} = 10^{-3} \times 10^{0.5}$. Because $10^{0.5} = 10^{1/2} = \sqrt{10}$, which is approximately 3, we have that $y \approx 10^{-3} \times 3 = 0.003$.

f) $\ln y = 3$ means $\log_e y = 3$; this is the same as $y = e^3$ (which is about 20).

Example 15-3: The definition of the pH of an aqueous solution is

$$pH = -\log [H_3O^+] \text{ (or, simply, } -\log [H^+])$$

where $[H_3O^+]$ is the hydronium ion concentration (in M).

Part I: Find the pH of each of the following solutions:
a) coffee, with $[H_3O^+] = 8 \times 10^{-6} M$
b) seawater, with $[H_3O^+] = 3 \times 10^{-9} M$
c) vinegar, with $[H_3O^+] = 1.3 \times 10^{-3} M$

Part II: Find $[H_3O^+]$ for each of the following pH values:
d) pH = 7
e) pH = 11.5
f) pH = 4.7

Solution:
a) $pH = -\log (8 \times 10^{-6}) = -[\log 8 + \log (10^{-6})] = -\log 8 + 6$. We can now make a quick approximation by simply noticing that $\log 8$ is a little less than $\log 10$; that is, $\log 8$ is a little less than 1. Let's say it's 0.9. Then $pH \approx -0.9 + 6 = 5.1$.

b) $pH = -\log (3 \times 10^{-9}) = -[\log 3 + \log (10^{-9})] = -\log 3 + 9$. We now make a quick approximation by simply noticing that $\log 3$ is about 0.5 (after all, $9^{0.5}$ *is* 3, so $10^{0.5}$ is close to 3). This gives $pH \approx -0.5 + 9 = 8.5$.

c) $pH = -\log (1.3 \times 10^{-3}) = -[\log 1.3 + \log (10^{-3})] = -\log 1.3 + 3$. We can now make a quick approximation by simply noticing that $\log 1.3$ is just a little more than $\log 1$; that is, $\log 1.3$ is a little more than 0. Let's say it's 0.1. This gives $pH \approx -0.1 + 3 = 2.9$.

> **Note 1:**
> We can generalize these three calculations as follows: If $[H_3O^+] = m \times 10^{-n} M$, where $1 \le m < 10$ and n is an integer, then the pH is between $(n-1)$ and n; it's closer to $(n-1)$ if $m > 3$ and it's closer to n if $m < 3$. (We use 3 as the cutoff since $\log 3 \approx 0.5$.)

d) If pH = 7, then $-\log [H_3O^+] = 7$, so $\log [H_3O^+] = -7$, which means $[H_3O^+] = 10^{-7} M$.

e) If pH = 11.5, then $-\log [H_3O^+] = 11.5$, so $\log [H_3O^+] = -11.5$, which means $[H_3O^+] = 10^{-11.5} = 10^{(0.5)-12} = 10^{0.5} \times 10^{-12} \approx 3 \times 10^{-12} M$.

f) If pH = 4.7, then $-\log [H_3O^+] = 4.7$, so $\log [H_3O^+] = -4.7$, which means $[H_3O^+] = 10^{-4.7} = 10^{(0.3)-5} = 10^{0.3} \times 10^{-5} \approx 2 \times 10^{-5} M$. [$10^{-0.3} \approx 2$ follows from the fact that $\log 2 \approx 0.3$.]

> **Note 2:**
> We can generalize these last two calculations as follows: If pH $= n.m$, where n is an integer and m is a digit from 1 to 9, then $[H_3O^+] = y \times 10^{-(n+1)}$ M, where y is closer to 1 if $m > 3$ and closer to 10 if $m < 3$. (We take $y = 5$ if $m = 3$.)

Example 15-4: The definition of the pK_a of a weak acid is

$$pK_a = -\log K_a$$

where K_a is the acid's ionization constant.

Part I: Approximate the pK_a of each of the following acids:
  a)   HBrO, with $K_a = 2 \times 10^{-9}$
  b) HNO_2, with $K_a = 7 \times 10^{-4}$
  c)   HCN, with $K_a = 6 \times 10^{-10}$

Part II: Approximate K_a for each of the following pK_a values:
  d) $pK_a = 12.5$
  e) $pK_a = 2.7$
  f) $pK_a = 9.2$

Solution:
  a) $pK_a = -\log (2 \times 10^{-9}) = -[\log 2 + \log (10^{-9})] = -\log 2 + 9$. We can now make a quick approximation by remembering that log 2 is about 0.3. Then $pK_a = -0.3 + 9 = 8.7$. Because the formula to find pK_a from K_a is exactly the same as the formula for finding pH from $[H^+]$, we could also make use of Note 1 in the solution to Example 15-3. If $K_a = m' \times 10^{-n}$ M, where $1 \le m < 10$ and n is an integer, then the pK_a is between $(n-1)$ and n; it's closer to $(n-1)$ if $m > 3$ and it's closer to n if $m < 3$. In this case, $m = 2$ and $n = 9$, so the pK_a is between $(n-1) = 8$ and $n = 9$. And, since $2 < 3$, the pK_a will be closer to 9 (which is just what we found, since we got the value 8.7). Given a list of possible choices for the pK_a of this acid, just recognizing that it's a little less than 9 will be sufficient.
  b)   With $K_a = 7 \times 10^{-4}$, we have $m = 7$ and $n = 4$. Therefore, the pK_a will be between $(n-1) = 3$ and $n = 4$. Since $m = 7$ is greater than 3, the value of pK_a will be closer to 3 (around, say, 3.2).
  c)   With $K_a = 6 \times 10^{-10}$, we have $m = 6$ and $n = 10$. Therefore, the pK_a will be between $(n-1) = 9$ and $n = 10$. Since $m = 6$ is greater than 3, the value of pK_a will be closer to 9 (around, say, 9.2).
  d)   If $pK_a = 12.5$, then $-\log K_a = 12.5$, so $\log K_a = -12.5$, which means $K_a = 10^{-12.5} = 10^{(0.5)-13} = 10^{0.5} \times 10^{-13} \approx 3 \times 10^{-13}$. We could also make use of Note 2 in the solution to Example 15-3. If $pK_a = n.m$, where n is an integer and m is a digit from 1 to 9, then $K_a = y \times 10^{-(n+1)}$ M, where y is closer to 1 if $m > 3$ and y is closer to 10 if $m < 3$. In this case, with $pK_a = 12.5$, we have $n = 12$ and $m = 5$, so the K_a value is $y \times 10^{-(12+1)} = y \times 10^{-13}$, with y closer to 1 (than to 10) since $m = 5$ is greater than 3 (this agrees with what we found, since we calculated that $K_a \approx 3 \times 10^{-13}$).
  e)   With $pK_a = 2.7$, we have $n = 2$ and $m = 7$. Therefore, the K_a value is $y \times 10^{-(2+1)} = y \times 10^{-3}$, with y close to 1 since $m = 7$ is greater than 3. We can check this as follows: If $pK_a = 2.7$, then $-\log K_a = 2.7$, so $\log K_a = -2.7$, which means $K_a = 10^{-2.7} = 10^{(0.3)-3} = 10^{0.3} \times 10^{-3} \approx 2 \times 10^{-3}$.
  f)   With $pK_a = 9.2$, we have $n = 9$ and $m = 2$. Therefore, the K_a value is $y \times 10^{-(9+1)} = y \times 10^{-10}$, with y closer to 10 (than to 1) since $m = 2$ is less than 3. We can say that $K_a \approx 6 \times 10^{-10}$.

Example 15-5:
  a)   If y increases by a factor of 100, what happens to log y?
  b)   If y decreases by a factor of 1000, what happens to log y?
  c)   If y increases by a factor of 30,000, what happens to log y?
  d)   If y is reduced by 99%, what happens to log y?

Solution:
  a)   If y changes to $y' = 100y$, then the log increases by 2, since

$$\log y' = \log(100\ y) = \log 100 + \log y = \log 10^2 + \log y = 2 + \log y$$

  b)   If y changes to $y' = y/1000$, then the log decreases by 3, since

$$\log y' = \log(\frac{y}{1000}) = \log y - \log 1000 = \log y - \log 10^3 = \log y - 3$$

  c)   If y changes to $y' = 30,000y$, then the log increases by about 4.5, since

$$\log y' = \log(30000\ y) = \log 3 + \log 10000 + \log y \approx 0.5 + 4 + \log y = 4.5 + \log y$$

  d)   If y is reduced by 99%, that means we're subtracting $0.99y$ from y, which leaves $0.01y = y/100$. Therefore, y has decreased by a factor of 100. And if y changes to $y' = y/100$, then the log decreases by 2, since

$$\log y' = \log(\frac{y}{100}) = \log y - \log 100 = \log y - \log 10^2 = \log y - 2$$

Example 15-6: A radioactive substance has a half-life of 70 hours. For each of the fractions below, figure out how many hours will elapse until the amount of substance remaining is equal to the given fraction of the original amount.
  a)   1/4
  b)   1/8
  c)   1/3

Solution:
  a)   After one half-life has elapsed, the amount remaining is 1/2 the original (by definition). After another half-life elapses, the amount remaining is now 1/2 of 1/2 the original amount, which is 1/4 the original amount. Therefore, a decrease to 1/4 the original amount requires 2 half-lives, which in this case is 2(70 hr) = 140 hr.
  b)   The fraction 1/8 is equal to 1/2 of 1/2 of 1/2; that is, $1/8 = (1/2)^3$. In terms of half-lives, a decrease to 1/8 the original amount requires 3 half-lives, which in this case is equal to 3(70 hr) = 210 hr. *In general, a decrease to $(1/2)^n$ the original amount requires n half-lives.*

c) The fraction 1/3 is not a whole-number power of 1/2, so we can't directly apply the fact given in the italicized sentence in the solution to part (b). However, 1/3 is between 1/2 and 1/4, so the time to get to 1/3 the original amount is between 1 and 2 half-lives. Since one half-life is 70 hr, the amount of time is between 70 and 140 hours; the middle of this range (since 1/3 is roughly in the middle between 1/2 and 1/4) is about 110 hours. The most general formula for calculating the elapsed time involves a logarithm: If $x < 1$ is the fraction of a radioactive substance remaining after a time t has elapsed, then

$$t = \frac{\log \frac{1}{x}}{\log 2} \times t_{1/2}$$

where $t_{1/2}$ is the half-life. (If you want to use this formula, remember that $\log 2 \approx 0.3$.)

NOTES

NOTES

NOTES

More expert advice from The Princeton Review

The Princeton Review can help you ace the MCAT, get into medical school, and make career moves that will let you use your skills and education to your best advantage.

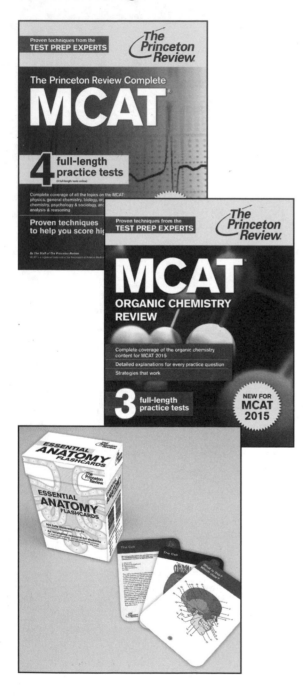

Princeton Review Complete MCAT
978-0-8041-2508-6 • $99.99/$112.00 Can.

MCAT Workout: Extra Questions and Answers to Help You Ace the Test
978-0-375-76631-2 • $23.99/$27.99 Can.

MCAT Elite: Advanced Strategies for a 45
978-0-375-42797-8 • $29.99/$35.00 Can.

MCAT Biology and Biochemistry Review
978-0-8041-2504-8 • $50.00/$58.00 Can.

MCAT Organic Chemistry Review
978-0-8041-2505-5 • $45.00/$52.00 Can.

MCAT General Chemistry Review
978-0-8041-2506-2 • $45.00/$52.00 Can.

MCAT Physics and Math Review
978-0-8041-2507-9 • $45.00/$52.00 Can.

MCAT Critical Analysis and Reasoning Skills Review
978-0-8041-2503-1 • $35.00/$41.00 Can.

The Best 167 Medical Schools, 2014 Edition
978-0-8041-2433-1 • $22.99/$25.95 Can.

Anatomy Coloring Workbook, 3rd Edition
978-0-375-76289-5 • $19.99/$23.99 Can.

Biology Coloring Workbook
978-0-679-77884-4 • $18.00/$27.00 Can.

Medical School Essays that Made a Difference, 5th Edition
978-0-8041-2584-0 • $13.99/$16.99 Can.

Planning a Life in Medicine
Ebook Only: 978-0-307-94500-6

Available everywhere books are sold and at PrincetonReviewBooks.com

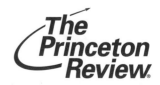